Purple Secret

PURPLE SECRET

Genes, 'Madness' and the Royal Houses of Europe

JOHN C.G. RÖHL, MARTIN WARREN

AND DAVID HUNT

BANTAM PRESS

LONDON · NEW YORK · TORONTO · SYDNEY · AUCKLAND

TRANSWORLD PUBLISHERS LTD
61–63 Uxbridge Road, London W5 5SA

TRANSWORLD PUBLISHERS (AUSTRALIA) PTY LTD
15–25 Helles Avenue, Moorebank, NSW 2170

TRANSWORLD PUBLISHERS (NZ) LTD
3 William Pickering Drive, Albany, Auckland

Published in 1998 by Bantam Press
a division of Transworld Publishers Ltd

A catalogue record for this book is available
from the British Library.
ISBN 0593 041488

Typeset by Deltatype Ltd, Birkenhead, Merseyside
Printed in Great Britain by
Mackays of Chatham plc, Chatham, Kent

Contents

Acknowledgements

We thank Her Majesty the Queen for her gracious permission to peruse some of the medical records in the Royal Archives, and Sheila de Bellaigue and Miss Frances Dimond for their kind assistance while we were working there. We also wish to reiterate our gratitude to HRH the Landgrave Moritz of Hesse for permission, granted in connection with an earlier project, to inspect the papers in the Hessisches Hausarchiv in Schloss Fasanerie. Much of the medical material on which this book is based was discovered not at Windsor or in Schloss Fasanerie, but in the family archive of the House of Saxe-Meiningen, and we are most grateful to the staff of the Thuringian State Archive at Meiningen – not least to its former director, Dr Hannelore Schneider and to Frau Katharina Witter and Yvonne Völker – for their patience and advice. We have also received generous help from Dr Franz J. Moegle-Hofacker of the Württemberg State Archive at Stuttgart, Dr Birgit Kehne of the State Archive of Lower Saxony at Hanover, Frau Anke Hölzer of the Manuscripts Department of the State Library of Lower Saxony, Herr Gerd Biegel of the State Museum of Brunswick, Frau Gerta Walsh of the Municipal Museum of Bad Homburg and Prof. Alfred Erck of Meiningen. Mr Nils G. Bartholdy of the State Archive at Copenhagen and Dr B. Woelderink, Director of the Royal House Archive at The Hague, were kind enough to answer our queries. We are also grateful to Mr Davenport Robertson, Librarian of the National Institute for Environmental Health Sciences in the Research Triangle Park, North Carolina, to Linda McCurdy of the

Duke University Library Special Collections, Suzanne Porter of the Duke University Center Library Historical Collections and above all to Alan Tuttle, Eliza Robertson and Jean Houston, indefatigable librarians at the National Humanities Center in North Carolina, for their near-miraculous ability to locate even the most esoteric text at very short notice. The National Humanities Center is altogether a most suitable place for putting the finishing touches to scholarly manuscripts.

In the course of our research for this book, we were given invaluable information and advice by numerous people, some of whom have asked not to be named. They will know who they are, and we thank them most warmly for their help. The late Prof. Claude Rimington, Prof. Sir Abraham Goldberg, Dr Geoffrey Dean, Dr John Mollon, Dr Donald Tschudy, Prof. Ian Christie, Dr John Ehrman, Lord Dacre of Glanton, Dr John Gurney, Dr Jenny Wormald, Prof. Jean Bernard, Dr Margaretha Honegger, Mr David M. Rohl, M. Philippe Rinsoz, Duke Conrad of Saxe-Meiningen and Prof. V. Jahnke all generously assisted us in various ways with information and comment. Our warm thanks are also due to Dr Marcelle Jay for her genealogical research, to Jadwiga Nicholson, our intrepid interpreter on our expedition to Poland, and to Dr Annika Mombauer for her help in reading eighteenth-century German manuscripts. Most of all we are indebted to Heather Nicholas for her unflagging detective work in reconstructing the medical biographies not just of kings and queens, but of sometimes quite obscure Royals as well. Without her selfless dedication and encouragement, the historical chapters of this book could not have been written.

For permission to obtain DNA from the shroud of King Charles I, we are deeply indebted to Mrs Marlies Bickersteth. For their generous help in arranging the opening of the grave of Princess Feodora of Reuss, we thank the Burgomaster and Deputy Burgomaster of Kowary, Mr Marek Jiruska and Mr Czeslaw Mikicki. We are also deeply indebted to the Stiftung Thüringischer Schlösser und Gärten and the Thüringisches Landesamt für Archäologische Denkmalpflege for allowing us to be present at the inspection of the graves of Duke Bernhard III of Saxe-Meiningen and his wife in July 1997, in the course of which we were able to obtain bone samples from the remains of Queen Victoria's granddaughter Charlotte.

We are particularly indebted to Profs. Tim Cox and George Elder, who have provided a wealth of information on porphyria and have made many very helpful suggestions. Dr Anna Evans has had the very difficult task of analysing the ancient DNA material and has done a remarkably thorough job. At various times she has been ably assisted by Dr Jenny Roper and Dr Kamal Dulai. Dr Henry Bellringer provided us with invaluable information about one particular case of porphyria. We appreciate his helpfulness and openness and also thank his daughter, Yasmine Cargill, for her help. There are many others too who have provided valuable pieces of information – such as Mrs Richard Hunter, Dr John Hadfield, Mr George Klouda, Mrs Jane Dexter, Dr Erika Hagelberg, Sheila Mitchell, Dr Sharon Wolf-Smith, Prof. Shoolingin-Jordan, Prof. Sir Tom Blundell, Dr Steve Wood, Prof. Stan Brown, Dr Jenny Houghton, Prof. Ray Bonnett and Prof. Ian Magnus.

We would also like to express our warm thanks to our agent, Mr Jonathan G. Harris, and to Sally Gaminara, Katrina Whone and our copy-editor Vicki Harris, for their generous help and support during the final preparation of the manuscript.

Finally, we are particularly indebted to the Wellcome Trust for funding much of this research.

Preface

In April 1813, the British Royal Family embarked on a search for the burial place of King Charles I, the exact location of which had long been a matter of speculation at the Court of St James. With the mind of King George III now irretrievably deranged, and the execution of the King of France on the guillotine still fresh in everyone's mind, this was perhaps not the most propitious of times for the Prince Regent and his siblings to be gazing upon the severed head of their ancestor, who had been decapitated at Whitehall on 30 January 1649. They therefore drew what comfort they could from the fact that, when the martyred monarch's grave was eventually discovered, his skeletal remains were found to be in remarkably good order. 'It was wonderful how much of it was perfect,' one of George III's daughters observed, 'the form of the face, the back of the head, the hair clotted with blood, and the head laid down on to the throat in the Coffin.'[1] Also present on that macabre occasion was Sir Henry Halford, the controversial physician who attended all the Royal Family, including George III, George IV, William IV and Queen Victoria, for many decades until his death in 1844; and when the 'valued relic' had been properly reburied, it emerged that Sir Henry had abstracted a bone from the Martyr King's coffin which he, the President of the Royal College of Physicians, liked to show to his guests at the dinner table. Charles I's errant bone was not restored to its rightful place until it was handed to the Prince of Wales, the future King Edward VII, at the end of the nineteenth century, who then personally laid it on his predecessor's casket in St George's Chapel.[2]

If King Charles's bone were still in the hands of the scientific and medical community today, in the age of molecular genetics, what would it tell us about inherited character traits and disorders in the dynasty that has occupied Windsor Castle and sat on the throne of England in genetic continuity since the time of William the Conqueror? Would we be able, after three and a half centuries, to decipher the message of the Royal Martyr's DNA? Would his bone hold the secret of Henry VI's madness; of Mary Queen of Scots' 'colicky' pains and vomiting; of her son James's debilitating illnesses, which were associated with the passing of urine the colour of dark red wine; of the physical and mental turmoil suffered by George III and several of his children, including the monarchs George IV and William IV and their brother the Duke of Kent, Queen Victoria's father? Such speculation might appear fanciful, but in the light of recent DNA tests which have posthumously unmasked the false Anastasia Romanov, analysed the medical condition of an Egyptian boy mummified thousands of years ago and solved the mystery of whether modern humans are related to the Neanderthals, it does not seem impossible. And this is especially the case if, as was proposed and hotly debated some three decades ago, the British Royal Family and several other European dynasties turn out to have been tormented by a serious metabolic disorder which can affect both the mind and the body and which is transmitted from generation to generation by a genetic mutation. Could Charles I's bone, if we still had it today, have helped to solve the riddle of the 'Royal Malady'?

In the 1960s, two British psychiatrists of German-Jewish origin, the mother-and-son team Ida Macalpine and Richard Hunter, shook the historical and medical professions with their suggestion that King George III's turbulent mental state was caused not by 'madness' or 'mania', as had universally been supposed, but by the rare hereditary illness of porphyria. As both Macalpine and Hunter died before they were able to complete their work, their retrospective diagnosis of the condition of George III, his forebears and descendants – they claimed to have traced the illness back to Mary Queen of Scots and her son James VI and I and forward to several of George III's children – remained unproven. It was accepted as probably true by most historians of the Hanoverian monarchy and by a majority of doctors and psychiatrists, but it also met with staunch and at times acrid opposition, and there is no denying that, on the basis of the then available evidence, the sceptics could make a good case.

This book seeks to complete the work which Ida Macalpine and Richard Hunter, through their untimely deaths, left unfinished. In an unusual crossover collaboration between two molecular geneticists and a historian, it combines meticulous research in the archives of Britain and Germany with the very latest techniques of DNA sequencing in an attempt to establish with certainty, one way or the other, whether porphyria was indeed the cause of Royal 'madness', and if so, what type of porphyria (for there are several) was involved.

Porphyria is a relatively rare condition. It is a name given to a group of largely inherited disorders which interfere with the ability of the body to make the red pigment in blood. The colour of blood is due to a compound called haem, whose role is to help transport oxygen around the various organs and tissues. Humans have to produce their own haem, and porphyria arises when something goes wrong with the biological machinery (the 'biosynthetic pathway') which manufactures this essential blood component.

Early nineteenth-century chemists were first to analyse the composition of blood. It was they who initially isolated the brilliant scarlet chemical which is nowadays called haem. By virtue of its colour they called it a porphyrin, which is Greek for 'red/purple', and it is from this that the term 'porphyria' was derived. Haem is a complex substance which is made from a number of smaller chemicals, pieced together like a molecular jigsaw. Porphyria is not due to a shortfall in haem production, but rather to an accumulation of some of the pieces of the molecular jigsaw ('intermediates') in blood and tissue. Different forms of porphyria are associated with different pieces of the jigsaw. The effect of some of these jigsaw pieces is drastic.

Clinically, porphyria has been classified into types which are associated with abdominal pain (acute porphyria), skin sensitivity (cutaneous porphyria) or those which cause both abdominal pain and skin sensitivity (mixed or variegate porphyria). The symptoms of porphyria include attacks of severe abdominal pain, peripheral neuropathy, temporary mental disturbance, sensitivity to sunlight and the production of discoloured urine. The peripheral neuropathy, literally meaning a disease of the nervous system controlling the body's non-conscious functions (heart, intestinal movement, sweating, etc.), causes not only general muscle weakness, numbness, constipation and difficulty in breathing and swallowing but also leads to profuse sweating, increased heart rate (tachycardia) and high blood pressure, all contributing to making the patient hypersensitive.

Because the symptoms of porphyria are multiple, and comparatively common when considered in isolation, patients in the past were quite often misdiagnosed. Thus porphyrics undergoing an acute attack with severe abdominal pain were diagnosed with appendicitis; those with a temporary mental disturbance were institutionalized. There is still no cure for this debilitating disease and, as in Georgian and Victorian times, the intervention of the uninformed physician can still be fatal.

Although some forms of porphyria can be acquired, for example by excessive alcohol consumption, or exposure to lead and certain chemicals, most forms of porphyria are genetically inherited; that is, the disease is due to a faulty gene. There are seven different genes which cause different hereditary forms of porphyria. The inheritance pattern in most cases is 'dominant', which means that the offspring of an affected individual have a 50 per cent chance of inheriting the faulty gene. A more detailed account of the science and medical basis of porphyria is given in the Appendix.

Although a clinical description of a disease can give an account of the symptoms associated with an attack, a better idea of the dangerous nature and severe discomfort which are allied with porphyria is gained from personal accounts. One such account is given below. The female patient was diagnosed as having acute intermittent porphyria (AIP) in April 1994 and the attack is thought to have been triggered after administration of an anti-malarial drug.

'Ten days after taking my first dose I experienced acute abdominal pain. My GP could find no reason for the pain and the hospital thought I had malaria. Four days after the onset of pain I was admitted to hospital for further investigations. Following a *grand mal* fit, found to be caused by hyponatraemia [low body concentration of sodium], the provisional diagnosis of porphyria was put to my husband. He contacted my parents and over the next few days they traced back and found that my father's sister had died of porphyria in 1959 (aged twenty-four).

'I remember very little of the next two weeks, and in that time my condition at first stabilized and got better but then deteriorated to the point where my husband was told to expect the worst. During all this time I constantly complained of pain (so I am reliably informed) and major complications set in such that I spent the next five days on a ventilator.

'Following extubation I developed peritonitis [inflammation of the membrane of the abdominal cavity], ascites [accumulation of fluid within the abdominal cavity], a pleural effusion [escape of fluid around the lungs] and intense pins and needles in my legs and feet. The porphyria was treated with haematin which brought it under control and after a month in hospital I was allowed home.

'Unfortunately, due to further complications I was readmitted to hospital after a week and I was treated with mefoxin (which I have since learnt to be contra-indicated for porphyria) and within five days the pain in my legs was so intense that I needed to use a wheelchair.

'With frequent massage and a lot of bullying I was up and walking, albeit slowly, with a stick and a limp within two months. Two years later I have had no recurrent attacks but I still walk with a limp and have an altered sensation in my right leg from the calf to the toes.

'I have given a brief outline of my problems and now I must consider my two children's future. I suppose the time is drawing near for them to be tested.'

The Royal Houses of Europe

*The names of the Kings and Queens of England
and Scotland are capitalized.
Except for the two children of George III
who did not survive beyond early childhood, all family
members mentioned in the text are shown.*

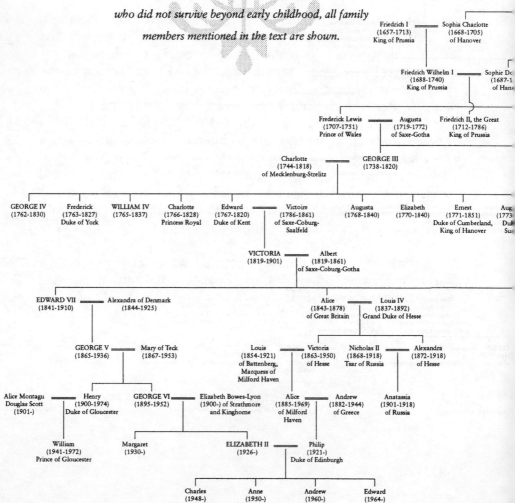

Friedrich I (1657-1713) King of Prussia === Sophia Charlotte (1668-1705) of Hanover

Friedrich Wilhelm I (1688-1740) King of Prussia === Sophie Do (1687-1 of Han

Frederick Lewis (1707-1751) Prince of Wales === Augusta (1719-1772) of Saxe-Gotha | Friedrich II, the Great (1712-1786) King of Prussia

Charlotte (1744-1818) of Mecklenburg-Strelitz === GEORGE III (1738-1820)

GEORGE IV (1762-1830) | Frederick (1763-1827) Duke of York | WILLIAM IV (1765-1837) | Charlotte (1766-1828) Princess Royal | Edward (1767-1820) Duke of Kent === Victoire (1786-1861) of Saxe-Coburg-Saalfeld | Augusta (1768-1840) | Elizabeth (1770-1840) | Ernest (1771-1851) Duke of Cumberland, King of Hanover | Aug (1773 Du Sus

VICTORIA (1819-1901) === Albert (1819-1861) of Saxe-Coburg-Gotha

EDWARD VII (1841-1910) === Alexandra of Denmark (1844-1925)

Alice (1843-1878) of Great Britain === Louis IV (1837-1892) Grand Duke of Hesse

GEORGE V (1865-1936) === Mary of Teck (1867-1953)

Louis (1854-1921) of Battenberg, Marquess of Milford Haven === Victoria (1863-1950) of Hesse | Nicholas II (1868-1918) Tsar of Russia === Alexandra (1872-1918) of Hesse

Alice Montagu Douglas Scott (1901-) === Henry (1900-1974) Duke of Gloucester | GEORGE VI (1895-1952) === Elizabeth Bowes-Lyon (1900-) of Strathmore and Kinghorne | Alice (1885-1969) of Milford Haven === Andrew (1882-1944) of Greece | Anatassia (1901-1918) of Russia

William (1941-1972) Prince of Gloucester | Margaret (1930-) | ELIZABETH II (1926-) === Philip (1921-) Duke of Edinburgh

Charles (1948-) Prince of Wales | Anne (1950-) Princess Royal | Andrew (1960-) Duke of York | Edward (1964-)

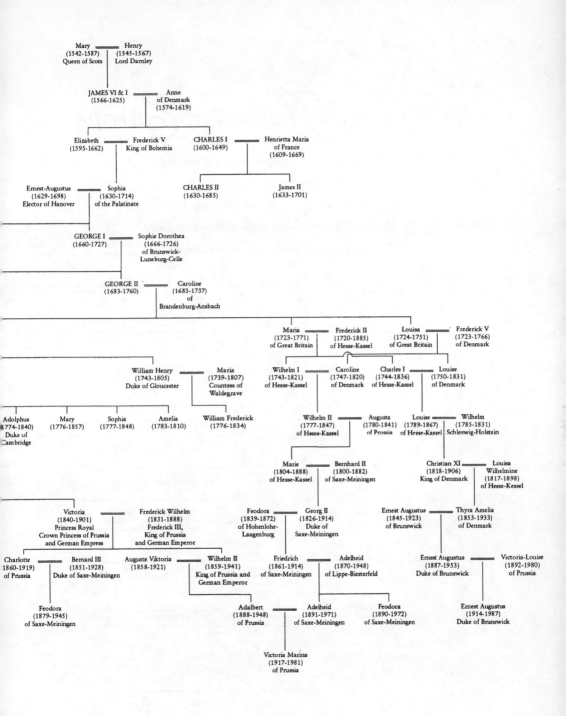

Mary
(1542-1587)
Queen of Scots
═══
Henry
(1545-1567)
Lord Darnley

JAMES VI & I
(1566-1625)
═══
Anne
of Denmark
(1574-1619)

Elizabeth
(1595-1662)
═══
Frederick V
King of Bohemia

CHARLES I
(1600-1649)
═══
Henrietta Maria
of France
(1609-1669)

Ernest-Augustus
(1629-1698)
Elector of Hanover
═══
Sophia
(1630-1714)
of the Palatinate

CHARLES II
(1630-1685)

James II
(1633-1701)

GEORGE I
(1660-1727)
═══
Sophie Dorothea
(1666-1726)
of Brunswick-
Luneburg-Celle

GEORGE II
(1683-1760)
═══
Caroline
(1683-1737)
of
Brandenburg-Ansbach

Maria
(1723-1771)
of Great Britain
═══
Frederick II
(1720-1885)
of Hesse-Kassel

Louisa
(1724-1751)
of Great Britain
═══
Frederick V
(1723-1766)
of Denmark

William Henry
(1743-1805)
Duke of Gloucester
═══
Maria
(1739-1807)
Countess of
Waldegrave

Wilhelm I
(1743-1821)
of Hesse-Kassel
═══
Caroline
(1747-1820)
of Denmark

Charles I
(1744-1836)
of Hesse-Kassel
═══
Louise
(1750-1831)
of Denmark

Adolphus
(1774-1840)
Duke of
Cambridge

Mary
(1776-1857)

Sophia
(1777-1848)

Amelia
(1783-1810)

William Frederick
(1776-1834)

Wilhelm II
(1777-1847)
of Hesse-Kassel
═══
Augusta
(1780-1841)
of Prussia

Louise
(1789-1867)
of Hesse-Kassel
═══
Wilhelm
(1785-1831)
Schleswig-Holstein

Marie
(1804-1888)
of Hesse-Kassel
═══
Bernhard II
(1800-1882)
of Saxe-Meiningen

Christian XI
(1818-1906)
King of Denmark
═══
Louisa
Wilhelmine
(1817-1898)
of Hesse-Kessel

Victoria
(1840-1901)
Princess Royal
Crown Princess of Prussia
and German Empress
═══
Frederick Wilhelm
(1831-1888)
Frederick III,
King of Prussia
and German Emperor

Feodora
(1839-1872)
of Hohenlohe-
Laagenburg
═══
Georg II
(1826-1914)
Duke of
Saxe-Meiningen

Ernest Augustus
(1845-1923)
of Brunswick
═══
Thyra Amelia
(1853-1933)
of Denmark

Charlotte
1860-1919
of Prussia
═══
Bernard III
(1851-1928)
Duke of Saxe-Meiningen

Auguste Viktoria
(1858-1921)
═══
Wilhelm II
(1859-1941)
King of Prussia and
German Emperor

Friedrich
(1861-1914)
of Saxe-Meiningen
═══
Adelheid
(1870-1948)
of Lippe-Biesterfeld

Ernest Augustus
(1887-1953)
Duke of Brunswick
═══
Victoria-Louise
(1892-1980)
of Prussia

Feodora
(1879-1945)
of Saxe-Meiningen

Adalbert
(1888-1948)
of Prussia
═══
Adelheid
(1891-1971)
of Saxe-Meiningen

Feodora
(1890-1972)
of Saxe-Meiningen

Ernest Augustus
(1914-1987)
Duke of Brunswick

Victoria Marina
(1917-1981)
of Prussia

CHAPTER 1

The Porphyria Controversy

I promise to eat my hat if the authors can produce
convincing evidence that they are right.
Dr Geoffrey Dean, April 1968

The Porphyria Theory

Was George III the mad King of England? There is no disputing the
fact that the mind of the King was deranged for several periods of
time during his sixty-year reign, a period of contrasting fortunes for
the country. When George III ascended the throne in 1760,
determined to exercise personal power, Britain had seized half the
world's trade and laid the foundation of her vast empire. His reign
witnessed the humbling loss of the American colonies, and yet by
the time of his death in 1820 Britain had defeated Napoleonic
France, she had acquired oceanic mastery and an expanding empire
and, in terms of world power, reigned supreme. It is clearly
important, when trying to assess the contribution he made to the
country's fortunes at home and abroad, that his character be
properly understood. But the medical condition of King George III
had many important implications not only for contemporary
politics and subsequent historical interpretation. His treatment by
the doctors was to bring psychiatry out of the closet and hasten its
recognition as an important branch of medical science.

Why was the King labelled as mad? During several episodes,
George was afflicted with 'flying gout', which travelled from his legs
to his head. He became weak, suffered from colic and insomnia,
and delirium ensued which caused him to talk rapidly and
incoherently and promoted his lascivious delusions about Lady

1

Pembroke. In historical terms, the monarch's bouts of temporary insanity destabilized the political equilibrium and, in the longer run, helped to establish the ascendancy of Parliament. The political turmoil it caused was most evident in the regency crisis of 1788, an episode which has recently been brought to the public's attention in Alan Bennett's play *The Madness of George III* and the resultant film, *The Madness of King George*. The story of the play and film revolves around the central dilemma posed by the King's illness: whether he should be considered as suffering from delirium or insanity and, depending on the diagnosis, whether Parliament should allow George to continue to act as king or install his eldest son as regent. The matter was temporarily resolved by George's rapid recovery, but the retrospective diagnosis of the nature of the King's complaint led to a great deal of speculation. The agreed outcome of this conjecture was that madness seemed the most likely explanation, and so the malignment of the King commenced, not to be corrected for over 150 years. In fact, the diagnosis of mania was incorporated into two separate reviews undertaken independently of one another by two American psychiatrists. The first, written in 1855, thirty-five years after the King's death, concluded that he had suffered from acute mania.[1] As an affective (psychiatric) disorder, mania is defined as a state of mind which rapidly undergoes changes in mood. During a manic attack, thought processes may be difficult to follow, speech becomes rapid and judgement poor, and delusions are not uncommon. Mania can also affect behaviour, leading to overactivity and sometimes violence. There is no doubt that the mental symptoms attributed to George III are characteristic of mania.

The problem with the diagnosis of mania was that, outside a small number of clearly delimited bouts of illness, George III appeared to be a normal, healthy individual with few of the vices often associated with royalty. He was interested in music and agriculture and had a high regard for the Church. He had a strong sense of morality and remained faithful to his wife, Charlotte of Mecklenburg-Strelitz, despite the fact that she was described as 'dim', 'dull', and as 'plain as she was ugly'.[2] He had fifteen legitimate children and was an adoring father. Moreover, there was no apparent family association with insanity; although mania fitted the *mental* symptoms exhibited by the King, it did not explain the origin and cause of the disorder, the accompanying *physical* symptoms, or the periodic nature of his attacks.

The conundrum appeared to be answered by the extrapolation of the mania theory to manic-depressive psychosis,[3] a mental illness involving alternating episodes of depression and mania. Such episodes are normally caused by specific events which are blown up out of all proportion. This diagnosis led to the assumption that George III's manic episodes were brought on by personal and political pressures. The trouble with this second interpretation, however, was that the King's mental breakdowns did not directly coincide with any major disturbance in his life.

Up until 1966, these two (closely related) interpretations were the only attempts to diagnose the King's ailment. Evidently the diagnosis of mania or manic-depressive psychosis appeared so sound that it did not seem worthy of challenge by either historians or medics. Not surprisingly, the predomination of such a view had disastrous consequences for the biographical interpretation of the King's character whose mind was declared to have been 'unsteady' and 'dark and cloudy'.[4] Given an apparently secure medical diagnosis, the view of the biographer/historian is slanted towards explaining the antics of the subject in terms of the expected symptoms, so much so that trivial information is given greater prominence than it would otherwise deserve. For instance, on the basis of the assumption that George III suffered with a psychiatric illness it was thought that he must have been mentally and emotionally retarded. Thus the story was accepted as fact that as a boy George was unable to read and write until he was eleven, and that even by the age of twenty he wrote like a child.[5] There seemed little point in challenging this view because it corresponded so well with the preconception of a mentally weak character. Yet later historians, doubting that George's mind became unhinged as a result of external pressures, were unable to find any substantiating evidence for such an interpretation of his childhood. Indeed, closer scrutiny of the early life of George III revealed that he was perfectly able to read and write, in both English and German, by the age of eight![6]

For decades, then, the medical file on George III looked as though it would remain closed, all the problems having seemingly been solved. The King, it was generally agreed, was a weak character who had to rely on his closest friends to steer him in the right political direction, he was sexually frustrated, inconsolable at the loss of the American colonies and disillusioned by the antics of his children and their lack of moral fibre. All these troubles, it seemed clear, provoked his manic attacks. And since the King was thought to have a mental illness, he was also looked upon as weak-minded – as 'Farmer George', the simpleton. All this was suddenly to change in 1966 with the propounding of the theory that King George III's 'madness' was due not to psychosis but to a rare inherited metabolic disorder. This hypothesis provoked a vigorous and often acrimonious debate among scientists, medics and historians, one that has never been satisfactorily resolved.

The fuse to this altercation was lit when two German-born British psychiatrists, Ida Macalpine and her son Richard Hunter, published a paper in the *British Medical Journal* (*BMJ*) entitled 'The Insanity of King George III: A Classic Case of Porphyria'.[7] Two years later, in 1968, after they had teamed up with the chemical pathologist Professor Claude Rimington, Macalpine and Hunter published a second paper expanding their previous article, entitled 'Porphyria in the Royal Houses of Stuart, Hanover and Prussia'.[8] This paper revealed their discovery of two living Royal Family members whom they believed to be porphyrics ('Patients A and B'). A further publication by Macalpine and Hunter, 'Porphyria and King George III', appeared in *Scientific American*.[9] In 1969 their research on the case, together with its subsequent influence on the development of psychiatry, was published in a major book entitled *George III and the Mad Business*, which was reprinted in 1991, 1993 and 1995.[10] The British Medical Association also produced the booklet *Porphyria – A Royal Malady*,[11] which contained the two *BMJ* articles with a brief historical interpretation of the significance of their findings and an expert medical description of porphyria.

All these papers and books were based on the novel idea that the King suffered from the inherited, metabolic disorder called porphyria, a condition which, it was argued, induced the observed mental derangement but which also caused a number of associated physical symptoms. Although the Macalpine and Hunter articles were thoroughly researched, their diagnosis was based on the very incomplete medical records and briefings then available. Despite this, they wrote as though the case had been proven, reflecting their own firm conviction that the King was a porphyric. It was the tone of their writing as much as the content that exacerbated the ensuing debate. To follow the controversy, we need briefly to highlight some of Macalpine's and Hunter's findings before we study the response which these elicited.

The Diagnosis of Porphyria in George III

Probably the most significant statistic which Macalpine and Hunter produced during their investigation into the illness of George III was that, up until 1810, when the King was in the eighth decade of his life, his mind had been deranged for a total of less than six months. He had four major attacks – in 1789, 1801, 1804 and 1810 – but the last attack was probably a series of attacks which became difficult to distinguish from the onset of senility. An attack in 1765, previously also thought to have involved mental incapacity, was shown to have been of a purely physical nature with no psychiatric involvement.[12] Thus, on the face of it, the patient had four attacks involving mental derangement which did not start until he was fifty years of age. The attacks did not coincide with any obvious political or emotional pressure and so the diagnosis of manic-depressive psychosis, whereby the monarch's breakdown was attributed to mental stress, could be discounted.

As psychiatrists, Macalpine and Hunter could not fit George's pattern of mental illness to any recognized psychiatric disorder. Obviously 'mania', a vague term used to imply rapid mood changes, could be applied, but for a character who had withstood such political disasters as the loss of the American colonies and the personal tragedy of the death of two of his children without any apparent breakdown, this seemed an unlikely diagnosis. The investigators therefore looked for an alternative explanation of the King's illnesses. They re-examined his periods of delirium more closely and found that in each case the mental illness was associated with physical symptoms which preceded the derangement of the monarch's mind. The most prominent of these physical symptoms included severe abdominal pain or 'colic', peripheral neuropathy and hypersensitivity. During the episodes of illness there were also some reports of discoloured urine. All these features are consistent with the onset of a form of porphyria called acute intermittent porphyria. This inborn error of metabolism is hereditary and is so called because the disorder manifests itself as sudden attacks with severe symptoms which have a comparatively short duration.

The historical evidence that George III had symptoms consistent with acute intermittent porphyria is very compelling. The authors argued that they could be confident of the diagnosis because 'attacks present an almost specific combination of seemingly unconnected symptoms'.[13] These symptoms appeared to be triggered by colds, coughs and a general feeling of malaise, and included pains in the chest, severe abdominal pain and constipation, tachycardia, hoarseness, painful weakness of the limbs, pins and needles (paraesthesia), hypersensitivity, pains in the neck, face and head, difficulty in swallowing (dysphagia) and flushing of the face (suffusion). Moreover, the King displayed encephalopathy (disease affecting the brain), agitation, very rapid and incoherent speech, hypersensitivity to light and sound, uninhibited behaviour, insomnia, rapid changes of mood and total delirium. Finally, Macalpine and Hunter found four references to discoloured urine: in 1788 the King's water was described as bilious, in 1811 as being of a deeper colour and leaving a pale blue ring, in 1812 as bluish and in 1819 as bloody.[14]

The diagnosis of a genetic disorder which is inherited in a dominant manner had two obvious important implications – the disease must have been inherited from one of George III's parents, and there was a 50 per cent chance that each of his fifteen children would also have inherited the complaint. However, porphyria is peculiar in that not everybody who inherits the agent responsible for the disorder develops the disease. We now know that the agent is a faulty gene, but in about 90 per cent of cases those who have the faulty gene remain asymptomatic or latent (that is, they do not exhibit any symptoms of the disorder). How this can happen is explained more fully in the Appendix, but the important implication is that the disorder can appear to skip generations, and thus parents or grandparents of victims may seem to be unaffected. In those who are unfortunate enough to inherit the faulty gene, porphyria can be brought on by certain drugs, by alcohol or diet. Notwithstanding these difficulties, Macalpine and Hunter searched for evidence of the disease among the immediate family of George III. They found no shortage of porphyric symptoms, with bilious attacks and gout in particular being recorded with high frequency. Of course, these could have been due to other things – poor hygiene and bad food preparation methods, for example – giving rise to genuine digestive complaints. Life one or two centuries ago was not as assured as it is today, at least in the West, and a brief illness could quickly develop into a fatal infection. Nowadays, we take the role of antibiotics for granted, and few of us appreciate the major influence that these compounds play in our general health. Without them, skin disorders, blood poisoning and a range of other bacterial infections would have a much higher pathological rate than they have today. Thus, in the seventeenth and eighteenth centuries, generalized complaints such as malaise, colic and weakness could be the result of myriad infections. None the less, Macalpine and Hunter claimed to have found the signs of porphyria in fourteen leading historical figures and to have traced its descendency from Mary Queen of Scots. Two of the more convincing accounts of porphyria from their file of affected members are given below.

By happy coincidence, in the course of their research on the history of psychiatry, Macalpine and Hunter had already come across James VI of Scotland (James I of England). James (1566–1625) had a complex medical history which was carefully recorded by his brilliant Swiss physician Sir Theodore de Mayerne.[15] In Mayerne's notes, Macalpine and Hunter found reference to the following symptoms:

- ☐ abdominal pain associated with vomiting and diarrhoea
- ☐ changes in mood
- ☐ fits of unconsciousness and delirium
- ☐ pain and weakness in the limbs
- ☐ insomnia
- ☐ respiratory difficulty
- ☐ sensitivity to sunlight and skin fragility
- ☐ production of dark urine which the King likened to Alicante wine.

From these symptoms Macalpine, Hunter and Rimington diagnosed porphyria, even concluding that James's last illness was due to that disorder. Their discovery seemed to provide an attractive break-through. The diagnosis of porphyria not only accounted for the King's illnesses and bouts of delirium and melancholy; it also provided a source for the faulty gene which George III would later inherit.

If a detailed description of King James's medical case could be obtained from the thorough accounts left behind by Sir Theodore de Mayerne, a similar debt of gratitude is due to Dr Johann Georg von Zimmermann, another Swiss physician and one of the greatest medical authorities of his day, who corresponded with Catherine the Great and was ennobled by her – and who was also doctor to several of George III's sons. According to the notes preserved in Zimmermann's papers in Hanover, the symptoms from which George III's son Augustus, Duke of Sussex (1773–1843), suffered included:

- ☐ sudden attacks or convulsions
- ☐ chest pains
- ☐ reddish/brown discoloration of the face associated with pain
- ☐ insomnia
- ☐ headaches
- ☐ weakness and tiredness
- ☐ breathing difficulty
- ☐ discoloured urine (amber or reddish) which accompanied the attacks and which disappeared as the attacks came to an end.

Zimmermann and his colleagues in Hanover also astutely noted that similar convulsive attacks occurred in Augustus's brothers the Dukes of York and Kent, and the doctors explicitly suggested a possible hereditary link.[16] The presence of symptoms of skin sensitivity in both James I and the Duke of Sussex persuaded first Rimington and then Macalpine and Hunter to change their original diagnosis of acute intermittent porphyria to variegate porphyria.[17] The only major symptomatic difference between these two disorders is that the latter is associated additionally with sun sensitivity. This change in diagnosis was perfectly reasonable given the difficulty of interpreting scraps of evidence hundreds of years old, but to the sceptics it looked like a sign of confusion and uncertainty, seeming to weaken their argument.

The Response of the Sceptics

Although many people contributed to the porphyria controversy, Macalpine, Hunter and Rimington had two main detractors, Professor C. E. Dent, head of the human metabolism unit at University College Hospital Medical School, and Dr Geoffrey Dean, the eminent physician who discovered variegate porphyria and showed that the disorder was rife in the Afrikaner population of South Africa. Dean had seen more variegate porphyria patients than any other physician and yet he did not recognize the symptoms described by Macalpine and Hunter. In the war of words exchanged by the proponents and debunkers of the porphyria hypothesis, Professor Abraham Goldberg, the leading British expert on porphyria, was left to act as arbitrator.

The new theory about King George III received a great deal of attention even in the daily press, as both *The Times* (7 January 1968) and the *Telegraph* (12 January 1968) and several overseas newspapers reported on it. The theory also prompted an article by the historian John Brooke on the 'Historical Implications of Porphyria' which was subsequently incorporated into the British Medical Association booklet *Porphyria – A Royal Malady*. This booklet was reviewed by another eminent British historian, Professor Hugh Trevor-Roper, who summarized his initial thoughts by stating that he found 'the medical argument both fascinating and convincing. No one can now continue to maintain that George III was a neurotic ... who took refuge from his responsibilities in madness.'[18] However, part of the reason for the initial acceptance of the theory was simply that those who disagreed with it had not fully aired their views, and they had several important and relevant points to make, most of which Macalpine sidestepped. Dent, for example, remained unconvinced by the diagnosis of porphyria, writing: 'Goodness knows what the disease was – the mental symptoms being so non-specific would fit many other diseases as well as porphyria,'[19] a view which was shared by many distinguished porphyria authorities. This point was taken further by two South African porphyria experts who asserted that not only was 'the evidence insufficient to support a diagnosis of variegate porphyria but in many cases it contradicts it'.[20] They even wondered aloud why the authors were so enthusiastic about their diagnosis, concluding: 'We were left with the impression that their researches and interpretation have been coloured by an understandable desire to sustain the thesis rather than to examine it.'[21] Geoffrey Dean was even less convinced and dedicated a whole chapter of his book *The Porphyrias: A Story of Inheritance and Environment* to debunking the theory.[22] He also wrote several letters to the *BMJ* stating that in his opinion the claim was 'highly unlikely' and certainly 'not proven'.[23] Later he rather rashly promised, as he wrote, 'to eat my hat if the authors can produce convincing evidence that they are right'.[24]

One of the major reasons why Dent, Dean and the South African physicians were unhappy with the diagnosis of variegate porphyria was that this disease in particular had been very well studied in South Africa. In general, as the critics repeatedly pointed out, the South African form of porphyria remains latent, and apart from some sun sensitivity acute attacks only occur when drugs such as barbiturates and sulphonamides are taken. This aspect was countered by Goldberg, who explained that variegate porphyria had increasingly come to be recognized in the UK and that attacks of porphyria could be provoked by factors other than modern drugs.[25] At the heart of Goldberg's point was a then poorly understood subject, genetic heterogeneity within a disease. We now know that different mutations or alterations within a gene can give rise to the same disorder but produce the disease with different emphasis on the main symptoms. Moreover, even the same faulty gene can behave differently between separate individuals, reflecting the varying genetic background in which the gene is expressed. It has now been reported many times that acute attacks of variegate porphyria do occur spontaneously, or can be induced by infections and diet.

With respect to King George III, as we have seen, Macalpine and Hunter found four reports of discoloured urine. At the start of an acute attack of porphyria, and during the attack, the urine of patients may be discoloured, usually becoming reddish-brown or very dark like Coca-Cola, as noted by Dean.[26] It may also appear bright red or orangey red, but in any case the unusual colour is due to the excretion of some of the porphyrin intermediates. However, two of the quoted references to discoloured urine in George III invoked a blue colour: 'bluish' in a document of 1812 preserved in the Royal Archives, and 'of a deeper colour – and leav[ing] a pale blue ring upon the glass near the upper surface' in notes written by the King's physician Sir Henry Halford in 1811. The discrepancy in the colour of the urine was debated fervently and ideas on colour perception and even bacterial infection have been forwarded.[27]

Nevertheless, it should always be borne in mind that urine colour by itself is not diagnostic of porphyria, as discoloured urine is a non-specific accompaniment of a wide variety of gastro-intestinal diseases. As Dent points out, highly concentrated urine passed after water restriction may appear discoloured.[28] Some people even pass red urine after eating beetroot. However, the presence of discoloured urine accompanied by abdominal pains, polyneuritis and psychiatric disturbance makes the diagnosis of porphyria very acceptable.

One of the strongest arguments against the porphyria theory was that if the condition could be traced back to Mary Queen of Scots, some thirteen generations, then there should be many members of the Royal Family with the disorder. Using Dean's wonderful study of variegate porphyria in South Africa as an example (where the marriage of a porphyric Dutch settler in 1688, Gerrit Jansz, to Ariaantje Jacobs, resulted in the propagation of the faulty gene into ten thousand present-day descendants), Dent argued that if porphyria were present in the extended royal family of Europe then there would be a considerable epidemic of overt porphyria nowadays.[29] Dean also argued the same case, stating that there would be many thousand royal porphyric descendants alive today, and then asked why Macalpine, Hunter and Rimington had found only two very doubtful descendants? A disgruntled Dent put the question of inheritance in a different form by sarcastically asking how the mutant gene could have had 'the uncanny knack for picking out the subjects in the direct line of succession: first son when available, otherwise whoever comes next'.[30] In her reply to such criticisms, Ida Macalpine did not really address these points as she was not interested in how many people had inherited the faulty gene, she was merely trying to strengthen her diagnosis of George III's illness 'by showing that this rare gene still exists in the family'.[31] 'Once the diagnosis of porphyria is established clinically and in the laboratory, the question of how many other members of the patient's family are affected is of scientific interest and useful for the possible prevention of attacks.'[32] A point which is also important to bear in mind is the difficulty of obtaining the necessary help and collaboration of family members in these studies. Asking Europe's most exalted families to provide stool and urine samples did not exactly meet with an alacritous or affable response.

The two living descendants described by Macalpine, Hunter and Rimington play a pivotal role in the porphyria controversy. By claiming to have found two living relatives with the disorder they argued first that porphyria did occur in the family, and second, that as the two patients in question were related to each other only through George II, they must have inherited the faulty gene from the Hanoverian line. In principle, this sounds like a strong argument, but unfortunately the data provided for the diagnosis of variegate porphyria in 'Patients A and B' were far from secure; in fact they were, as we shall see, positively weak. As Dent was quick to point out, more information on A and B was needed, particularly with regard to 'the type of porphyria together with the family evidence so that sporadic or inbred porphyria from another branch of the family could be eliminated'.[33] More specifically, the adversaries of the porphyria theory eagerly pointed out many more weaknesses in the diagnosis of patients A and B. The critics obviously realized that by demonstrating the frailty of the diagnosis they could discredit the entire porphyria theory.

The diagnosis of Patient A was based on the opinion of an unnamed 'distinguished physician' and no biochemical data were given. As Dean pointed out, 'I have known many distinguished physicians to make a mistake in the diagnosis of porphyria.'[34] This aspect was emphasized further by others. 'No clinical or biochemical data on Patient A are available for assessment, and as porphyria is often erroneously diagnosed it leaves us hesitant to accept this diagnosis.'[35] Needless to say Dent was even less impressed, arguing that the diagnosis demanded 'more than the fragmentary description quoted ... Without this we cannot have full confidence in the diagnosis of a distinguished physician dealing with a VIP.'[36]

Patient B did not fare much better at the hands of the antagonists. The patient was reported to have produced discoloured urine at various times over the years and to have suffered from colic and constipation. Macalpine, Hunter and Rimington had managed to procure both urine and stool samples for biochemical analysis, but although they claimed the results were indicative of porphyria, in reality the readings were only on the high side of normal. 'The symptoms [of B] would do reasonably well [for porphyria] but the reported faecal porphyrin concentration given make this diagnosis unlikely'[37] was the conclusion reached by one group of South African experts. Dent also pointed out the weakness in the biochemical readings from Patient B: 'The data needs more consideration,' he wrote, 'at best it is marginal.'[38] Dean was more forthright, stating bluntly: 'The values for B are not at all diagnostic of variegate porphyria.'[39]

One of the criticisms levelled at the porphyria theory was that its proponents had not tried to fit the observed symptoms to other diseases or disorders. This allowed their detractors to say that 'the authors are unjustifiably reluctant to accept alternative explanations'.[40] Many of the symptoms of porphyria can obviously be caused by a range of illnesses, from general gastroenteritis to kidney infection. Dent had his own alternative explanation for many of the symptoms displayed by George III. 'They could have been produced by his doctors, for instance, by excessive purgation and that the so-called paralyses, for instance, could have been due to low potassium – a common complication of excessive purgation.'[41]

Macalpine had anticipated such an objection and responded in her usual sprightly fashion. 'It is interesting to speculate – as we have done quietly too – which of the King's treatments made him actually iller and not better. Purgation, as you say, may well have been responsible for a lot of mischief, but it could not have been a precipitant of an attack because it was used after the outbreak of the symptoms.'[42]

As the articles in the *BMJ* were also reported in the national press, they of course came to the attention of porphyria sufferers. Dent was particularly worried about the effect the articles would have on his patients, especially as they mentioned so many sudden deaths. He recorded the feelings of one such patient 'currently pregnant who was exceedingly upset when she read your recent accounts of this hereditary disease'.[43] Presumably that patient's anxiety was aroused in particular by the suggestion made by Macalpine, Hunter and Rimington that porphyria was responsible for the sudden death of Princess Charlotte, the only child of George

IV. She died unexpectedly in 1817 of an undiagnosed problem, shortly after giving birth to a stillborn son. However, the anxiety among porphyrics was not universal, and indeed many took the opposite view. For example, Professor Cochrane, himself a latent porphyric, wrote to thank Macalpine and Hunter for making porphyria better known and even to some extent glamorous. As he pointed out, with porphyria the main risk to the patient is misdiagnosis or delayed diagnosis, and 'I think that these two papers have substantially reduced these risks.'[44] Goldberg also found that his patients were not upset at reading the articles and reported that, 'indeed, most of them showed considerable interest and even sneaking pride that they might have a *royal malady*'.[45]

Much of the bitterness of the debate on the porphyria theory could have been avoided had Macalpine written her articles in a less assertive, more hypothetical manner. The tone of the letters which appeared in the *BMJ* in the six months after the second article was published was frequently acrimonious, as was that of the privately conducted correspondence between the chief participants. In a letter written by Dent to Macalpine, for example, he cynically asked why she was trying to separate royalty from madness, 'why you were so anxious to remove the *taint* of mental disease from the Royal Family. Our psychiatrists are always telling us that mental disease should be considered exactly like any other disease and under no circumstances should it be thought to be any sort of disgrace.'[46] To which Macalpine vehemently responded: 'We were not aware of being *anxious* to remove the *taint of madness* from the Royal Family. As historical statement this has been printed again and again. We simply drew a conclusion from our study to contradict and so correct an error. Perhaps we should have put *taint* in quotes in order to avoid the impression it made on you as if we considered mental illness a disgrace.'[47]

Macalpine, in particular, was concerned about the harsh words that were being used about Claude Rimington in connection with the data he had presented on Patient B. Rimington and Dent worked in the same college hospital, but they had little time for each other, and Macalpine sensed that something of a personal vendetta might be at work against Rimington. She referred to Dent, Dean and the other experts on the South African disease as 'the axis' and wondered whether the vitriolic nature of some of the criticism was prompted by professional jealousy.[48] To try and counterbalance the spate of critical letters appearing in the *BMJ*, she contacted Dr A. Gajdos in Paris, asking if he would write a short though authoritative letter to the journal in support of Rimington.[49] Sure enough, the following month, a letter from Gajdos appeared in the *BMJ* stating that he was much impressed by the gigantic work which had led the authors to the conclusion of the possibility of variegate porphyria in the royal houses of Europe. The authors, he declared, 'deserve congratulation and encouragement', yet criticisms published in the *BMJ* 'seem to have been written with the opposite intention, even pointedly so'.[50] In an attempt to cool the debate, the letter concluded that 'although discussion of opposing views can only further our knowledge in every field . . . we must avoid that discussion becomes dispute'.[51]

The Debate Today

With the death of Ida Macalpine in 1974 and that of her son in 1981, the porphyria controversy came temporarily to an end without having reached a satisfactory conclusion. Some eminent medical authorities the world over write as if the hypothesis the two authors advanced had been proven beyond doubt, while others ignore their findings altogether.[52] One British psychiatrist, himself a sceptic, has informally estimated that 'perhaps 95% of psychiatrists nowadays' accept the theory as fact.[53] In the historical world, too, there is uncertainty and confusion, with one biographer of Mary Queen of Scots confidently asserting that the Stuart Queen's pain and emotional distress was caused by porphyria inherited from her father,[54] while another eminent historian of the period tells us that the thought of porphyria never crossed her mind.

Meanwhile the porphyria debate, though now less intense, still rumbles on. When the *Guardian* published an article on Alan Bennett's play and film, describing the playwright's misgivings on taking liberties with King George – which were needed, he explained, to thicken the plot[55] – one reader wrote to affirm that the play and film would 'provoke a wry smile from those who recognise the ineradicability of fashionable myth'.[56] The correspondent expanded his reasons, citing how Geoffrey Dean had exploded the whole porphyria myth with 'a series of articles so devastating that no one should ever again have paid the theory a moment's attention'.[57] This rather blinkered authoritarian statement is another misrepresentation of the truth which only serves to emphasize the polarity which the debate on the porphyria theory had caused. A second letter expressed exactly the opposite view, reassuring Alan Bennett that he need not worry about the cause of the King's 'madness', as it was indeed porphyria.[58] The writer explained that, while researching his biography of Kaiser Wilhelm II, he discovered a cache of letters written by the Kaiser's eldest sister, Princess Charlotte of Saxe-Meiningen, to her doctor, Ernst Schweninger, on her own distressing medical condition. These letters, from a great-great-granddaughter of George III, describe all the classic symptoms of variegate porphyria.

As Abraham Goldberg has always urged, the retrospective diagnosis of porphyria in King George III should be treated as a hypothesis or a theory. The symptoms which afflicted the King are consistent with this diagnosis, but for the diagnosis to become fully acceptable, more evidence of the existence of the disorder within the royal houses of Europe needs to be sought.

CHAPTER 2

On the Trail of Living Descendants

I sometimes give my fancy wings
And eyes to see the souls of things.
Claude Rimington, 1987[1]

A retrospective diagnosis of any ailment in a deceased person is dependent upon the available recorded evidence, which in historical figures is nearly always circumstantial. In the case of George III and porphyria, the hereditary nature of the disorder allowed Macalpine and Hunter to clamber up and down the family tree to search the medical records of George's forebears, relatives and descendants in an effort to show the presence of the disease within the wider Royal Family.[2] This part of their research was less convincing and, with only a few exceptions, Macalpine and Hunter seemed to many to have included in their porphyria file any Royal who was afflicted by an unexplained illness.

A good example of this tendency is their diagnosis of porphyria in the fourth son of George III: Edward, Duke of Kent, the father of Queen Victoria. Their diagnosis included the account of his sudden death on 23 January 1820. Shortly beforehand, on 7 January, the duke had caught a cold, possibly from his infant daughter Victoria, who had a sore throat and was restless.[3] Despite the discomfort of his infection, Edward insisted on looking after the horses but came back soaked and chilled. His cold developed, became violent and turned still worse during the next few days. His doctor was called and realized that the duke, who was now delirious and vomiting and had developed a high fever and a severe pain in his chest, was in a grave condition. As was often the case, however, the intervention of the physician only made matters worse. Dr Wilson recommended

17

the application of leeches, blistering and cupping. As the duke showed no sign of improvement, the removal of more blood was ordered. No less than six pints of blood were taken from him, a quantity which one royal physician felt, in retrospect, had been insufficient![4] Not surprisingly, then, by 19 January Edward was weaker still, had a very high fever, a severe cough, and pain in his side, and was delirious. These symptoms are all entirely consistent with pneumonia, yet Macalpine and Hunter looked upon the hoarseness and respiratory difficulties as evidence of porphyria.[5] The diagnosis of pneumonia is now supported by a study of his autopsy report which we were allowed to view in the Royal Archives at Windsor. It describes how the right lung was 'enlarged', 'heavy', 'in a complete state of suppuration, or abscess, it being entirely gorged with pus or matter'. The left lung was inflamed and charged with blood. In conclusion, the report states: 'The previous symptoms of his Royal Highness's disorder so accurately described by Dr Wilson . . . perfectly accorded with the appearances of the Lungs on dissection, particularly of the right side, and most evidently proved the immediate cause of . . . death.'[6] We are not saying that Edward did not have porphyria, as we have every reason to believe that he passed the disease on to his daughter and into the Saxe-Coburg line (now the House of Windsor), but the diagnosis of porphyria as the cause of death on this evidence is so weak that it detracts from the more convincing evidence of porphyria in James I and VI and in Augustus, Duke of Sussex, which we outlined in Chapter 1.[7]

Macalpine and Hunter realized that, to prove the existence of a hereditary form of porphyria within the Royal Family, they would have to provide a clinical diagnosis of porphyria in living family members. In the 1960s, porphyria was clinically diagnosed by the presence of certain chemical intermediaters (porphyrins) in urine and faeces, even though such chemicals are generally only excreted during an attack. Readings of this kind are still taken today, but enzyme measurements and DNA sequencing are also undertaken which allow for a more accurate diagnosis. As the royal families of Europe are closely interrelated, Macalpine, Hunter and Rimington potentially had a large patient base in which to try to identify porphyria. If their theory was correct, then many of these living descendants of George III should have the disorder. Although they were forewarned by their friends of the problems of obtaining the appropriate samples – 'I doubt whether Royal persons would cooperate by collecting their urine and faeces,' wrote one such colleague[8] – they did eventually uncover the two living relatives whom they reported as porphyric in their second *BMJ* paper. (This number had risen to four by the time their book on George III was published.) The problems of obtaining the necessary samples did prove to be a major frustration to Macalpine, as evidenced by her remarks: 'The greatest difficulty seems to be the squeamishness of living members to supply the necessary goods',[9] and 'How I look forward to the time when we no longer depend on Royalty.'[10] Rimington also acknowledged the difficulty, wistfully reflecting on one occasion: 'How I wish some of our critics could see the sort of reply one gets to a polite request.'[11] However, bearing in mind that the 'polite request' involved the provision of a specimen of early morning urine and stool, it is not too surprising that they had difficulty in obtaining the appropriate co-operation from European royalty.

The identity of the two then living relatives who were co-opted into the study was naturally kept secret. In fact, Patient A did not even know that she was included in the study. Both patients had a family lineage which could be traced back to the Hanoverian Kings of England. Little information was given, however, about the diagnosis of porphyria except that it was consistent with variegate porphyria. As discussed in Chapter 1, Patient B was reported to have had elevated levels of porphyrin in her excrement but the levels which were reported in the *BMJ* paper were only on the high side of the normal level. No readings were given for Patient A; all we are told is that an examination by a 'distinguished physician' had been conclusive. However, as Dr Geoffrey Dean points out, 'even distinguished physicians can misdiagnose porphyria'.[12] Thus the diagnosis of porphyria in the living relatives, like that in several of the historical figures, remained far from convincing.

So, who *were* Patients A and B, and was there any further evidence to suggest that they really were porphyrics? Did they have any children, and if so had they inherited the disorder? If the disorder was still present in the family line, would relatives be willing to co-operate with us in determining the genetic lesion which was the cause of their illness?

Ida Macalpine and Richard Hunter

The mother-and-son combination responsible for the porphyria hypothesis made a unique family team, as they were both eminent psychiatrists with a strong interest in the history and evolution of their chosen profession. It was this awareness of and interest in historical 'madmen' that led them to study George III and to extend their research by investigating the occurrence of the disorder in some of the other royal houses of Europe. Unfortunately both Macalpine and Hunter are now dead, having succumbed to a disease much more common than porphyria, cancer.

Ida Macalpine was born in Nuremberg on 19 June 1899, the daughter of Sigmund and Mathilde Wertheimer. After qualifying as a doctor she married Ernst Hirschmann (German for 'Hunter') but was divorced after only a few years. They had two sons, Richard being born on 11 November 1923. The menace of Nazism in Germany persuaded Ida Hirschmann to emigrate to England, where she had an uncle, in 1933.[13] To obtain permission to work as a physician in Britain, Dr Hirschmann took a Scottish medical qualification, the triple conjoint Colleges' examination, in Edinburgh. She adopted the name Macalpine and subsequently specialized in psychiatry and took up an appointment at St Bartholomew's Hospital in London.

Macalpine's friends and colleagues described her as quite remarkable – tall and slim in build, with dark hair and a thin friendly face. She was a determined lady with a typically Jewish quality, it was said, of always trying to make things better. She had a gentle and compassionate personality but people could misunderstand her because she was so positive. This may explain why she was not held in the same esteem by all who met her. For instance, one eminent historian who wished to remain anonymous recalled how a colleague of his had called on Macalpine and Hunter, presumably to discuss George III, 'and his account to me was so hilarious, and his picture of them so comic, that neither he nor I could take their theories seriously. Macalpine – as you may know – was the mother of Hunter, and, according to my colleague, totally dominated him; and she was dotty. All this may merely illustrate our prejudices, but it discouraged me from spending more time [on the porphyria theory].'[14] Those, on the other hand, who knew Macalpine well felt that if she had lived in England all her life she would probably have been rewarded with a prominent position within the medical establishment, such was the depth of her knowledge and understanding.

In 1974, Macalpine was diagnosed as having lung cancer. The condition was inoperable and she declined the opportunity of chemotherapy, preferring to bow to the inevitable. She died on 2 May 1974, at the age of seventy-four. Her obituary again stressed how she was of quiet character, gentle, persuasive, very hardworking and meticulous, and always ready to give help and advice to those in trouble or seeking information on the history of psychiatry.[15]

Both of Macalpine's sons also went into medicine. Richard went to Cambridge and was described as one of the cleverest students in his year, very personable and a dependable friend and colleague. He qualified from St Bartholomew's in 1946 and, although he first took up surgery, he later found his niche in psychiatry. He was appointed to the National Hospital, Queen Square, as senior registrar in 1957 and later in 1960 as physician in psychological medicine. He had always been interested in medical history and together with his mother he began a thorough exploration of the history of psychiatry. Over the years, this led to the acquisition of a large number of books on psychiatry, yielding a remarkable private library comprising several thousand volumes. After Richard's death, this collection was purchased by Cambridge University Library. It was this literary treasury which allowed Macalpine and Hunter to write their authoritative account of *Three Hundred Years of Psychiatry, 1535–1860* which was published in 1963.

Richard Hunter's knowledge of medical history and his enthusiasm for the subject made him a popular lecturer, although his ideas were not always appreciated by his colleagues. He was described as kindly, modest and generous but as having little patience with those who did not share his views.[16] In 1975 he married and became a family man, devoted to his wife and three children. However, shortly after being diagnosed with cancer of the pancreas, and despite major surgery, he died in 1981 at the age of only fifty-eight.

Claude Rimington

Claude Rimington was born in London in 1902 and studied science at Cambridge, where he came to appreciate the importance of basic scientific research. Although always interested in medicine, his curiosity for biological chemistry attracted him into the academic life. He took his PhD in Cambridge in 1928 and eventually, after the Second World War, was appointed to the chair in Chemical Pathology at University College Hospital Medical School in London, where he set up a laboratory which specialized in the study of the biochemistry of porphyrins and the porphyrias. Rimington's major contribution to the whole porphyrin field was the elucidation of the structure of one of the haem intermediates, porphobilinogen. It was largely in recognition of this work that he was elected a Fellow of the Royal Society (FRS) in 1954. Rimington was always enthusiastic about his science, was devoted to his work and proved inspirational to those with whom he came into contact. He is quoted as saying: 'My whole life has never been planned. I just followed opportunities as they came up, and yet, it has really been quite interesting. And I have been fortunate because I have always been able to do what I am interested in: that is something to be eternally grateful for.'[17]

Rimington far outlived Macalpine and Hunter. After retiring from University College Hospital Medical School in 1968, he eventually took up residence in his holiday home at Askeröy in Norway. However, in 1984 he eagerly seized the opportunity of continuing his research into porphyrins, specifically their application to cancer treatment in a process called photodynamic therapy, as a 'guest' scientist at the Norwegian Radium Hospital in Oslo. By this time he was eighty-two years old, yet he was still able to show his enthusiasm for this comparatively new subject. He continued to work on this topic until his death in August 1993, his ninety-first year.

Finding Patients A and B – Where to Start?

If George III really did suffer from a genetically inherited form of porphyria and had passed it on to his descendants, then it should be possible to identify the faulty gene by extracting DNA either from deceased known sufferers or, more easily, one would think, from one of his living descendants. In order to obtain DNA from a living family member, our obvious starting place was to discover the identity of Macalpine and Hunter's Patients A and B. Although a family tree was included in their paper in the *British Medical Journal* outlining the descent of A and B from the Hanoverian line, it was deliberately obscure in order to disguise their identity; it merely showed that A and B were respectively six and five generations removed from George III's grandfather, George II. We, however, needed to discover the actual identity of these two patients. We had to know their exact lineage and ideally more details on the diagnosis of their illness. What Macalpine and Hunter had also failed to do was to show a family history of the disorder in the case of either A or B. Obviously, if we knew their identity then we could also address this point. Of course, Macalpine and Hunter felt no need to show a family history because they were convinced that their historical research had demonstrated this sufficiently. This argument is logically flawed, however, because there is always the chance that the porphyria in a living relative may be a spontaneous new case of the disorder, a chemically acquired form of the disease, or have been derived from a different family line.

Our starting point was therefore to locate Macalpine's and Hunter's research notes which might help us identify the two (or four) mystery patients who they believed had had the disease. Some of Macalpine's correspondence and notes relating to the events up to the publication of her second paper on the Royal Malady had been filed away in an open cardboard box in the vaults of Cambridge University Library, and from these dust-covered notes and files we were able to piece together not only the identity of Patients A and B, but also how Macalpine came to hear about them, as well as the evidence for the diagnosis of porphyria. Reading these notes also gave us an insight into the enthusiasm and dedication with which Macalpine, Hunter and Rimington pursued their quarry. The tension and excitement which their detective work generated made compelling reading.

By 1965, Macalpine and Hunter had already formulated their hypothesis that King George III had suffered from porphyria rather than from any recognized mental illness. As the country's most famous 'mad' patient he had caught their interest from their earlier research on the history of psychiatry. As psychiatrists, they were not happy with the diagnosis of mania, and when their research revealed that prior to his final illness the King was mentally deranged for a total of only five or six months, their suspicions were aroused further still. The realization that the King's bouts of 'madness' were preceded by physical symptoms led them to believe that they were dealing with a physical illness which caused mental aberrations. The nature of the symptoms – severe abdominal pain, peripheral neuropathy and discoloured urine combined with a disturbance of the mind – allowed them to make the porphyria diagnosis. They became more convinced after hearing Abraham Goldberg, even then one of the country's leading authorities on the disease, give a lecture in London on the acute porphyrias, and they wrote to him shortly thereafter asking about some of the finer medical aspects of the disease.

Goldberg, who was knighted for his services to medicine in 1983 and now lives in retirement in Scotland, remembers Macalpine and Hunter well. When Macalpine and Hunter published their initial article on porphyria and George III, Goldberg wrote to them noting how their article seemed to have been well received but stressing that they needed to pursue the historical side further if their ideas were to gain general acceptance. Undoubtedly, he was worried by the tone of their writing. He has always felt, and still feels, that the diagnosis of porphyria to explain the King's illness is reasonable, but that it should be treated as a theory only. When the present authors spoke to Sir Abraham in 1997, he likened the diagnosis to the unique Scottish judicial verdict of 'not proven'.

In his reply to Goldberg, Richard Hunter revealed that 'meanwhile we have managed to trace a number of members of his [George III's] family, both forebears and descendants, whose medical history seems highly suggestive – some even having portwine coloured urine noted by thorough physicians. In confidence, we have also been approached by living members who are now under investigation.'[18] It is to these living relatives that we now turn our attention.

Patient B

The reference to living descendants relates to contacts Ida Macalpine had made with the head of the House of Hanover, Duke Ernst August of Brunswick, in 1966. From some accounts it appears that the duke was genuinely interested in the porphyria story but, as we shall see later, he also had a wicked sense of humour. The duke told Macalpine that an elderly relative who regularly came to stay with him had many of the symptoms of porphyria, including the production of red urine. Through the efforts of the duke, and presumably with the co-operation of the old lady's physician, Macalpine and Hunter were promised both urine and stool samples. Although not named explicitly in the correspondence, it is clear that the patient was an aunt of the duke.

At the end of 1966, Macalpine informed Rimington that she had been promised samples from a German princess and would collect them in person and bring them to his London laboratory for analysis. Rimington was renowned as one of the world's leading experts on the separation and characterization of the various known intermediates in the porphyrin metabolic pathway. However, he had recently become convinced that he had found a new way to diagnose variegate porphyria – that 'X-linked porphyrins' (porphyrins which have become attached to small protein molecules) were diagnostic of this disease. In retrospect, this measurement turned out to be something of a red herring. Porphyrins can form chemically reactive compounds which can link to small proteins which are excreted in the faeces, but how and in what proportion this happens is still not known. Thus, *any* porphyria which leads to a build-up of porphyrin will give rise to X-linked porphyrins, and so the latter cannot be reliably used as an indicator of a particular type of porphyria. Rimington's misplaced trust in the X-porphyrin reading was to be a major flaw in the diagnosis of Patient B in the follow-up paper.

Early in January 1967, Macalpine informed Rimington that 'the old lady, whose maid had noticed red urine over many years, had another attack, was very ill and her urine was portwine coloured. 'May I come to your laboratory to be instructed and equipped on how to carry the samples,' she asked, as she was about to travel to Germany to collect the precious evidence.[19] Rimington supplied the necessary information and instructions, adding: 'How aggravating that the red urine passed by the old lady in Germany was not saved and sent for some definitive chemical test.' Realizing the importance of actually having specimens to examine, Rimington observed: 'Perhaps 1967 will turn out to be *breakthrough* year – I do hope so.'[20]

The samples from Germany arrived safely but the results were inconclusive, since, although they showed the presence of coproporphyrin, protoporphyrin and X-linked porphyrin, the readings 'were not strikingly raised', as Rimington himself noted, the values being at the upper end of normal.[21] However, in Rimington's view, the X-linked porphyrin value was elevated. Furthermore, this suggested to Rimington that the type of porphyria from which the princess was suffering was not acute intermittent porphyria but variegate porphyria. With the clinical evidence in hand, Rimington convinced Macalpine that the original diagnosis of George III needed to be changed to variegate porphyria and that evidence for variegate porphyria in the relevant historical figures should be sought. As the only major symptomatic difference between acute intermittent porphyria and variegate porphyria is photosensitivity, Macalpine and Hunter began to scour the archives for cases of skin fragility, blisters and rashes.

All in all, the diagnosis of porphyria in Patient B is very weak. The clinical tests failed to provide the necessary evidence and the only basis for believing that the princess was porphyric is provided by the testimony of her maid concerning the periodic production of red urine. Our understanding is that Patient B died unmarried with no children. For this reason, and also because, unlike his father, the present head of the House of Hanover and his advisers have been singularly uncooperative in our historical investigations, we have been unable to pursue this line of enquiry.

There is a mysterious postscript to the tale of Dr Macalpine's visit to Hanover, however, which needs to be told. She actually brought two patient samples back from Germany. The second sample, of urine, was found by Rimington to be 'weakly positive'.[22] Although again rather inconclusive, this result no doubt helped to convince Macalpine that she was indeed on the right track, having now discovered, so she believed, a third living Hanoverian descendant with the disorder. But whose was the urine she had brought back with her? Duke Ernst August had led her to believe that the sample he had given her was his own, and as he was a direct descendant of George III on both his father's and his mother's side the 'weakly positive' sample appeared to be an important breakthrough. In actual fact, however, as the irascible duke informed John Röhl on a visit to Calenberg in 1985, the sample was not his own but his first wife's, Princess Ortrud, by birth a princess of Schleswig-Holstein-Sonderburg-Glücksburg, who was not descended from George III. Whatever the duke's motives were in playing this rather cruel practical joke on the prying Macalpine, apart from deftly sidestepping her request for a sample of his own urine, the last laugh, as so often, was on him. For Princess Ortrud of Hanover, though not descended from George III, *was* descended from George II through the Hesse-Kassel line.

Patient A

In an attempt to find more royal porphyria patients, Macalpine, Hunter and Rimington wrote to various friends and colleagues asking if they had come across any such cases. One of those who replied was Alfred Vannotti (b. 1907), Professor of Medicine at the University Medical Polyclinic in Lausanne, Switzerland. Vannotti was a highly respected authority on porphyria and had written a book on the subject in French which Rimington, with his expertise in languages, had translated into English.[23] Rimington was under the impression that Vannotti had some connection with the Greek Royal Family, and he felt that he might be able to tease some information out of him. In fact, the information that Vannotti provided was to act as the major evidence for the occurrence of porphyria in a living Royal.

In May 1967, Vannotti wrote to Rimington with information concerning one of his former patients.

Princess Adelaide of Prussia, wife of Prince Adalbert of Prussia, third son of the last emperor Wilhelm of Germany, was treated by me during the war for a bronchopneumonia. She had very dark urine and often abdominal pains. I examined twice the urine of the patient and I found a big amount of coproporphyrin, uroporphyrin and porphobilinogen. Unfortunately, the results of these analyses, which were done in the 'Policlinique' were lost; so I cannot give you the doses, but it was not doubtful that the patient suffered from an abdominal form of porphyria. There were no neurological, no cutaneous symptoms, but practically I saw the patient only during one month. Since then I had no news from her and I don't know if she died and how. She had a daughter; I was told she was married in USA.[24]

As can be imagined, this news caused great excitement – a living relative examined by an authority on porphyria with elevated levels of coproporphyrin, uroporphyrin and porphobilinogen in her urine, the classic diagnostic hallmarks of variegate porphyria. Both Macalpine and Rimington were bursting with further questions: 'What were her symptoms?' they wanted to know.

Was it her first attack or at what age did she suffer her first attack? Had she then or previously any cutaneous manifestations such as fragility of the skin or abnormal pigmentation? Was there any indication of a precipitating factor such as the use of barbiturate sleeping tablets? Was anything recorded concerning family history, similar illness among relatives, or any follow-up investigation undertaken? What has been her subsequent clinical history?[25]

However, as Vannotti had only seen the patient for a relatively short period of time some twenty-five years earlier, he was unable to answer most of their questions. Macalpine feverishly tried to find out as much as she could about Princess Adelaide from other sources. A trip to the German Embassy in London provided the next excitement. 'Eureka!' she wrote. 'Her address is Villa Mandragore, La Tour de Peilz, near Montreux.'[26] There was more good news, as Macalpine had discovered the whereabouts of Princess Adelaide's children: 'She has a daughter living in Washington and a son in Stuttgart and I will try and find their medical attendants,' she

28

reported.[27] Macalpine of course realized that, if their mother had the disease, there was an excellent chance that at least one of her children would also have inherited the disorder.

When Vannotti was told Princess Adelaide's address he recalled that an acquaintance of his, a Dr Paul Niehans, was a close friend of the family.[28] Vannotti set about trying to contact Niehans to see if it was possible for him to obtain the samples which Rimington wished to analyse. Unfortunately, although Vannotti made contact with Niehans, this proved to be a mistake, as Macalpine recounted to a colleague. 'Vannotti found a friend of the titled lady and asked him to procure specimens. This man [Niehans] was so stupid to ask whether she would receive me!! And she said no thank you.'[29] As Vannotti explained to Rimington later, 'the reason why Princess Adelaide will absolutely not collaborate is – I think – she is afraid her name could be published in a scientific paper'.[30] Significantly, however, Niehans did inform the researchers of the immediate cause of the princess's attacks: 'They were induced by barbiturates and . . . the Princess has been advised never to take such drugs again.'[31]

Although samples were never obtained for analysis, the diagnosis of porphyria in Princess Adelaide is quite good. Vannotti was highly regarded and despite the fact that the records of the analysis done during the war had been destroyed,[32] it is likely that he would remember details of so prominent a patient. We asked Sir Abraham Goldberg whether he would rely on a diagnosis by Vannotti. 'Quite definitely, yes,' was his reply. Furthermore, the fact that the attack was provoked by the administration of barbiturates is further evidence that it was porphyria. The urine analysis is strongly indicative of variegate porphyria. On this fairly secure basis, Princess Adelaide became Patient A in the article on porphyria in living family members.

One thing Macalpine, Hunter and Rimington were unable to do at that time was to study the medical history of Princess Adelaide. Fortunately, once her true identity was established it became possible to locate some of her correspondence and, from this, piece together some of her ailments. These records, preserved in the Thuringian State Archive at Meiningen in east-central Germany, reveal the agony which the disease inflicted upon her in the early years of her life.

The Archival Record

Princess Adelaide, or Adelheid ('Adi') in German, was the daughter of Prince Friedrich ('Fritz') and Princess Adelheid ('Ada') of Saxe-Meiningen. Adi was inseparable from her sister Feodora, often referred to as Feo II to avoid confusion with their slightly older cousin, the daughter of Friedrich's elder half-brother Bernhard and of Charlotte, the Kaiser's sister. Like Charlotte and her daughter Feo I, the two sisters Adi and Feo II had a close, almost filial relationship with the half-British third wife of Duke Georg II of Saxe-Meiningen, Helene ('Ellen') Baroness Heldburg,[33] and it is largely due to this coincidence that we are able to reconstruct the medical biography of all four of them.

Both Adi (1891–1971) and her sister gave cause for concern at an early age. On the advice of Ellen Heldburg's brother Dr Reinhold Franz, their backbones and shoulder-blades were examined and measured, presumably because of back pain, as early as 1904, when they were in their mid-teens. Though no abnormality was found, both girls were advised to lie flat on the floor for forty-five minutes each day.[34] Two years later it was their emotional state that gave rise to concern. Feo made 'terrible scenes' for her parents, she shouted and screamed, cried all day and became like a shadow of her former self, her frightened father said, and he feared that Adi, who was 'more emotional still than Feo', would be even worse once she had recovered from a recent physical illness. 'She has been ill and is in bed again now with stomach pains, headache & nausea, but without a temperature,' he informed the baroness on 3 May 1906.[35] Relations between the two girls and their parents became seriously strained, and their physical condition, too, deteriorated with the onset of puberty. The family doctor ordered Adi to take a good deal of exercise in the fresh air but at this time expressed the optimistic view that 'with the right treatment she will grow out of all her troubles. She has simply grown too fast. Naturally very special care must be taken of her.' Feo was dispatched to spend the summer with her grandfather and Ellen Heldburg at Meiningen. 'She is suffering from anaemia, and in consequence from palpitations ['*Herzklopfen*'] when she climbs the stairs and so on.'[36]

Only a few weeks later the family physician sent Adi for a rest in the Bavarian Alps. 'Since Adi is at the stage of rapid development, more than Feo, the doctor is very much in favour of peat baths,' their father explained.[37] This new treatment, which was repeated the following summer, had been suggested by an alarming new symptom: Adi had to 'contend constantly with a kind of eczema ['*Flechte*'] on her head. The roots of her hair are said to be diseased.'[38] In the family doctor's opinion, 'Adi was *absolutely* in need of peat baths every year on account of her weak mucous membranes.'[39] In March 1907, it was Adi's turn to recuperate on the estates of her grandfather in the company of Ellen Heldburg, who took the opportunity to call on her brother to give the princess a thorough examination.[40] Unfortunately we do not have Dr Franz's diagnosis, but we do know that it was deeply disturbing and pessimistic. As Fritz Meiningen wrote to his stepmother, 'what he said about his diagnosis of Adi's condition has really shocked us. If only she can grow out of it.'[41]

The girls were now being examined more and more frequently in an effort to get to the root of their disease. Feo in particular suffered from a stomach disorder and was thought to be 'unfortunately extremely sensitive with her body'. On 5 June 1908, a doctor in Hanover gave her a thorough examination and found the organs themselves to be in good order. 'He too thinks, in agreement with G[eheim] R[at] Franz, that it is only a matter of anaemia, and he does not think there is a stomach ulcer. He will get in touch with G. R. Franz. He also thinks that a sojourn at [Bad] Schwalbach would be advisable. The constantly recurring pains & the lack of resistance [to infection] are very depressing. Both things naturally worry us a great deal.'[42]

In the summer of 1911 Adi was sent for an extended 'massage cure' by a Swedish woman in Hanover. The reason her mother gave for this treatment is again significant: it was intended to alleviate the princess's 'flatulence & colic pains'.[43]

In the very last days of July 1914, with war only days away, the Kaiser's third son Prince Adalbert wrote passionate letters first to Ellen Heldburg and then to Adi herself proposing marriage to the young princess. Adi rushed to Wilhelmshaven where Adalbert was serving on the *Prinz Regent Luitpold* and they were married on 3 August, as the German Army was storming into Luxembourg and Belgium.[44]

Early in January 1916, Princess Adelheid of Prussia, as she now was, began to complain of feeling sick and extremely weak. On 28 January she reported to Ellen Heldburg that the doctor had ordered her to take iron and to lie down for an hour each day 'because I am anaemic'. He also recommended that she should spend some time resting in the mountain air.[45] As she got worse she moved to Meiningen. By mid-February 1916 her illness had developed into a serious 'inflammation of the kidneys' with a high temperature.[46] Her husband and her mother-in-law the Kaiserin both asked to be kept in touch daily; Prince Adalbert sent Dr Karl Holzapfel from Wilhelmshaven to be with her.[47] When Adalbert was able to visit her at the end of the month, Adelheid's temperature was down to 36.2°C, though she was still very pale and felt a little dizzy and weak. She had been given Adaline, and some Tokaya wine to strengthen her. 'If only this anaemia could be treated more successfully!' Adalbert sighed.[48]

When she eventually left there at the end of April 1916, it was for a clinic in the spa town of Bad Neuenahr, just south of Bonn. She was permitted to go for gentle walks, but not to climb uphill 'since the daytime samples [of urine?] examined by the Prof. show a significant difference from the nighttime samples, suggesting that every exertion may be harmful!' She was receiving arsenic injections, presumably for dermatological problems, felt well and was even getting rosy cheeks.[49] Her initial optimism was misplaced, however. Less than two weeks after her arrival at Neuenahr, Adi was again complaining of exhaustion and expressing frustration at her lack of progress. Like all her earlier doctors, the professor at her clinic diagnosed her as severely anaemic with abdominal disorders.[50]

Ten days later, Adelheid suffered a 'feverish attack' so alarming that her husband was summoned to her side. The doctor was forced for the moment to abandon her 'cure' and rather helplessly suggested that lying on the balcony in the fresh air might do her some good.[51] Not until 27 May was she able to report some improvement in her condition, saying she was allowed to go for walks again and now suffered her 'attacks of weakness' or 'waves of tiredness' only sporadically. Her appetite was improving, and she was beginning to look better, too.

With defeat and revolution in 1918 and the death of the baroness shortly thereafter, the correspondence breaks off and we lose sight of Princess Adi until she resurfaces as Professor Vannotti's patient in Lausanne during the Second World War. His clinical diagnosis of her condition as 'abdominal [acute] porphyria' is entirely consistent with the medical history we have been able to reconstruct on the basis of the archival record for the dozen years between the onset of puberty and the early years of her marriage. That record now enables us to answer some of the questions Macalpine and Rimington posed in 1967 and Vannotti was unable to answer:

☐ Adelheid's first 'life-threatening' attacks, like her sister's, occurred in 1908, and they were followed by numerous further attacks, notably during the First World War, when she was obliged to spend several months in a clinic at Bad Neuenahr.

☐ The doctors consistently diagnosed her as suffering from severe anaemia, but they were aware of other – abdominal and cutaneous – symptoms that they seemed unable to account for. Reinhold Franz appears to have warned as early as April 1907 that her condition was grave and possibly incurable.

☐ It was at about that time that she developed an unsightly eczema on the scalp and problems with her mucous membrane that would suggest variegate porphyria rather than acute intermittent porphyria as the cause of her suffering.

☐ As for her relatives, we have seen that her sister Feo (II), the later Grand Duchess of Saxe-Weimar-Eisenach, had symptoms not dissimilar to those plaguing Adi.

Princess Adelheid survived her autocratic and arrogant Hohenzollern husband by several decades, cutting a lonely and at times eccentric figure, and finally dying in her eightieth year, alone in the beautiful Villa Mandragore on the shores of Lake Geneva on 25 April 1971. The notice of her death inserted by her children in the local newspaper gives only the faintest hint of the struggle she had undergone: she had passed away, it said, *'après une maladie courageusement supportée'*.[52] Several of her relatives have confirmed to us that she was indeed suffering from porphyria, one member of the family saying: 'What you write . . . enables me with hindsight to make sense of all those dark hints and all that secretiveness. It goes to confirm your researches.'

Following the Line of Patient A: The Search for Her Daughter

Since Meiningen was behind the Iron Curtain in Communist East Germany, such archival evidence would not have been available to Macalpine, Hunter and Rimington in the 1960s, even if they had known of its existence. Given the lack of absolute evidence for porphyria in Princess Adelaide – no clinical readings were available to support the claim – they turned their attention to her children instead. As mentioned earlier, Macalpine had discovered that in 1961 the princess had a daughter living in Washington and a son in Stuttgart. They never made contact with the son. The daughter, Victoria-Marina, was to cause them as much frustration as her mother.

The editor of the *British Medical Journal*, Dr Martin Ware, was just about to travel to Washington. After explaining the background and the importance of Adelaide's daughter to their research, Macalpine persuaded him to search for Victoria-Marina's address on his visit. On 18 June 1967, Ware wrote to Macalpine from his hotel in Washington: 'Just a line to say I've located your Princess, via the husband (Captain Patterson) from whom she is now separated. He thinks she will cooperate and he goes to see her in two weeks time armed with a photocopy of the George III article. She is now called Countess Victoria-Marina Lingen, and her address is 7801 Mocking-Bird Lane, Scotsdale, Arizona.'[53]

Ware suggested that Macalpine should not try to contact the princess immediately so as to give the husband time to explain the situation to his estranged wife. Macalpine telexed back immediately, her excitement reflected in a porphyric pun: 'Splendid achievement, we are tickled purple!' Of course, the main issue on Macalpine's mind was how to obtain the appropriate samples. There was also a problem in having the samples sent on such a long journey from the other side of the Atlantic, since there was a danger that they might either deteriorate or be lost altogether. To overcome this hurdle, Rimington set up a collaboration with a friend in the

United States called Dr Cripps. When the time was right, Macalpine would arrange for the sample to be sent direct to Cripps's laboratory.

The interest in Countess Lingen[54] must have been heightened by some of the other information her husband had provided. He had told Macalpine and Rimington about an illness she had had four years earlier during which she was admitted to the NIH hospital in Bethesda, just outside Washington DC. This led to an interesting and revealing correspondence between Rimington and Dr Donald Tschudy, a physician specializing in porphyria at the hospital.[55] Tschudy listed the reasons why she had been admitted.

> She is a descendant of Queen Victoria as you probably know. She was a patient of Dr John Fahey and was shown to have Waldenström's macroglobulinaemia [presence of excessive amounts of an immunoglobulin within the blood] with thrombocytosis [increase in the number of platelets], anaemia and hyperproteinemia. There was a bleeding dithesis which was studied, but no diagnosis of haemophilia or other cause for bleeding apart from the macroglobulinaemia could be made. Other diagnosis: 1) menorrhagia [heavy periods] and metrorrhagia [bleeding from uterus other than due to period], questionable etiology, 2) chronic sinusitis, 3) mild peripheral neuropathy, 4) post-phlebitic syndrome, 5) questionable mass, right breast. She had other vague symptoms which were thought to be hysterical and the neurologists left the question of peripheral neuropathy unanswered, if present it was certainly of a mild degree.[56]

On the burning issue itself, he could not help, commenting ruefully: 'Wouldn't it be ironic if she has porphyria and we missed it? My only excuse would be that she was not my patient and I did not examine her. No chemical tests for porphyria were done, but she was given [a number of potential porphyric drugs] with no detrimental effects.'[57]

Rimington was most excited by the disclosures that Donald Tschudy had made and remarked on the countess's bizarre medical history. Although he agreed that there is no known association between Waldenström's macroglobinaemia and porphyria of any variety, he could not help feeling that many of the other symptoms which Tschudy had enumerated – for example menorrhagia (not uncommon in porphyria), chronic sinusitis and mild peripheral neuropathy – were highly indicative of variegate porphyria. Furthermore, to Rimington, the suspicion of hysteria was also quite suggestive. These indications sufficed for the countess to become the fourth positive case alluded to in the Macalpine-Hunter book when it was published. However, the London researchers were acutely aware of the urgent need to obtain samples from Countess Lingen, since if her recent confinement in the hospital had been due to porphyria she might still, they believed, have the tell-tale elevated levels of porphyrins in her excrement.

After the necessary delay, the indefatigable Macalpine wrote to the countess, asking whether she would be willing to participate in the study. She explained that she would send containers which the countess could then forward to Dr Cripps for analysis. Though the countess had indicated that she would be willing to provide the necessary samples, nothing more was heard from her. After one month of frustration, with no news from America, Macalpine dropped a note to Cripps to ask how the investigation was progressing. 'Unfortunately no good news,' Cripps replied.[58] The specimen containers had been sent to the countess, he explained, but after waiting two weeks for a reply Cripps had telephoned her. She had replied that she had received the containers, but had decided not to go through with the experiment.

There is no doubt that this news came as a severe disappointment to the researchers. They were relying on a positive result from either Princess Adelaide or her daughter to provide the clinching evidence of porphyria in a living relative. It was left to Macalpine to reply to Cripps in the hope that something might yet be salvaged from their efforts. 'What a pity the lady will not play,' she wrote. 'We even thought of a private eye! Please keep on trying. We had a lot of trouble with members refusing and I am told that porphyric patients are in this respect usually reluctant or is it that they fear mental implications and therefore rather not know?'[59]

The researchers were never to receive the precious samples from either Princess Adelaide or her daughter. Although they tried to trace the countess's local physician in Scotsdale, this line of investigation also failed. Overall, then, Macalpine, Hunter and Rimington had to make do with the readings that they had measured from Patient B's samples, and to quote Vannotti (not by name but by referring to him as a distinguished physician) on the fact that he had diagnosed Princess Adelaide as porphyric. These meagre results mask the immense trouble to which they had gone to try to find patients and the difficulty which surrounded the process but also the fact that no hard evidence for the occurrence of porphyria in a living family member had actually been found. Despite Rimington's theory, in Patient B the level of X-porphyrin was not significant and the values of coproporphyrin and protoporphyrin were within normal limits. Thus we are left with the diagnosis by Vannotti of Patient A which, although it can be trusted, is not absolute as the actual reading of elevated porphobilinogen and porphyrins had been discarded. Furthermore, Vannotti had been the princess's physician for only one month and that had been during the war which had ended more than twenty years earlier. Notwithstanding the lack of evidence, Vannotti's diagnosis is consistent with variegate porphyria and the confirmation of the diagnosis via Dr Niehans, the princess's own physician, that the attack was triggered by barbiturates is quite compelling. It is also strongly supported by the evidence we have unearthed in the archives and statements made to us by her close relatives. The case for porphyria in her daughter, Victoria-Marina, is less conclusive and she appears to have suffered a number of complex illnesses.

The Trail Peters Out

From September 1967 onwards, Macalpine concentrated on writing the follow-up paper. She had acquired an enormous amount of historical information and her ability as an archival researcher is most impressive. It is not her historical scholarship but her interpretation of the ailments based upon it which can be disputed. Clearly, in all the historical figures that Macalpine had researched, she was looking for symptoms of porphyria. Thus anybody who suffered with general malaise, headaches, muscle weakness or gout immediately fell under suspicion.

A draft copy of their research article on the widespread occurrence of porphyria in the European royal families was prepared and sent to Abraham Goldberg. It is interesting to note that as early as September 1967 Goldberg suggested to Macalpine that 'as a general point, you should be a little less definite about your claim'.[60] These words of wisdom were not taken on board and the porphyria story was written up as fact rather than as a hypothesis in need of further verification.

Although the correspondence on the occurrence of porphyria throughout the royal houses of Europe continued after the publication of the paper, it was now rather mundane. Macalpine did for a while pursue the possibility of acquiring samples but again with little success. There is, however, one intriguing footnote to a letter from Macalpine to Rimington which reads: 'I have heard nothing more from Bodley Scott's patients. I trust you would let me know in case Goldberg has something up his sleeve!'[61] Sir Ronald Bodley Scott was the head physician of the British Royal Family. However, although Goldberg discussed with Bodley Scott the possibility of porphyria in the House of Windsor, and Bodley Scott confirmed to him that the Royals would be willing to be examined, no samples were ever obtained. This is because, according to Goldberg's own account, he felt that, in the absence of any physical sign of the disease, there was no point in analysing the family.

The recollections of a junior member of the royal medical household are slightly different. He points out that, as a haematologist, Sir Ronald Bodley Scott was well qualified to deal with porphyria. He asserts that Bodley Scott did in fact screen all the immediate and several distant members of the Royal Family, sending their samples to Goldberg in Glasgow for analysis. Although the junior doctor did not know the outcome of Bodley Scott's researches, it seems that the tests did put the royal minds to rest. Other members of the royal medical household have been keen to confirm this view, insisting that they have heard of no evidence of any living member of the Royal Family producing any symptoms or signs compatible with porphyria. As we shall show, one very interesting case was being overlooked.

CHAPTER 3

'Madness' and King George III

Whenever God of his infinite goodness shall call me out of this world,
the tongue of malice may not paint my intentions in those colours she
admires, nor the sycophant extol me beyond what I deserve.

King George III

The health of leading figures has always been of great interest to historians because of the direct effect that ill-health has on the individual in both thought and deed. Whereas the outcome of physical illnesses is comparatively easy to assess, the consequences of mental illness on historical characters requires complex interpretation, not least because mental illness can be so difficult to define. For instance, at what point does depression become a mental disturbance, or when should mood swings be defined as manic depression, and at what point does bizarre behaviour become schizophrenia? Where is the line drawn between a peculiar personality trait and a mental disorder?[1]

Perhaps the term 'madness' has an attraction for historians precisely because it is imprecise and can cover a host of disorders. In this account we shall define 'madness' as a drastic change in character and personality. What is the cause of madness? It is known that there are genetic predispositions to mental disturbance, but the susceptibility to such a condition is not dependent upon a single gene; rather, several genes are involved, which is why these complex neurological traits are referred to as 'multifactorial' disorders. Outside of physical damage to the central nervous system, mental derangement can also be caused by infection and metabolic imbalance, as is the case with porphyria. The whole area of mental disturbance comes under the auspices of psychiatry and, as with all branches of medicine, requires lengthy and detailed training if it is to be properly understood. An even deeper quagmire exists in the area of retrospective psychoanalysis, the understanding of mental disorders based upon the teaching of Sigmund Freud. Psychoanalysis pays particular attention to the influence of unconscious forces in a person's emotional and mental life. The application of psychoanalysis to historical figures is contentious because the unconscious forces are deduced from the available information on the upbringing of the individual, while an assessment of the individual's personality is based on the interpretation of biographers. In their reappraisal of George III, and in light of Manfred S. Guttmacher's theory of manic depressive psychosis,[2] both Sir Lewis Namier[3] and Sir John Plumb[4] correlated psychology with history to produce a character sketch in which the King was represented as being susceptible to both personal and political pressure. As we shall see later, a very different conclusion has been reached by later historians who have eschewed Freudian preconceptions.

Although George III is traditionally viewed as England's mad king, he is by no means the only monarch to be tagged with this description. In fact, European history in general seems to be replete with monarchs whose minds buckled under the pressures of authoritarian power. A recent American study of the *Mad Princes of Renaissance Germany* examined over thirty cases of serious royal insanity on record for that region in the sixteenth century alone.[5] There are no grounds whatever for supposing that German princes were any more susceptible to madness than any other monarchs. In Sweden the mad King Erik XIV, whose brother had also gone insane, had to be imprisoned in 1569, and in Hungary Princess Elizabeth Bathory (1560–1614) also descended into the black hole of insanity.[6] Vivian Green's fascinating account of *The Madness of Kings* demonstrates the enormous influence which the mental health of leaders has had on world events over the last 2500 years, from the Roman emperors to the bloodthirsty dictators of our own day.[7]

In the interests of balance and fairness, then, and to set the case of George III in its proper perspective, we should look at genuinely 'mad' monarchs and compare their illnesses with George III's, whose sanity was most likely temporarily disturbed by a transient metabolic imbalance. To this end we shall briefly explore the medical history of two related medieval monarchs, Charles VI of France and Henry VI of England, before turning our attention to the Hanoverian king.

Charles VI (1368–1422)[8]

King Charles VI of France suffered numerous attacks of mental derangement which occurred with ever greater frequency and duration as he got older. Charles was the son of King Charles V (the Wise) of France and Jeanne de Bourbon. On his mother's side, there appears to be a family history of mental instability and she herself suffered with a severe breakdown, possibly post-natal depression, shortly after the birth of her seventh child in 1373. The first episode of mental derangement suffered by Charles VI occurred in April 1392, shortly after he was struck down by a mysterious 'unheard of disease'. The symptoms, including fever, dizziness and anxiety, and his delirium persisted for several months and reached a climax in August, while he was on an expedition to avenge the murder of one of his friends. The illness resulted in the King's becoming completely deranged, so much so that he killed four or five of his own knights. After being restrained by his guards, Charles apparently suffered a *grand mal* seizure and went into a coma for two days.

The King's illness, which started back in April, may have been due to typhoid, but encephalitis has also been suggested. Encephalitis is an inflammation of the brain, usually as a consequence of infection or allergic reaction. Whatever Charles VI's illness might have been, and although he made something of a recovery from his 1392 episode, it clearly affected his central nervous system, as during the next thirty years, until his death in 1422, he suffered repeated attacks of insanity. During these attacks his mind became cloudy and deluded. He did not recognize himself as King and at times believed that he was made of glass, even inserting iron rods in his clothes to protect his delicate frame. There seems little doubt that the monarch was by now a schizophrenic. This severe mental condition is characterized by a fragmentation of normal thought processes and a removal from reality and emotion. Delusions and hallucinations are common and the patient feels that his thoughts and actions are controlled by others, in this case epitomized by the

41

fact that many thought the King was under the influence of witches and sorcery. The disorder can start in adolescence or young adulthood, and it is interesting to note that Charles's first major attack took place when he was twenty-four years old. Schizophrenia normally runs a progressive course, as was also observed with the King's condition. Although schizophrenia does not generally show a simple pattern of inheritance, it is certainly influenced by genetic factors and there is often a familial association with the condition. In contrast to the mental disturbances which affected George III, the bouts of madness suffered by Charles VI did not apparently coincide with any physical illness.

One of the consequences of Charles VI's condition was the political disorder which it caused in France. The in-fighting and the political vacuum which resulted from his incapacity meant that the country was poorly prepared when the army of King Henry V landed in France in 1415 to recover the French kingdom. Despite being ravaged by a severe outbreak of dysentery, the English Army defeated a much larger French force at the battle of Agincourt. By 1419 the English were victorious and, by the Treaty of Troyes, it was arranged for Henry V to marry Charles's daughter, Catherine, and succeed Charles VI as King of France. As it turned out, Henry V died in 1422, two months before Charles VI. Henry's son, Henry VI, thus became sovereign of both England and France at the age of nine months.

Henry VI (1421–71)[9]

It has been suggested that Henry VI was born with a congenital mental weakness; certainly he did not have the strong will required to rule over both England and France. Admittedly, it cannot have been easy for a child to be groomed for the kingship of two countries which had been at war with each other for nearly a hundred years. During Henry's childhood, his uncle the Duke of Gloucester was appointed Regent in England whilst another uncle, the Duke of Bedford, was appointed Regent in France. Despite Henry's claim to the French throne, Charles VI's son, Charles VII, contested the succession and fighting between the two claimants soon broke out. In comparison to the fragmented French opposition against the English armies of Henry V, this fresh outbreak led to an increased show of patriotism on behalf of the French people which was manifested most evidently in the appearance of Joan of Arc. Although she led a spirited resistance to the English, she was eventually captured and burnt at the stake at Rouen. Henry VI was crowned King of France in 1431, when he was ten years old, but by 1453 the English had lost all of their gains and at the end of the Hundred Years' War in 1453 only Calais remained in English hands.

The loss of the war was obviously a major blow to Henry VI and shortly afterwards he went insane, drifting into a 'state of severe melancholia and depressive illness' in the summer of 1453. He relapsed into a state of withdrawal, unable to reason, unaware of his surroundings, and was not even able to dress himself. He lost his memory and did not know of the birth of his son Edward. Henry did not recover from this mental breakdown for two years, and even after he was thought to be well again, there is evidence to suggest that he suffered a relapse in early 1456. As with his grandfather, Charles VI, there is no suggestion that the derangement of his mind was due to any extenuating physical illness. The appointment of Henry VI's cousin, Richard Duke of York, as Protector of England during the King's illness was to lead to his eventual downfall. After Henry had recovered from his mental aberration, Richard was reluctant to give up his power. Supported by the Yorkists, Richard fought against Henry, who was upheld by the Lancastrians, a confrontation which resulted in the Wars of the Roses. Although Richard was killed in the Battle of Wakefield in 1461, his son continued the fray until the Lancastrians were eventually beaten at the Battle of Tewkesbury in 1471. Henry VI (whose son Edward was killed at Tewkesbury) was eventually murdered.

As a grandson of Charles VI, there is a chance that Henry VI would have been predisposed to schizophrenia, and in fact catatonic schizophrenia has been suggested as the cause of Henry VI's breakdown. This condition is marked by severe motor disturbances, causing the patient to become mute and lethargic and adopt odd postures, with the limbs being moved passively into positions which are then retained. The genetic predisposition to schizophrenia may be of importance, but it is also possible that Henry suffered from manic-depressive psychosis. Whatever the cause, the major illness which affected Henry VI is very different from the repeated episodic attacks which affected George III. There is no record of physical illness in the medieval monarch and, apart from the inference of peripheral neuropathy reflected in Henry's lethargy, his illness would not appear to have been life-threatening.

As Henry VI and his son had been killed, this royal line was not to pass its possible predisposition to schizophrenia into the later British Royals. Rather, they were to inherit a faulty haem biosynthetic gene, probably from the Stuarts, which then passed from them to the Hanoverian line. Most markedly, the effects of this gene were to manifest themselves in George III.

George III (1738–1820)[10]

George III succeeded his grandfather George II as King of Great Britain and Ireland in 1760. His father, Frederick Lewis, had died unexpectedly in 1751 after picking up what appeared to be a minor cold. This propelled the young Prince George into the role of king-in-waiting. His grandfather was sixty-eight at the time and it was hoped that he would last at least until the young prince came of age. Fortunately, George II survived until the prince was twenty-two years old, but what effect the psychological pressures of being heir had on the prince's mind is difficult to gauge. It certainly did not overtly appear to affect him and his general health seems to have been good.

However, in June 1762, the King, now aged twenty-four, suffered from what appeared to be a persistent feverish cold. The illness constricted the King's chest, making breathing difficult. It was uncomfortable enough for him to complain of pain and stitches. Whether because of worries about the similarity with the fatal illness of the monarch's father, or because of a more general concern that the illness might be consumption (i.e. tuberculosis), the royal physicians took the infection seriously. The King was blooded seven times, had three blisters, and was prescribed asses' milk, thought to be a remedy for consumption. The King was also given a laxative, which he referred to as his 'manna', indicating that perhaps he was also constipated. During the illness, his pulse was elevated and after nearly two weeks of feeling poorly George reported that he still had a slight cold and chest pains and was tired.

The doctors, although undoubtedly pleased with the recovery, were concerned that the infection would reappear in the winter with fatal consequences. Fortunately, the King was to remain free from illness for the next thirty months.

Although George III appeared to make a full recovery, the reappearance of a similar infection in 1765 rekindled the original worries about consumption. This time the illness occurred in winter, starting on 13 January as a violent cold with 'stitches' in the chest. Once again he was blooded and cupped to reduce the fever. Cupping, the method employed for drawing blood from a laceration by using the vacuum generated by a warm cup over the wound, was particularly painful. The illness appeared to clear up within several days, but a month later, on 25 February, the King was again blooded because of a feverish cold. A week later, on 3 March, he was still unwell with a fever, pain in the chest and a rapid pulse, although he appeared to be in good humour. His illness led to a certain amount of weight loss. On 9 March, although still of a cheerful disposition, George requested peace and quiet to complete his recovery, but by 22 March he was still complaining of a cough and chest pains and, consequently, was cupped again. The predilection of his physicians for this agonizing – and completely useless – procedure must have been one of the reasons for the King's growing distrust and dislike of the medical profession. By the end of March, the monarch appeared to have recovered from his illness, but the fever was to return at the end of May. During this period of the attack his pulse was quick and he suffered from insomnia, sleeping only a couple of hours for several nights. Although the King was soon reported to be well once more, another feverish attack occurred at the end of July with symptoms similar to those he had had before, with the result that he was blooded yet again. As in 1762, the physicians feared a return of the illness in the winter, but apart from a brief cold and fever in February 1766, during which the King received the accustomed blood-letting, there was no sign of consumption.

During the bouts of illness from 1762 to 1766 there was no mental incapacity and at no point was the King's mind deranged. Later suggestions that the King was insane during his 1765 illness were an assumption based on rumour rather than on historical fact. Disproving the myth of the King's 1765 insanity was one of the most impressive pieces of historical research undertaken by Macalpine and Hunter.[11] However, the pattern of illness, whereby George III's condition would suddenly relapse just as he seemed to be improving, was to be repeated in his later illnesses.

The First Attack of 'Madness', 1788–9

In general, the King remained in good health for the next twenty-two years. It was not until a week after his fiftieth birthday, on 11 June 1788, that George was afflicted with a smart bilious attack. The discomfort was so severe that he was forced to take to his bed, which was the only place he could adopt a 'tolerable posture'.[12] Sir George Baker, one of the King's doctors and President of the Royal College of Physicians, was called and he immediately prescribed a purgative to help clear what he presumed to be blockage of the intestine. Eighteenth-century physicians were limited in the treatments they could offer their patients. They generally prescribed either emetics (to promote vomiting), purgatives and enemas (to promote defecation) or opium-based painkillers such as laudanum. Most of their other procedures caused more harm than good, as is witnessed by their frequent use of leeches and cupping. As the distinguished chronicler of the time, Sir Horace Walpole, noted, 'A disorder that requires no physician is preferable to any that does.'[13] It seems very likely that George's physicians, rather than alleviating his symptoms, merely exacerbated them.

The King's complaint was described as 'disagreeable and indeed alarming' by his daughter the Princess Royal, who noted that her father was badly indisposed from 3 a.m. to 8 p.m.[14] In fact the attack was prolonged, as the King was retained at Kew House for two weeks due to his colic. Queen Charlotte attributed the illness to the dryness and heat of the season, and it was generally decided that a holiday would benefit the King, especially as the parliamentary session was drawing to a close. Earl Fauconberg offered him a house at Cheltenham, where the mineral water was reported to be an excellent remedy for bilious complaints. Baker recommended a month of convalescence, and the royal party set off on 4 July 1788. The holiday appeared to do the trick. 'The waters are more efficacious than I could possibly have expected, for while they removed byle in a very gentle manner they strengthen the stomach and are a gentler bracer to the constitution,' the King reported.[15] On 16 August the royal party returned to Windsor with the King apparently restored to health.

However, on 17 October 1788, at 7.25 in the morning, the King was struck down with another bilious attack. He was bent double with stomach pain and his breathing was difficult and uneasy. The pain continued for most of the day until he had emptied his bowels. He informed his physician, Sir George Baker, that he had been suffering recently from muscle cramps in his legs and rheumatism in all his limbs, making him lame. He also had a rash on his arm which caused his daughter Princess Elizabeth to remark on its 'very red' appearance and how the rash formed 'in great weals as if it had been scourged with cords'.[16] On 18 October 1788, Baker noted 'some yellowness in the eyes and urine bilious' (presumably referring to its dark appearance), although he also noted that both the eyes and the urine had returned to a more normal colour by the next day. On 20 October the King was very ill in the night, with the return of the acute abdominal pain and a very rapid pulse. He found it extremely difficult to concentrate and his general lack of muscle tone made him easily tired. Two days later the monarch's rapid pulse had not abated and he was constipated. Baker saw the King that afternoon and was taken aback by his very peculiar mood as he was detained for three hours and bombarded with a range of repetitious questions. The meeting so worried Baker that he considered the King's condition in a state 'bordering on delirium'.[17] A further two days, and George's condition was still a concern for his physicians, especially as he 'was weak and somewhat lame' and continually troubled with insomnia.[18]

By 26 October it was reported that the King was talking rapidly with a hoarse voice. He was hardly sleeping at all and was remarkably agitated. When Baker visited him on 27 October, at the request of the worried Queen, he found George III talking incessantly, 'making frequent and sudden transitions from one subject to another'. He was still lame, suffering from rheumatic pain and was 'continually sitting and rising'.[19]

During the next few days the King's rapid speech continued and he appeared very agitated. Moreover his vision was confused, his hearing was failing and he was beginning to lose his memory. George's condition did not improve, and by the beginning of

November he was still troubled by lameness, muscular weakness, failing sight, agitation, confusion and insomnia. He talked incoherently and was in a state of delirium. On 5 November, Baker reported that the King was 'under an intire alienation of mind'.[20] The next day Baker noticed that the monarch's pulse was 120 and he was still delirious. He was bled again, but of course to no avail. When Baker himself was indisposed due to illness, Dr Richard Warren, a well-known 'society' doctor (that is, one who was paid to tell his patients what they wanted to hear) and physician to the Prince of Wales, was called in on the case. Warren was loathed by George and was refused admittance to the sickroom, so he listened and observed the King from a strategic vantage point behind the door. Horrified by what he saw and heard, Warren made straight for the Prince of Wales and told him that the King's life was in danger and that he was suffering a 'seizure upon the brain', and that 'if he did live, there was little reason to hope his intellect would be restored'.[21] The implications of this diagnosis were obvious to the prince and his political supporters, the Whigs, led by Charles James Fox. The King would have to be 'sectioned' and the prince installed as a caretaker monarch. Warren's intervention can thus be looked upon as the beginning of the Regency Crisis.

George III's condition continued to worsen and Baker reported to the Prime Minister, William Pitt the Younger, 'that the King's delirium continued through the whole day'.[22] On 9 November a rumour spread that the King had died. In fact, though he was still alive, he was very seriously ill after several convulsions which had resulted in a coma. The following day, the King was only semiconscious and still extremely ill. He was not sleeping but was talking incessantly throughout the night and completely delirious. He had now been ill for a month and his doctors still had no idea as to the nature of his malady. The royal physicians, who were responsible to both the Royal Family and the government, were in an unenviable position. They had an unmanageable and unpredictable patient and yet had no idea how to treat his condition as none of them had ever come across anything quite like it before. Not only the Court and the politicians but also the general public wanted to know what was wrong with the King, and so the physicians were forced to write public bulletins, which were generally banal and meaningless and merely added to the general sense of frustration.

Once it became general knowledge that the King's mind was deranged, stories and rumours flew about London. It was suggested that while in Cheltenham the King had tried to race against a horse. George was also said to have got out of his coach in Windsor Great Park and addressed an oak tree, believing it to be Frederick the Great, the King of Prussia, even shaking hands with the lower branches.[23]

By now there were no fewer than seven royal physicians who argued amongst themselves as to the cause and prognosis of the King's illness. On 29 November 1788, the King was moved from Windsor to Kew, where the doctors felt the greater privacy would facilitate a more rapid recovery. On his first night at Kew, the King was both agitated and violent, although his mood would rapidly change. His overall condition, however, simply did not improve, and by the end of November it was decided that the Reverend Francis Willis, 'who has great skill and experience in treating this unhappy malady', be sent for.[24] Dr Willis was a clergyman who had set up a madhouse in Lincolnshire and had been awarded a medical degree by the University of Oxford. As he relied on the help of his sons in its management, Willis's asylum could be looked upon as a family enterprise.

Willis believed that the King's madness could be controlled by intimidation, coercion and restraint. As he explained to one of the ministers, patients had to be broken in, like 'horses in a manège'.[25] When the monarch behaved violently or inappropriately, he was placed in a straitjacket and sometimes also tied to his bed, and was only released when he repented of his ways. By now there was a clear divide in the attitude of the royal physicians, which reflected their political beliefs as much as their medical training. Warren and Baker were of the opinion that the King was insane, an argument which was used by the Whig Opposition, who pressed for the introduction of a regency under the Prince of Wales. Willis, on the other hand, viewed the illness as delirium and felt that the King would make a complete recovery, the argument used by the Tory government to remain in power and put off the proposed Regency Bill. However, as the King was obviously gravely ill, the government knew it would have at least to contemplate such an eventuality.

As early as 20 October 1788, Parliament had considered what

should be done if George III's condition did not improve. Without the King, the Prime Minister would not be able to control the House of Commons and would have to submit to the Opposition. The longer the King's illness continued the greater the political uncertainty became, and some resolution of the crisis was imperative. On 3 December 1788, the Privy Council decided to question the royal physicians under oath, to help Parliament reach a decision on the question of a regency. When Parliament convened the next day, it was decided that both the House of Commons and the Lords would appoint committees to question the physicians further. This was, in part, a stalling procedure to allow extra time for the King's recovery. The committees met on 8 and 9 December 1788, and the lack of consensus among physicians quickly became apparent. Baker and Warren felt that the King's present condition was unrelated to his fever and inferred that he was now insane. Their colleagues were more optimistic, indicating that a full recovery was possible. Willis was the most dogmatic, declaring: 'I have great hopes of his recovery.' It was his evidence which helped to prevent the Opposition from imposing a regency straight away.[26]

By the middle of December there was some improvement in the royal patient's condition and he was allowed to walk in the garden at Kew and to see the Queen. However, shortly afterwards the King had a relapse, blisters were applied to his legs and he was straitjacketed again. The record of his symptoms bears a familiar ring: muscular weakness, incoherent speech, an elevated pulse and abdominal pain. Moreover, his delusions took on an explicit theme when he began to display amorous intentions towards Lady Pembroke, a long-standing family friend. However, outside of his delirium, he was able to recall these lascivious thoughts and apologized most profusely for them. None the less, when his more confused periods returned, so too did the explicit, embarrassing references to Lady Pembroke. As noted by his attendants, she became 'his favourite delusion'.[27] George III's lust for Lady Pembroke during his illness, and his dislike of the Queen, were to provide the basis for the Freudian theory that the King was frustrated in his marriage and that this contributed to his mental instability.

Even in this long period of illness in 1788–9, George's mind was not deranged all the time; as with the pattern of his physical symptoms, his mental state oscillated between total confusion and perfect lucidity. When his attacks were severe he talked gibberish, but as they subsided he would have prolonged periods when he made perfect sense. For instance, when he was first introduced to Dr Willis, the King remarked: 'Sir, your dress and appearance bespeaks you of the church, do you belong to it?' And when Willis replied: 'I did formerly, but lately I have attended chiefly to physicks,' the monarch retorted: 'I am sorry for it. You have quitted a profession I have always loved, and you have embraced one I most heartily detest.' Dr Willis countered: 'Our saviour went about healing the sick,' but the King retorted just as quickly: 'Yes. But he was not paid £700 a year for it!'[28] Once, during their later exchanges, George suggested to Willis that Dr Warren would make a suitable patient for his asylum in Lincolnshire, and later still, on hearing that his gardener was preparing a basket of exotic plants for Dr Willis, the King quipped: 'Get another basket – and pack the doctor in it.'[29]

As Christmas 1788 approached, King George was in a very poor state: he was sleeping for only a few hours, his pulse was very rapid (120 beats per minute), he was delirious, hoarse and constipated. However, by the end of the year he was over the worst of the attack and even started to show signs of improvement. This was just as well, since the House of Commons was becoming increasingly concerned about his condition and a regency seemed to many the only sensible course of action. To expedite a formal decision on the regency question, the Commons committee arranged another meeting with the physicians for 6 January 1789. The doctors again voiced different opinions, with Warren claiming that there was no sign of improvement, whereas Willis expressed not 'the least doubt of his recovery', although he would not hazard a guess as to how long it would take.[30]

After a brief relapse in early January 1789, the year in which political turmoil and social unrest in France would spiral out of control, George III suddenly appeared to make a significant improvement. Although still predisposed to bouts of delirium, weakness and pain, the general trend from mid-January to the beginning of February was of increased periods of lucidity. Despite the arrival of a restraining chair, to which he was strapped on Willis's orders, the general improvement in his health produced a sense of optimism in some of his doctors.

By the beginning of February 1789, his pulse had dropped, the abdominal pain had abated and he was much less agitated. By mid-February, the Whig Opposition acknowledged that the King's health had improved and the Regency Bill, which was due to have its third reading in the Lords, was shelved. On 26 February 1789, the medical bulletin read: 'There appears to be this morning an entire cessation of His Majesty's illness.'[31] King George had recovered and was to remain in good health for the next twelve years.

The Later Attacks, 1801 and 1804

A smaller-scale version of the King's illness of 1788–9 which sparked the Regency Crisis occurred in early 1801. The manner in which the illness started, the symptoms and the recovery all bear a remarkable similarity to the 1788–9 episode. On 3 February, George suffered with cramps all over, was hoarse and constipated, had little sleep, felt nauseous, complained of abdominal pain and excreted dark urine. He reported to his incoming Prime Minister Henry Addington that he had a severe cold. By 17 February, the King's manner was described as 'hurried', and shortly thereafter it became apparent that 'His Majesty's mind was not in a proper state'.[32] On 21 February the King was delirious and on the 23rd he lapsed into a coma. The Willises were summoned again to help the monarch regain his mind through their strategy of coercion. By now the King had a pulse of over 140 beats per minute and he was dangerously ill. On 25 February, out of his coma but still feverish with an elevated pulse, his disorder was rather oddly described as 'turning to black jaundice', which has been interpreted as meaning that the King's urine was again very dark.[33] At this stage of the illness, George was very confused and could neither read nor write. His sexual fantasies about Lady Pembroke had also returned.

By the beginning of March, however, the King was on the road to recovery, his fever had receded and his constipation had been successfully treated with calomel (mercury). As with the illness of 1788–9, his recovery was interrupted by several relapses. For instance, on 2 March he descended into a state of delirium and sleeplessness with a racing pulse of 136 beats per minute. Two days later the crisis abated as the King's mind became lucid again. By 6 March, his pulse had slowed to seventy-two beats per minute and, although he was still not sleeping well, his appetite had returned. By 11 March, George was reported to be well again and on the 14th he was able to receive the Prime Minister. Thereafter he steadily improved and remained free from illness for nearly three years.

As with the illness of 1801, the attack in 1804 was much less severe than that in 1788–9, although its course and symptomology followed an almost identical path. In the third week of January 1804, the King caught a cold and felt generally unwell with a certain amount of rheumatic pain. His limbs were weak and his foot had become swollen. Although he appeared to improve in general health over the next few weeks, he relapsed in the second week of February, as the bilious colic and fever returned with a vengeance. By now his mind was affected and he was greatly agitated. However, on 17 February he was reported to be out of danger and recovering well. The Willises had been sent for again but they were barred by the Royal Family from seeing the King and a new mad-doctor, Dr Samuel Simmons, was called in on the case. Simmons was just as harsh as Willis and sons and was not averse to using the straitjacket to restrain the sovereign. Indeed, the King's behaviour, which could at times be uncontrollable and violent, required its use to protect Simmons and the other physicians. Fortunately, by the end of February, the King seemed quite well again, and from this point on, although weak, his abdominal and rheumatic pain, together with the rapid pulse, abated. Occasional mention is made in the medical record of agitation and hurried speech, but on the whole the King was now in remission.

The Final Episode, 1810

The illness of 1810, which was again characterized by general malaise, abdominal and rheumatic pain, muscle weakness, rapid pulse, insomnia, delusions and excretion of dark urine, was different in one respect from the earlier attacks in that the King now suffered short-term memory loss and displayed all the hallmarks of the onset of senility. This final illness started on 25 October 1810, George reporting that he had a headache and cold. His mind had become agitated and he was sleepless. By 29 October his conversation was unconnected and Dr Simmons was called but, as he was not allowed complete management of the King, he returned home.

On 2 November 1810, King George became violent and disorderly and had an elevated pulse. He was restrained in a straitjacket, medicine was administered and leeches applied. The King's health subsequently improved, but by mid-November his fever, insomnia and elevated pulse had returned. By the end of that month, he had abdominal pain and was constipated. Although the physical symptoms eased a little, his mind remained cloudy and confused. Towards Christmas 1810 his condition worsened as the abdominal pain intensified, his agitation increased, his pulse quickened to 120 beats per minute, he remained constipated and had little sleep, and his urine was dark.

By the end of December 1810 the physicians were worried about another symptom – he 'continually adjusted the bedclothes' and 'sorted and moved his papers'.[34] George III was never to recover from this bout of illness and his condition undulated between relative calm and severe attacks. For instance, on 15 July 1811 it was thought that the monarch was dying – he was confused, agitated, violent, sleepless and had a very rapid pulse. During this stage of his illness, the Regency Bill was passed at last and the Prince of Wales (later King George IV) took the oath of office on 6 February 1811.

By the beginning of 1812, George III's physicians were of the opinion that he was unlikely ever to recover from his illness. His memory had become badly affected and it was apparent that senile dementia was setting in. At the same time, however, the King was still affected by periodic bouts of abdominal pain. In January 1812, for example, he was sleepless, extremely agitated, his face was flushed, his voice hoarse and his urine dark. The King's life for the remaining eight years faded into grim obscurity as the dementia took hold. Blind from cataracts and deaf, playing his harpsichord, he cut a pathetic figure in these final years. At 8.32 p.m. on 29 January 1820 his long life, mercifully, came to an end.

George III, Porphyria and the Historians

It is a tribute to the painstaking medical historiography of Macalpine and Hunter that all the major biographers of George III writing after 1969 base their account of his illnesses on this research. John Brooke not only wrote the article 'Historical Implications' which appeared in the British Medical Association booklet *Porphyria – A Royal Malady*, but he has also written probably the most authoritative biography of King George III, which was published in 1972.[35] His account portrays the King as a strong-willed character, stubborn at times, but a man who upheld his beliefs, loved his God and his country, was devoted to his wife and family and took an unprecedented interest in science and agriculture. Though Brooke makes clear that George III was neither a great king nor a great man, he is insistent that he was not a 'madman'.

Brooke welcomed the porphyria hypothesis with such alacrity because, to him, it confirmed what he had always believed, namely that George III was not a mentally and emotionally weak character predisposed to breakdowns under the pressure of authoritarian power. Quite the reverse, he viewed the King as an almost obstinate monarch who, for some unknown reason, suffered a series of mental aberrations. The explanation of these aberrations in terms of a rare metabolic disorder provided him with the connecting piece to complete his character analysis. In comparing the two possible diagnoses of George III, Brooke points out that manic-depressive psychosis 'can only be maintained by making assertions that are not true' and 'ignoring the physical symptoms', whereas a diagnosis of porphyria 'does not violate the facts of history' and does account for the King's physical and mental symptoms. As he puts it, when taking into account the porphyria theory, 'the myth of George III's insanity is exposed'.[36]

Stanley Ayling, whose biography of George III also appeared in 1972, accepts the diagnosis of porphyria without question. So convinced was he that he wrote without hesitation: 'The first attack of porphyria occurred in 1762.'[37] As with John Brooke, Ayling was relieved that the Freudian psychoanalytic interpretation of George III as a sexually frustrated psychotic could at last be discounted. Ayling acknowledges the immense debt of gratitude historians of

George III owe to the research of Macalpine and Hunter. He points out that the Willis collection, relating to the King's illness of 1788–9 alone, amounts to forty-seven volumes!

In her account of *George III at Home*, which was published in 1975, Nesta Pain found the evidence for porphyria quite convincing. Macalpine and Hunter, she writes, 'seemed to have made out an overwhelming case for their belief that George III suffered from porphyria, and that a number of other members of his family suffered from it as well'.[38] However, she also points out that the theory was not universally accepted, as 'informed opinion remains divided'. On the question of whether the 'madness' was caused by a metabolic imbalance or manic-depressive psychosis, she asks, 'Does it matter?' This question was also addressed several years earlier in the correspondence columns of the *British Medical Journal*, one participant in the debate asserting, 'A madman is a madman, whether or not his madness reflects schizophrenia, manic depressive psychosis, general paralysis of the insane, cerebral arteriosclerosis, or porphyria.'[39]

But the diagnosis *does* matter, and this for several reasons. From a biographical point of view the difference between the various diagnoses leads to a vastly different interpretation of character. After all, it was George III himself who demanded to be remembered for what he was, writing: 'Whenever God of his infinite goodness shall call me out of this world, the tongue of malice may not paint my intentions in those colours she admires, nor the sycophant extol me beyond what I deserve.'[40] Was he to be remembered as a mentally unstable character prone to breakdowns when the going got tough, or as an understanding man with high moral principles who was unfortunate enough to have inherited a metabolic disturbance? From a medical point of view, the presence of a potentially fatal 'faulty' gene within a family is of the utmost concern, as precipitating agents which might trigger a porphyric attack need to be avoided.

In his biography of George IV, Christopher Hibbert also draws attention to the retrospective diagnosis of porphyria made by Macalpine and Hunter. Although he acknowledges that the diagnosis for George III has been questioned, he states that 'most historians of the period find it convincing'.[41]

The porphyria theory is not only accepted but is expanded upon by Antonia Fraser in her highly successful biography of Mary Queen of Scots. She finds that the illness offers a rational explanation for the illnesses of Mary and her son, King James I and VI, which fall within the broad symptomology of porphyria. However, she goes further still and argues that 'the mysterious hysterical manner of the death of James V' is also suggestive of porphyria, and concludes that Mary may therefore have inherited the disease from her father.[42] It is clear that the imaginative theory advanced by Ida Macalpine and Richard Hunter about the nature of George III's illness has ramifications not just up and down the family tree of the British Royal Family, but for the history of many other royal houses, too.

Evidence of Porphyria in Some of the Relatives of George III

Our understanding of the threat that porphyria posed to the monarchies of Europe will be enhanced if we survey some new research on two of George III's contemporary relatives in the German lands, King Friedrich Wilhelm I of Prussia, known as the 'Sergeant King' (1688–1740), and the Elector Wilhelm I of Hesse-Kassel (1743–1821), the ruler who sold his conscripts to the English for their war against the American colonists. Both men were considered by Macalpine and Hunter to be likely porphyria sufferers, though the evidence available in their day was so scanty that they wrote no more than a few lines on each.[43] The new evidence on the medical condition of both monarchs is of more than passing interest to our enquiry, and not only because the establishment of porphyria-like symptoms in two of George's blood relations would tend to confirm the diagnosis of porphyria in his own case. Since the Prussian King, the Hessian Elector and George III were all descended from common ancestors, the three cases together should provide us with a strong indication of the line through which the disease had been passed down to them. Furthermore, we have a special interest in the two German cases because both Friedrich Wilhelm I of Prussia and Wilhelm I of Hesse-Kassel were direct ancestors of Patient A, Princess Adelaide of Prussia.

King Friedrich Wilhelm I's mother was Sophie Charlotte of Hanover, the sister of King George I of England. His wife was Sophie Dorothea, the sister of George II, and *their* elder son was destined to enter the history books as Frederick the Great. The House of Hohenzollern at this time was therefore linked almost as closely as the British Royal Family to the Hanoverian line, that 'exemplary collection of oddballs', as one historian has termed them.[44] Girlish as a child, Friedrich Wilhelm grew up to be fat and squat, uncouth and uncivilized, grizzly and full of uncontrollable rage – in short, one of the least attractive figures in the history of European monarchy. He was certainly one of the cruellest, forcing his son to look on while he had his closest companion beheaded. Historians regard him as the founder of the Prussian military state and indeed of the Prussian 'national character' with its emphasis on frugality, hard work and obedience to authority. He more than doubled the size of the Prussian Army and subordinated the entire population to the requirements of the military, and yet he never risked that army in a war, leaving this well-drilled military machine for his son to use to seize Silesia from his Austrian neighbour. As the French ambassador famously observed, after the reign of Friedrich Wilhelm I Prussia was less a state with an army than an army with a state. The one luxury the Sergeant King did allow himself was his '*Lange Kerls*' – the enormously tall soldiers he recruited all over Europe and whom he loved above all other things.[45]

Not surprisingly, Friedrich Wilhelm's eccentric character has attracted the attention of medical historians and psychologists. The former have concluded that his physical symptoms were caused by gout and hydrophilia (dropsy), illnesses they declare to have been hereditary in the Hohenzollern family into the middle of the nineteenth century.[46] Psychohistorians, on the other hand, have deployed post-Freudian object-relations theory to diagnose the King as a dangerous 'borderline' personality.[47] While both interpretations are interesting, they clearly fail, both singly and in combination with one another, to account for many of the monarch's most striking symptoms. Recently two scholars, Professor Claus A. Pierach, a porphyria expert at the Abbott Northwestern Hospital in Minneapolis, and Erich Jennewein of Saarlouis in Germany, taking their cue from the work of Macalpine, Hunter and Rimington, have posed the explicit question 'Was the Prussian King Friedrich Wilhelm I suffering from Porphyria?', and have provided a strongly positive answer on the basis of a painstaking examination of the medical record. The following is a brief account of their research.[48]

The Sergeant King suffered his first attack, which was nearly fatal, in 1707 when he was nineteen years old. He had a sudden onrush of high temperature, colic, circulatory problems and a skin rash, together with a host of mental symptoms variously described as outbreaks of rage, fainting fits, restlessness, fantasies and depression. The symptoms continued for four months and then disappeared. Eleven years went by before the next acute episode, in 1718. After feeling unwell for several months, Friedrich Wilhelm, in the words of Pierach and Jennewein, 'suffered a classic porphyric attack which took him to the edge of the grave'. He was putting a regiment through its paces when, as he himself wrote, he was 'covered all over with smallpox-like variolae'. Again he had a fever, suffered *'une colique néphrétique'*, his heartbeat raced and his hands were lame. Not until the Surgeon-General prescribed ipeca-cuanha did the fever and the pains begin to subside, but the King would never be well again. The skin on his legs and feet in particular was constantly inflamed – the abscesses were at times described as 'phlegmons', at others as 'erysipelas' – and a source of pain. His rabies-like attacks of 'madness' became more furious: he beat strangers in the streets of Berlin and Potsdam as well as the doctors and servants at Court, and once made as if to kick the British ambassador before thinking better of it. He was seized by 'black melancholy' during the day and by murderous nightmares at night. In an attack of 1729, when he was forty-one, he was completely lame in both legs and arms, insisting on being pushed around the palace in a wheelchair with his arms resting on crutches. 'The poor King had terrible pains, and black bile which had poured itself into his blood, caused him to be in an evil mood,' his daughter recorded. On one occasion his wife found him alone with a noose around his neck, very close to death.

The King's severest attack, with the exception of the fatal illness of 1740, occurred in 1734 and lasted for more than seven months. Pierach and Jennewein were able to reconstruct the course of this episode in detail on the basis, among other contemporary sources, of the journal kept by the monarch's personal physician, which is held in the Prussian Secret State Archive. The attack began with 'podagra [gout] in the left hand'. This was followed by more threatening symptoms: Friedrich Wilhelm had difficulty in breathing, his face took on a bluish-red colour, the skin of his legs filled with water and was covered in 'phlegmons or erysipelas ulcers', his blood, when let, thickened into a 'nice red mass'. His body was hideously swollen up to the navel and he could not walk or sleep; he went for periods of up to thirty minutes, it is reported, without being able to draw breath. His face was described by one ambassador as being 'completely dark blue' in colour. On top of that, the doctors noted, his 'membra genitalia are swollen, he is unable to p . . . . .'. The King had fainting fits, his face made compulsive movements, he was beginning to lose the faculty of speech, he lost the use of his arms and legs, he suffered from 'spasmum diaphragmatis' and flatulence and spasms in the stomach and intestines. He was nauseous and had a burning sensation in his abdomen. His excrement was 'yellow and white' and had an 'exceptionally foul smell'. His pulse was alarmingly fast – and then again 'slow and sluggish'. He had feverish panic attacks, nightmares, pains in the chest and around the heart, headaches, pain in the legs. And on no fewer than five occasions in the period between mid-October and mid-December 1734, the doctor records that the King's urine was 'very red'.[49]

Red urine was also a prominent symptom of Friedrich Wilhelm's final illness in 1739–40, which is likewise carefully chronicled, this time by the King's surgeon Dr Pallas, his courtier Pöllnitz and the imperial ambassador Demeradt, and Pierach and Jennewein have again made careful use of these archival sources. When the illness began in the autumn of 1739, the King went lame and suffered from attacks of breathlessness and feelings of suffocation. He had abdominal pain and felt pressure on the chest. Again he lost the use of his right hand. He was unable to sleep. He spent his time being pushed around in his wheelchair, insisting that he must not be left alone, and yet he was so violently abusive that all those with him were driven to despair. All medicines proved useless. The doctors sighed that they 'knew not what name to give' to the monarch's malady. By February 1740 the pains in the chest were so severe that the King was no longer able to lie down. Oedema reappeared on both legs, which were badly swollen, while the rest of his body was reduced to skin and bone. His son, on the threshold of 'greatness', wrote of the King's condition at this time: 'The blood was black and as thick as pitch . . . His mood is worse than ever . . . He is unable to pass water, in short it is the Status mortis.' And yet the King did not die for another three and a half months. By March 1740, Demeradt was reporting a 'constant burning sensation and cruel pains in the intestines and indeed all the innards, as well as a very savage attack of heat mounting towards the head'; it was as if the monarch were rotting away from the inside. As Dr Pallas, who spent every night from 6 to 26 April 1740 at the King's bedside, reported to his colleague in the mornings: the patient had slept no more than one and a half hours, he had coughed and vomited, his feet were swollen, he had a fever and was delirious, he had 'burning feelings in the chest and stomach', he was 'unable either to cack or urinate', he had 'cried out with violent pain in the left knee', he had 'complained throughout the night of pain in the right side, especially the abdomen' and 'the colon', and – on 20 April – his urine was 'very red'.[50]

The Sergeant King died five weeks later, at the age of fifty-two. The post-mortem examination revealed ulcerous lungs and a 'cirrhotic' pancreas, but the kidneys were 'in fairly good shape' and stomach and intestines were 'found to be in their natural condition'. Pierach and Jennewein conclude: 'An analysis of Friedrich Wilhelm I's symptoms without doubt suggests porphyria, particularly as there is no other diagnosis which would account for such a confusing profusion of symptoms. If he really did have porphyria, then variegate porphyria, which is associated with both cutaneous and nervous symptoms, suggests itself as the most likely type.'

George III was only two years old when Friedrich Wilhelm of Prussia died, but Wilhelm I of Hesse-Kassel was his exact contemporary; indeed, in George II of Hanover and England they had a common grandfather, Wilhelm's mother being Princess Mary (1723–72), the sister of George III's father Frederick Lewis (1707–51). Whereas in George's reign, not least because of his long periods of 'madness', Parliament continued to gain power at the expense of the Crown, Wilhelm's rule became a byword for arbitrary tyranny and unenlightened despotism. By 'renting' thousands of his troops to his cousin George III for the war against the 'rebels' in America, Wilhelm not only rendered his own country defenceless but became, with a little help from his neighbour Meyer Amschel Rothschild in Frankfurt, the richest prince in Germany, lending vast sums to the Prince of Wales and the Duke of Clarence, among others. Though married (to his cousin Caroline of Denmark), Wilhelm's private life was every bit as scandalous as that of his Hanoverian relatives in England: he had four children by one mistress, four by another and six by the next, all of them raised to the nobility and kept at public expense. The recent research on him is quite different from the work of Pierach and Jennewein on the Sergeant King of Prussia. It consists of a meticulously edited translation (from French into German) of the Hessian Elector's own memoirs, which were based closely on his diaries.[51] Even though Wilhelm's descriptions of his illnesses are anything but scientific or detailed, this autobiography is nevertheless an intimate and authentic chronicle of someone suffering from a variety of puzzling symptoms similar to the illness afflicting Friedrich Wilhelm I of Prussia and, as we shall see in the next chapter, several of the children of George III. As one reviewer of Wilhelm's memoirs put it, his life was overshadowed by 'incredible physical suffering. Reports of abscesses in the ear, raging headaches, diarrhoea, rheumatism and gout, the loss of his teeth, colic, infection and wounds of all sorts fill page after page of the diary.'[52]

In late 1770, we read for the first time of an attack that might possibly have been porphyria. Wilhelm records that he had felt unwell throughout that summer. Then, when his wife discovered his affair with Marianne von Wulffen, he lost his ability to sleep and his 'blood became more and more agitated'. On 14 November 1770 a serious ague or shivering fit set in, followed by a 'night of agony. Bile entered my stomach and my blood. My servant Müller gave me an emetic but for which I would have been lost.' As the prince was now 'dangerously ill', Dr Socin was summoned from Hanau. 'My nights were very bad and, tormented by fear of death, I began to lose consciousness.' In a state of delirium he asked to be carried from one room to another. The scenes his wife made brought on a relapse just as he seemed to be getting better. Finally, though he could 'neither think nor walk, and the previous night had been full of the most terrible symptoms', he decided to join his mother in Hanau. 'I was nothing but skin and bone', Wilhelm wrote, 'and was so completely emaciated that no one recognized me.' There, on the banks of the River Main, he made something of a recovery, was able to climb the stairs again and to ride out in his carriage. But then he 'caught cold and was plagued by such severe rheumatism that I could move only with the most dreadful pain'. The acute phase of the attack ended at the beginning of 1771 with a bloodletting; the illness had lasted six weeks. 'Even today I cannot thank God the Almighty enough for saving me from the terrible danger in which I found myself,' he wrote.[53]

Another episode followed in 1778 and again seems to have been brought on by stress and excitement, if of a different kind. Although Wilhelm had just received the news that his Hessian regiment had capitulated to the Americans at Saratoga, he had a burning passion to take part personally in a war and had written to Frederick the Great begging to be allowed to join the War of Bavarian Succession as a 'volunteer'. The suspense while he was waiting for the King's reply quite literally almost killed him. 'I was so obsessed that my health began to suffer,' he recalled. 'I couldn't sleep, I couldn't eat. I became more ill by the day: My stomach was full of bile and I had a violent fever.' When at last Frederick's invitation to join him in Silesia arrived, Wilhelm was 'delirious' with joy.

Not only was he to be gravely disappointed by the Prussian King's humiliating treatment of him, but physically, too, the long trip proved to be a disaster. On his way to war he was struck down by a 'violent fever' and a 'dreadful' attack of diarrhoea.[54] In the middle of the campaign he was laid low for over a week by 'abdominal pains which caused me terrible suffering'.[55] In August 1778, the Prince had an attack of what his servant Müller thought – probably correctly – was dysentery. 'In the night the illness got worse, and was accompanied by terrible pains.' Wilhelm was finally persuaded to allow himself to be taken to the field hospital, where he spent a night of torment, 'for the most part thrashing around on the floor in pain. An inner fire consumed my innards and a burning fever brought my blood to the boil.' On the journey back to Hanau his condition went from bad to worse. 'I was unable to leave my bed,' he remembered. 'I hardly dared to eat the little that I needed to stay alive. The tiniest crumb of bread I ate caused me unspeakable pain inside.'[56]

Six years later, in May 1784, Wilhelm had an 'extraordinarily stubborn' attack of malarial-like intermittent fever lasting for several weeks. He attributed its onset to the summer heat, which had led him to discard his clothes and expose himself for too long to the sun. The attacks returned 'with extreme violence' on several further occasions, but then disappeared when, 'against the express wish of my brother Karl', his doctor gave him chincona (quinine). Peace and quiet, and a careful diet, had also helped, he realized.[57]

From this point on, 'gout' in various guises becomes the most common term used by Wilhelm to describe his painful illness and – interestingly – that of his two brothers and his younger son as well. In March 1784 he records that Karl fell seriously ill with 'gout which almost paralysed all his limbs for several weeks'. This attack of 'violent gout pains' is of especial significance since, as Wilhelm notes, it was accompanied by a 'surfeit of viscous bile' which occasioned terrible suffering. For a number of years now, Prince Karl had been under the influence of the notorious alchemist and swindler the Count de Saint-Germain (who now called himself Welldone), and it was to the effect of his medicines on Karl's 'nerves' that Wilhelm attributed his brother's sorry state.[58]

In the spring of 1785, Wilhelm himself complained of headaches and a sore throat, but the pain soon travelled down to his feet, he says, to become 'the beginning of the podagra [foot gout] from which I have suffered ever since'.[59] Ten years later, in June 1795, he had another 'violent attack of gout', which this time 'lasted only eight days because it was summer and only one foot was affected'.[60] Then, 'On 1 December [1796] I had an attack of gout more violent than ever before.' The stress he was under made his suffering worse, he believed, so that 'for the first time in my life it lasted for four weeks'. The following February the 'gout' returned, again in the form of 'podagra'.[61] In the final days of the year 1800, he recorded another attack of gout, this time in his right hand, which plagued him for eight days.[62] He was to be plagued with gout in various places for the rest of his life.[63]

We cannot be certain that the 'gout' of which Wilhelm of Hesse-Kassel complained really was gout or some other metabolic disorder. There was, at that time, no differential diagnosis that would have distinguished gout from other kinds of pain and paralysis in the arms, hands, legs or feet. What is clear is that the Elector suffered throughout his life from numerous other symptoms that do not form part of the characteristic pattern taken by gout – colic and diarrhoea, abscesses in the head and ears, burning pains in the stomach and intestines, nausea and vomiting, heat rashes, malaria-like intermittent fever, shivering fits or ague, and so on. It is not without significance that his brothers and sons had very similar symptoms, and that one of his sons died of a sudden attack that some thought might have been caused by poison. This unusual combination of symptoms certainly makes porphyria seem a possibility. Though there is, in Wilhelm's own account – we do not have the account of his doctors – no direct record of discoloured urine, as there is in the case of George III and the Sergeant King, we should perhaps direct our attention to those numerous references, both in his own case and in that of his brother, to 'bile' entering the stomach and the bloodstream. If such lay diagnoses were based on observation, then the 'viscous bile' must have been noticeable either in his urine or his stool.

Wilhelm of Hesse and George III of England were second cousins, but there is also evidence of unexplained painful illness in the King's blood relations closer to home. George III's younger brother William Henry, the elder Duke of Gloucester (1743–1805), also suffered from strange symptoms and died a premature death. On a visit to the German states in 1770 the duke, who had complained of being unwell for several weeks, suddenly fell acutely ill in Vienna on 17 September, being 'seized with a pain in his side'. Though he 'soon recovered' after the doctors had blistered him, his health was henceforth precarious. At Leghorn the following year, the Victorian historian Percy Fitzgerald tells us, 'the duke was seized with a most serious illness, and for a time his life appeared to be in danger; but he happily recovered'.[64] On his 'disastrous wedding tour' through Italy with Maria Countess of Waldegrave (1739–1807), 'the duke was always ill' and from time to time 'really in great danger', despite his liberal intake of burgundy, claret and peppermint. In June of the following year, at Trent, he again fell ill and became so emaciated that two physicians were rushed over from England to his sickbed. Though on their instructions the duke 'sucked the breasts of some healthy country women that were sent for from the mountains', even this imaginative remedy brought little improvement, and they gave up hope of saving his life. 'His royal highness passed a very bad night, in great pain, no sleep, weak beyond expression; in short, in all human appearance the poor amiable duke can live but a very short time.' In fact, however, William Henry recovered and made the journey back to London, apparently quite restored to health.[65] His final illness, which began in the summer of 1803, was complicated by his deliberate deception of his doctors. As Queen Charlotte noted, 'We are in hourly expectation of the news of the poor Duke of Gloucester's Death. His sufferings must have been dreadfully Painfull; but ... I understand that he was not quite open with His Physicians, & that some Complaint He kept a Secret for three days, to which the Medicines which they administered at that time were almost fatal.' It is unfortunate for our purposes that the Queen did not record what the complaint was.[66]

The Duke of Gloucester's son William Frederick (1776–1834), George III's nephew and son-in-law, died in December 1834 after an illness which, according to an interesting note by John Wilson Croker, 'began with a bilious inflammation but ended in the *family* complaint, and the immediate cause of death was the bursting of a scrofulous swelling in the head'.[67] It is to the evidence of the 'family complaint' in George III's children that we must now turn.

CHAPTER 4

The 'Family Complaint':
The Fifteen Children of George III

We have been informed that the whole of the
Royal Family are liable to spasms of a violent description.
The London Medical Repository, 1828

George III, whose 'madness' one historian has attributed to sexual
frustration, had no fewer than fifteen children, only two of whom
failed to reach maturity. If the King was suffering from a dominant
genetic disorder such as porphyria, we should expect several of his
offspring to be afflicted with the same malady. The children's
correspondence with one another and with their friends and
relations, courtiers and doctors provides us with an intimate
collective portrait of their lives. It also contains evidence that some
of them had inherited 'the *family* complaint'.[1] Macalpine and
Hunter believed they had found convincing evidence of porphyria
in four of George III's sons and in Princess Charlotte, George IV's
daughter, but they did not pursue their quest with respect to the
older George's six daughters.

By exploring the medical history of the six daughters and seven
surviving sons of George III in the order in which they were born,
focusing in particular on such symptoms as might be consistent
with porphyria, we should be in a position to determine whether
George III's genetic mutation survived his own death in 1820. We
shall be on the look-out especially for tell-tale signs of discoloured
urine, of course, but also for evidence of fragility of the skin which
might indicate variegate porphyria. Needless to say, we shall also
have to be watchful for the symptoms of other diseases that might
account for what at first sight looks like porphyria.

George, Prince of Wales, Later Prince Regent and King George IV (1762–1830)

In his two-volume biography of King George IV, which is based on extensive research in the Royal Archives and other record offices as well as on this monarch's published correspondence, Christopher Hibbert describes the 'violent and sudden attacks of illness' from which his dissolute subject suffered in the following terms:

> His usual symptoms, accompanied by 'great agitation of spirits', were high fever, a racing pulse, weakness in the arms and legs, severe abdominal colic and what he himself referred to as 'violent bilious attacks', 'a violent stoppage of the bowels', 'severe spasms on the neck of the bladder', and 'violent inflammatory attacks' on the lungs. From an early age he seems also to have suffered from gout and 'some degree of rheumatism' and these complaints appear to have been exacerbated in times of stress . . . He insisted on being blooded with alarming frequency . . . took a great deal of laudanum accompanied by medicines to make him sweat, and tried cures at Bath and Cheltenham. But he discovered no satisfactory treatment.[2]

After such a detailed and impressive enumeration of George's symptoms, Hibbert's conclusion – 'It is possible that, like his father, he was a victim of porphyria' – seems if anything overly cautious. Certainly he is right to state, as he does in the second volume of his biography, referring to the work of Macalpine and Hunter, that 'the Prince's symptoms seem consistent with such a diagnosis [of porphyria], though he was never subject to the extreme mental derangement which characterized his father's case'.[3] A similar judgement is passed by another biographer, Cecil Daphne Woodham Smith, who writes: 'King George IV . . . was probably, like his father George III, the victim of the group of diseases called porphyrias, not then diagnosed or understood . . . The disease is hereditary; Mary Queen of Scots brought it into the English Royal Family.'[4]

No one was more aware than George III's eldest son that his own periodic attacks of illness were similar to those of the 'mad' King. This was hardly surprising, since from their earliest childhood, he and his siblings had two doctors in constant attendance whose chief aim, in the words of Mrs Papendiek, a contemporary of Queen Charlotte's, was 'to watch the constitutions of the royal children, to eradicate, or at least to keep under, the dreadful disease, scrofula, inherited from the King', the symptoms of which included ugly swollen glands and purplish oedema on and under the skin of the neck.[5] Like several of his brothers, the younger George was convinced that his constitution was in some way abnormal, both physically and mentally. '*Mine is a very nervous* and so far a *delicate* fibre,' the then Prince of Wales confided to Dr John Turton in 1799, 'consequently the disorders of the body in general *with me* owe their source to the mind. (This God knows has for sometime, and a long time too, been too much the case with me, and then any little addition, such as a casual cold, or even any indisposition, no matter how trifling, contributes much to the unhinging the whole system.)'[6] Precisely because of his fear that he was a victim of the 'family complaint', George went to considerable lengths to hide the real nature of his illness from all but his closest and most trusted friends.[7]

There can be no doubt that he was seriously ill, indeed close to madness and death, on a number of occasions, and not all of his multifarious symptoms can be accounted for in terms of his drunkenness, gluttony, drug abuse and sexual excesses. Records show that, while in his late teens, he was forced to stay in his bedroom for a fortnight, as his face was covered with red, eruptive blotches that were 'dreadful to behold'.[8] Around 1786, he suffered 'one of his violent paroxysms of fever' that alarmed Dr Warren, not least because the prince's pulse 'resembled a machine completely disorganised'.[9] Again in 1787, he was 'suddenly taken ill with an inward complaint . . . which returned so violently . . . as to keep his physicians in anxious suspense'.[10] If, as frequently happened after bouts of heavy drinking, he had to take to his bed with a violent fever, he did not hesitate to take a lancet to open up his own veins.[11] When he became violently ill with 'an inflammation of the stomach', not everyone was willing to attribute this to hard drinking.[12] He also developed unsightly swollen glands which he tried to hide with a high collar and the doctors sought to cure with sea-bathing.[13] In 1791 he fell 'very seriously ill indeed' with a 'violent complaint' which left his nerves 'in a shattered state'.[14] After spitting blood and fainting, he was said to have ulcers on his lungs.[15] A couple of years later he admitted to having been *'very ill indeed'*, and it is little known *how ill'*.[16] In 1799 he confided to his mother that his 'old enemy, the *bile'* had returned to torment him and that he was extremely ill with a 'violent bilious attack'.[17] Taking the waters at Bath had, however, he believed, lessened 'the frequency as well as the violence of my spasmodic attacks . . . which tormented me so much of late'.[18] In 1800 he complained of 'a violent stoppage of the bowels' with excruciating abdominal pain.[19] In February of that year George was rumoured to be dying.[20] His extraordinary behaviour at the time of his marriage to Caroline of Brunswick led to widespread and persistent rumours that the Prince of Wales was insane – rumours which never subsided.[21] There were indeed times when he himself felt he was going mad, took great quantities of the opiate laudanum and insisted on being bled – on one occasion losing no less than thirty-six ounces of blood in three days.[22] Lady Elgin wrote to the Queen of the 'terrible infirmities' suffered by the Prince of Wales. She had found him 'in the most violent agitation and distress of mind and body' with 'a violent cramp and bowel complaint', she reported.[23]

If the signs of near-madness were thus plentiful, their cause remained a mystery. In 1804 it was said that the prince was in a 'fever of uneasiness' and 'talking all day without ceasing'. Interestingly, he had at this time 'just recovered from an illness in which his life was despaired of for two days', and it was widely feared that his extreme agitation might lead to a return of the disease, whatever it had been.[24] In September 1806, on hearing the news of the death of his political ally Charles James Fox, he flung himself on the sofa, burst into passionate tears, utterly lost his appetite and even his taste for wine, and could not sleep for weeks. He looked old and pale, and his strength failed him completely. His former apothecary, Walker, found his pulse 'quite thin, low and weak' and thought him 'seriously unwell'.[25] This attack of weakness, which brought him very close to death, continued for several months. He drank the strongest tea, which was iced in a vain effort 'to allay an internal heat'.[26] George's entire appearance changed, his face becoming 'very old and wrinkled' and his eyes dull 'as if he suffered mental and corporeal pain'. As late as May 1807, everyone was struck by how 'very ill he looked'.[27] The prince himself complained that for weeks he had been 'persecuted by the most horrible and spasmodick attacks in my head . . . The agony I suffer is hardly to be credited,' he wrote.[28] His behaviour, especially in his romantic escapades, continued to verge on the insane and, as Lady Bessborough complained after warding off the most unwelcome attentions of 'that immense, grotesque figure': 'I really believe his father's malady extends to him, only takes another turn.'[28]

Such views became commonplace in late 1811 when, shortly before assuming the unrestricted regency, George was struck down by yet another bout of abdominal pain and paralysis of the limbs. Few observers believed the official line that he had twisted his ankle while doing the Highland fling, particularly when they learnt that he lay *constantly on his stomach in bed*, suffering from 'violent pain' and 'spasmodic affection' in spite of taking a hundred drops of laudanum every three hours. This attack, too, lasted for many weeks and brought on intolerable 'pains in his arms and fingers' and 'the loss of power in them'. His friend and doctor, Sir Henry Halford, thought the Prince Regent might be suffering from palsy, whereas George himself believed the attack in the arm to be 'paralytic'. He was, he complained, at times 'incapable of moving a single joint' in his 'whole frame'. He was also virtually unable to sleep, in spite of taking as many as 250 drops of laudanum a day; only 'a great quantity' of hemlock alleviated his insomnia.[30]

During this episode of 1811, there were once again disturbing suspicions that the Regent's mind had given way. George's younger brother, the Duke of Cumberland, sarcastically opined that the official story about the twisted ankle was 'all sham' and that the real problem lay elsewhere, namely 'higher than the foot and . . . a blister on the head would be more efficacious than a poultice on the foot.' The only thing wrong with the prince, he proclaimed, was that 'he *was* mad'. One of his doctors, Sir Walter Farquhar, said that George suffered 'such agony of pain all over him it produces a degree of irritation on his nerves nearly approaching to delirium', and William Fremantle expressed the view that the prince's mind was affected to the point where he was 'totally incapable, for want of nerves, of doing anything'. Lady Bessborough now wondered: 'What will become of us, if as well as our King our Regent goes mad? It will be a new case in the annals of history.'[31]

By mid-December 1811, the danger appeared to be over and George, though still extremely nervous, felt able to return to

London. As Colonel Sir John McMahon could report at the end of the year, 'The *P.R.* is in general health perfectly good, and all unpleasant remains of his sprain are entirely gone, but spasmodic tinglings of his hands and arms are not yet quite removed.'[32] He explained to Mrs Creevey that whereas in the past 'he used to be always *chilly*, [he] was now never so – that he never had a fire even in his bedroom, and slept with one blanket and sheet only'.[33] One year after this attack, however, he again complained that he was unable to hold a pen, and that he had the *'greatest pain and difficulty in writing, having the gout all over him but particularly in both his hands'*.[34] The 'gout', he complained, was robbing him of the use 'both of my senses & my poor hand'.[35] After another attack in 1814 which 'began by a spasm . . . in his bowels' and continued with great pain, a racing pulse and vomiting, Sir Henry Halford said he had never seen the prince so ill in all his life, and warned that another 'such attack' could be *'fatal'*.[36] Once again, the pain seemed to go hand in hand with mental turmoil. Several political leaders expressed their alarm at the Prince Regent's 'state of agitation beyond description' and thought his 'perturbation of mind' to be 'beyond anything [they] had ever seen'.[37] As Thomas Creevey wrote to his wife in 1814, 'all agree that Prinny will die or go mad. He is worn out with fuss, fatigue and *rage*.'[38] George's behaviour only gave credence to such fears. When he was given the news of Wellington's victory at Waterloo, for example, he had to drink a beaker of brandy to overcome his fit of giggles. Although his assertions that the victories over Napoleon were the result of his own personal exertions on the battlefield and at sea may well have been meant as a joke, they only added to the growing belief that the Regent was suffering from 'hallucinations'.[39]

In September 1817, another episode of illness occurred which again almost resulted in George's death. As Lady Holland recorded: 'We have been near losing our Regent, and as the physicians mistook his disorder, they have probably curtailed his length of life, for the disease was treated at first as inflammatory and they took 60 ounces of blood. When [Dr Matthew] Baillie saw him he declared it to be spasm, and gave laudanum and cordials.'[40] Deeply shocked by the unexpected death of his only child, Princess Charlotte, George's condition deteriorated further. As he himself described his mysterious illness in a letter to his mother on 16 December 1817:

I do not know under what denomination to class the attack, or by what name regularly to define it and call it, for it seems to me to have been a sort of mishmash, Solomongrundy, Olla podrida kind of business in itself that is quite anomalous; a good deal of rheumatism, as much of cold, with a little touch of the bile to boot, not a very pleasant mixture on the whole, and composed of as unpleasant ingredients, as can well be thought of or imagined. In short all this potpourri has rendered me both bodily as well as mentally very unfit.[41]

At the time of George III's death in January 1820, his eldest son, 'rheumatic and gross', was 'dangerously ill' with 'pleurisy' and unable to attend the funeral. His symptoms quickly 'assumed an alarming aspect', and were accompanied by insomnia, a racing pulse and pains in the chest. The doctors pronounced him close to death and drained more than seventy ounces of blood (three and a half pints) in the belief that 'he must have died if he had not been blooded'.[42] On many occasions, not excluding his coronation, he behaved in a manner so inappropriate to his position that rumours again circulated widely about his sanity.[43]

After his accession, George IV's condition went from bad to worse. In 1821 Sir Astley Cooper was called in to remove a sebaceous tumour on the King's head, an operation which turned out to be more dangerous and painful than anticipated.[44] His 'rheumatic gout' was now more painful than ever. 'We left the King very ill,' Princess Dorothea von Lieven wrote to Prince Metternich in 1821. 'He is tortured by gout and employs the most violent remedies to be rid of it. He looks ghastly; he is plunged in gloom; he talks about nothing but dying. I have never seen him so wretched.'[45] His 'irritability of temper' was becoming 'intolerable' to all those around him.[46] In January 1823, Princess Lieven found him 'aged a great deal', and limping noticeably.[47] He now had another very serious attack of 'gout' – this one accompanied by periods of high temperature and 'erysipelas' (that is, a red rash) on one foot – which left many convinced that he would be dead by the end of the year.[48] He complained of 'accessions' of 'flying gout' and lameness, and many remarked on how ill he looked, and on his 'incessant perspiration'.[49] From other records we know that he was also suffering from 'irregularity of the pulse, occasional pain about the praecordia, sensation in the left arm and sudden breathlessness'.[50] In 1823, Emily Cowper noted: 'The King is in a strange state of health now. He suffers dreadfully from rheumatic gout so as hardly to be able to turn in bed without screaming . . . I cannot help feeling that his life is very precarious – one thing after another always starting up and keeping him so weak and ill.'[51] Later that year, Greville recorded that 'various instances of eccentricity' had persuaded him that 'the King is subject to occasional impressions which produce effects so like insanity that if they continue to increase he will end up by being decidedly mad'.[52] The newspapers, too, now openly speculated on whether the King might be suffering from hereditary madness.[53]

As Hibbert writes of the 'Windsor Recluse', towards the end of his life George IV's 'reluctance to show himself in public was . . . becoming almost obsessive. Rather than risk the cruel gibes that were unfailingly directed at his stout body and swollen legs, his now hobbling gait and the face whose ageing appearance grease-paint could only partially disguise, he chose to remain in secluded retirement as much as he possibly could.' He went to extraordinary lengths to avoid contact with other human beings, ordering his servants not to stare at him and forbidding visitors to Windsor to look up at the windows lest he might be passing. Before he went for a drive he had the streets cleared so that no one might see his ravaged countenance.[54]

In his final years, King George IV is described as 'lying at full length in a lilac silk dressing-gown, a velvet nightcap on his head, his huge bare feet (for he has gout) covered with a pink silk net'. His clothes were grubby, he slept badly at night and rarely got up before dinner.[55] He was often in excruciating pain, in different parts of the body. In 1826, Sir William Knighton told Canning, the Foreign Secretary, that the chief seat of pain was in the bladder and the penis. 'Nothing can exceed the pain of such attacks,' he wrote, which he diagnosed as 'gout, principally confined to the neck of the bladder and all along the course of the urethra'.[56] In the summer of 1827, George's knees, legs, ankles and feet swelled 'more formidably and terribly than ever', and he had to be carried up and down stairs and wheeled about in a merlin chair.[57] His 'flying gout' severely affected his left arm and both legs.[58]

In addition to his usual gout and rheumatism, at Christmas 1827

George suffered a 'feverish attack, attended with great tightness and oppression upon the chest', which was made worse by 'very acute pain in the back and loins and one arm'. He was still unable to stand, let alone walk, in February.[59] He had to be roused repeatedly from a state of 'something like sleep' during meetings of council at which he had no fewer than seventeen leeches stuck to one knee.[60] In the summer and autumn of that year, his right arm was so 'full of gouty inflammation' that it was 'as large as two hands' – his valet could not get it into the sleeve of his coat. He had 'attacks of spasms' and suffered from piles, inflammation of the bladder and the symptoms of dropsy.[61] In May 1829 there was 'violent irritation which is only subdued by laudanum and always returns when the effect of the opiate is gone off'.[62] He claimed he could eat only after imbibing unbelievable quantities of cherry brandy.[63] He went blind in one eye and it was believed he would lose sight in the other.[64] Many, not excluding the King himself, once again feared that he was on the verge of madness.[65] 'He is in great fright with his father's fate before him,' wrote the diarist Charles Greville on 16 September 1829, 'and indeed nothing is more probable than that he will become blind and mad too; he is already a little of both.'[66] Lord Ellenborough also heard that the King was 'ill, if not mad. In fact this excitement in which he is may lead to insanity.'[67] The Duke of Wellington and the other ministers were so concerned that his violence and irritability might drive the monarch over the edge into madness 'that they were obliged to let him have his own way for fear he should be ill'.[68]

In early 1830, George IV's insomnia and mental confusion grew even worse, as did the pain in his bladder and 'his dreadful spasms of breathlessness'.[69] Sir Henry Halford, who by this time had attended the Royal Family for over three decades, registered that the present King's distress was worse than anything he had witnessed even when his brothers the Dukes of Clarence and Sussex were suffering 'under their attacks of spasmodic asthma'.[70] In mid-April, his doctors reported that the King had suffered a 'bilious attack, accompanied by an embarrassment of breathing' which had left him extremely agitated. 'Under His agonies of embarrassment', Halford informed the Duke of Wellington, 'partly from the necessity of support, partly from an apprehension, which belongs peculiarly to disorders of the heart, His Majesty would not relinquish his hold of my hand.'[71] As the monarch struggled against attacks of breathlessness, and was unable to lie down because of the fluid in his lungs, he went wholly without sleep until the doctors managed to rig up the pillows in his bed chair in such a way as to permit him to sleep holding his head in his hands.[72] He was still taking enormous quantities of laudanum.[73] His agitation was made worse by the realization that his symptoms were identical to those from which his brother the Duke of York had died just three years earlier. As Halford put it in his report to Wellington of 3 May: 'There is such a similitude in His Majesty's present distress & embarrassment, to that which the King witnessed in His latest visit to the poor Duke of York, as it is evident occurs to His Majesty's own mind, & increases His apprehension of Himself.'[74]

George IV also had sores and watery blisters – the doctors called them anasarca – all over his body.[75] He was 'black in the face and the ends of his fingers [were] black', Ellenborough recorded.[76] Halford's diagnosis was that fluid which had so far been directed outwards, to the skin, was now finding its way into the King's chest and abdomen, with fatal consequences. After witnessing the monarch's 'tremendous struggle' to get out of bed 'for a purpose' on the evening of 29 April 1830, he informed the Prime Minister: 'I have now to say that I fancy the effusion *is going on*, & tho' the stream *has been* diverted to the surface of the body hitherto, with some temporary relief, yet it seems to me, more than probable, that the internal cavity of the chest, has not escaped, & is not likely to escape an addition to its incumbrances.'[77] The following day seemed to bring confirmation of the physician's worst fears. 'It was hardly possible to be more distress'd than the King was, all yesterday,' Halford told Wellington. 'The King has every indication of water within the membrane which invests the heart – and of a small quantity within the chest, and I am not clear that there may not be some in the cavity of the belly. The legs are very much swollen, and I fear we have now had all the advantage which could have been expected from the external swelling, & that the interior may become henceforward more embarrass'd.'[78]

Soon, however, Halford had better news to report. On 7 May Benjamin Brodie was called in to puncture the King's legs and the soles of his feet so as to drain away the fluid that had accumulated there, and for a time the monarch's overall condition improved. As Halford informed the Prime Minister:

> Mr Brodie has made the drains, by puncture, more effectual – and undoubtedly since the deposit has been made under the skin, and since that deposit has found an exit, His Majesty's symptoms have been less severe. The paroxysms of difficulty of breathing not recurring so frequently nor with so much struggle & hazard when they do occur. His Majesty has eaten his food well moreover, and tho' we cannot command sleep to the extent we might wish, His Majesty obtains short refreshments of it, from time to time – and His system is sufficiently supported to maintain itself – and our remedies upon His Gigantic constitution work satisfactorily.[78]

Unhappily, the respite lasted for a few days only. On 9 May the doctors registered the King's 'great distress and embarrassment' – he suffered attacks of 'more than ordinary terror' – and reported that, in spite of the new leg punctures and the fact that he had stopped his 'frequent potations', his waist was very swollen, which led them to conclude that 'the effusion continues, probably'.[80] Though further quantities of water were drained from the legs in the next few days, bringing temporary relief, Halford warned that 'the principal malady in the organs of the chest' was as grave as before, and that the King was manifestly growing weaker.[81] Not until 17 May 1830 could Halford write that, though George was still 'very languid & irritable', the 'diminution of His Majesty's bulk is very considerable', giving rise to the hope 'that the cavity of the belly has been drained as well as the chest'.[82]

George IV died on 26 June 1830. The post-mortem examination which was performed by Halford, Tierney, Cooper and Brodie reveals several clues as to the nature of the King's final illness. Though his body had an emaciated appearance, 'a very large quantity of fat was found between the skin and the abdominal muscles' and also in the abdomen itself. To their surprise, the doctors found no more than an ounce of water in the abdomen. They were also struck by the condition of several of the King's organs. 'The Stomach and Intestines . . . were of a darker colour than natural in consequence of their containing mucus tinged with blood; and in the Stomach was found a clot of pure blood, weighing about six ounces. The Liver was pale and had an unhealthy granulated appearance,' they recorded, and whereas the spleen, the pancreas, the prostate gland, the kidneys and the bladder as such were not diseased, the colon had formed 'unnatural adhesions to the bladder accompanied by a solid inflammatory deposit of the size of an orange. Upon a careful examination of this tumour, a sac or cavity was found in its centre which contained an Urinary Calculus of the size of a filbert and this cavity communicated by means of a small aperture with the interior of the Bladder at its fundus.' On opening the chest, the medics measured two pints of water in the right side and almost four pints on the left. The lower edge of each lobe of the lungs had a remarkable fringe made up of fat. 'The mucous membrane lining the Air Tubes was of a dark colour in consequence of its vessels being turgid with blood.' The pericardium surrounding the heart contained half an ounce of fluid, 'but its opposite surfaces in several parts adhered to each other from inflammation at some remote period'. The heart was surrounded by a large quantity of fat, and the organ itself, which was much larger than usual, was 'so tender as to be lacerated by the slightest force'. The valves of the aorta were 'ossified throughout their surface and the inner coat of that blood vessel presented an irregular surface and was in many parts ossified'. Confirming Halford's earlier diagnosis, the doctors concluded:

> The original disease of His Majesty consisted in the ossification of the valves of the Aorta which must have existed for many years, and which by impeding the passage of the current of blood flowing from the heart to the other parts of the body occasioned effusion of water into the cavities of the Chest and in other situations. This mechanical impediment to the circulation of the blood also sufficiently explains those other changes in the condition of the body which were connected with His Majesty's last illness as well as all the symptoms under which the King had laboured.[83]

Though aortic-valve stenosis was certainly the cause of the monarch's final illness, leading to a huge accumulation of fluid in his skin and chest, and though a gastric haemorrhage was very probably the immediate cause of his death, as the doctors believed, these conditions obviously cannot explain the terrible suffering to which he was subjected throughout his life. Can we come to any conclusion other than that the chief cause of his violent cramps and spasms, bilious attacks, headaches and mental disturbance, lameness and paralysis of the arms and hands, unsightly sores and scrofulous rashes on the skin, was variegate porphyria inherited from his father? The view that we are dealing here with a hereditary 'family complaint' receives strong confirmation from the fact that so many of his sisters and brothers had almost identical symptoms.

Frederick, Duke of York (1763–1827)

During his final illness, as we have just seen, George IV 'constantly thought of his Brother the Duke of York', who had died three years earlier, and stressed 'the similarity of their symptoms and was always comparing them'.[84] Though we know a good deal less about the condition of George III's second son, there are several hints in the royal correspondence which enable us to say that, alongside other illnesses, Frederick too seems to have inherited the family malady.

When he became ill at the age of twenty, Frederick was put in the care of the renowned Swiss physician Dr Johann Georg von Zimmermann, the physician to the British Royal Family at Hanover, who sent reports on the case to the duke's father in London. Four years later, on 16 and 21 July 1787, Zimmermann submitted further reports on Frederick's condition, this time to Queen Charlotte. Unfortunately, neither of these two sets of what were undoubtedly intelligent records could be traced in the Royal Archives at Windsor. Though Zimmermann's own notes on his examination of Frederick and several of his brothers are kept in the public State Archive of Lower Saxony in Hanover, and though some of these notes were made available to Macalpine and Hunter in the 1960s, the present authors were denied access to these two-hundred-year-old medical records by the present head of the House of Hanover and his advisers.[85] We do know from Zimmermann's other correspondence with the English court, however, that for two years after the first serious attack in 1783, and possibly longer, the young Duke of York suffered from 'terrible cramps and spasms' in the stomach, which Zimmermann thought might be alleviated by taking the waters at Bad Pyrmont.[86] In 1784, Frederick caught a 'feverish cold . . . of the aguish kind' which was attributed to the 'excessive heat' of summer.[87] In 1787 and 1788, in his letters to the duke's equerry General Richard Grenville, Zimmermann recalled numerous occasions on which both he and Grenville had 'trembled' for Frederick's health, and expressed his astonishment that the young duke had withstood all the crises of the past few years. Referring in particular to episodes which had occurred at Lüneburg and Hanover, he said he hoped a recent accident at Lille would not 'reactivate the old disposition' which had been banished by Grenville's careful management. He, Zimmermann, did not doubt that 'our excellent Prince will survive if he at last makes up his mind seriously to avoid all that is noxious to him', but warned that, if he failed to do so, 'His Royal Highness will face a woeful and wretched future, as I have always said and as I have not omitted to warn His Majesty'.[88]

In the summer of 1789 Frederick was afflicted with a severe skin rash – a 'very large eruption all over his countenance' – which Dr Warren at first thought was measles, but which was soon complicated by other symptoms such as abdominal pain, a severe tightness of the chest, and a 'very violent intermitting fever', indicating an illness of a different kind.[89] In later years, too, we read of his being 'extremely ill indeed' with 'spasms' and his usual 'stomach complaint'. 'You talk of an attack of bile,' his elder brother wrote to him in 1820. 'I also have had my share of it . . . and my old enemy the gout flying about me.'[90]

Despite these indications that he might have had variegate porphyria, Frederick's death in 1827 is still attributed by historians to 'dropsy', and indeed his last illness bears few signs of a porphyria attack.[91] Victorian observers blamed the 'decay' which had set in some years before the duke's death on his 'character and the laxity of his life'. He liked to play cards all night, and this refusal to take up a recumbent position of rest led, it was thought, 'to a fatal dropsy and corrupt state of the blood'. When at last he did attempt to lie down, Frederick 'could not do so, as a feeling of suffocation came on'. For months before his final 'long and painful struggle', he never entered a bed, but – like his brothers George and Augustus – slept in a padded easy chair with a leg-rest built specially for him, making sure that 'anti-spasmodic medicines' were always within reach.[92]

In August 1826 he moved to Brighton, but there the swelling of his legs only got worse, a serous fluid oozing out of the distended skin. The duke was in 'excruciating pain throughout great parts of the day'. As water began to accumulate in his abdomen, too, he was rushed from Brighton to London in five and a half hours. The operation of 'tapping', which was performed on 3 September, succeeded in draining twenty-two pints of water from his body, but nevertheless the doctors had to tell him that he would not live for more than a few weeks. By 22 October 'his appetite had totally failed him, and other symptoms were equally unfavourable'. Six days later 'his royal highness appeared very weak, and had some attacks of nervous faintness; which, together with other unfavourable symptoms, satisfied the physicians that the danger was becoming more imminent'. He complained of severe 'inward pain', and rapidly lost ground. His doctors were shocked at the 'extraordinary change' that took place in him from one day to the next. 'He appeared extremely feeble, and under great uneasiness from pain, but otherwise composed,' one of them recorded on 30 December 1826. In early January 1827, he 'passed a very restless night, with occasional attacks of faintness and spasm', his pulse became feeble and irregular, his breathing more difficult, 'but yet there were no symptoms of rapidly-approaching dissolution'. He died on 5 January without any apparent pain.[93]

William, Duke of Clarence, Later King William IV (1765–1837)

Though William IV's medical history has not been fully explored, and though Macalpine and Hunter overlooked him as a possible royal porphyric, there is evidence in the biographies to suggest that he might well have suffered from the same disorder as his father and two elder brothers. Philip Ziegler, who had access to the records in the Royal Archives, informs us that even in his twenties the prince 'suffered from a series of fevers; prickly heat caused him intense irritation and stopped him sleeping; large blotches formed on his skin, giving place to inflamed boils when he moved to a cooler climate; rheumatic pains racked his right side and thigh until he was no longer able to stand'. William's health was hardly improved by excessive drinking and frequent attacks of venereal disease, which his doctors treated with mercury.[94] In the autumn of 1787, while on naval duty in Quebec, the prince went down with a mysterious 'tropical fever' which caused him 'several nights of delirious raving'.[95] As he grew older, his chief complaints were pains in the legs ascribed (as ever) to gout, and annual attacks of (sometimes life-threatening) asthma in the summer.[96] In June and July 1810, for example, when William was so ill that he thought he was dying – 'I have not been so ill for five years,' he wrote to one of his sons – he described his illness as 'my usual and annual complaint'.[97] Significantly, it was at this same time that he developed 'a very painful whitlow [an inflamed sore with suppuration] on one of the fingers of his right hand' which made it impossible for him to hold a pen.[98] In May of the following year Mrs Jordan, William's mistress (and the mother of ten of his children), wrote to her eldest son: 'Your father is yet very well but June is not yet over and I really dread its arrival', and sure enough, on 16 June 1811 she explained that the duke had been unable to write, since 'for this fortnight past [he has] been suffering very much with one of his usual attacks of asthma and gout', adding that 'one of his eyes is a good deal *inflamed*' as well.[99] The next summer brought on a very similar attack, Mrs Jordan confessing that though there were hopes that the duke would this time escape a severe attack, she had her 'own *opinion* and *fears* on that subject' and had sent for the 'asthma doctor'.[100] As another of his biographers describes the curious rhythm of William's illness: in early summer, the King was 'habitually unwell. This seasonal infirmity manifested itself physically with gout and asthma, sometimes accompanied by glandular swellings, and mentally with periods of intense excitement. As his body returned to normal, so his mind grew calmer. But a full restoration to physical and mental health was seldom achieved before midsummer.'[101] Indeed, there were many occasions in the winter months, too, when the duke was 'very seriously indisposed'.[102]

When the eccentric William came to the throne in 1830, many thought he was as mad as his father and the elder brother who had preceded him. As George IV lay dying, Sir Henry Cooke reported that 'the general bet is that Clarence is in a strait-waistcoat before the King dies'; Thomas Creevey also thought a straitjacket might soon be necessary; and Greville, who had long observed signs of 'incipient insanity' in William, noted in his diary that the new monarch 'bids fair to be a maniac'.[103] The 'exaltation' of coming to the throne at the age of sixty-five was so great, Greville believed, that William 'nearly went mad, and distinguished himself by a thousand extravagances of language and conduct, to the alarm or amusement of all who witnessed his strange freaks; and though he was shortly afterwards sobered down into more becoming habits, he always continued to be something of a blackguard and something of a buffoon'.[104]

Seemingly unable to control his temper, William IV would grow 'literally purple with rage' and hurl incoherent abuse at those around him. Shortly after William's accession, Greville noted that the new King 'is going much too fast, and begins to alarm his Ministers and astonish the world. In the morning he inspected the Coldstream Guards, dressed (for the first time in his life) in a military uniform and with a great pair of gold spurs half-way up his legs like a game-cock – although he was not to ride, for, having chalk-stones in his hands, he can't hold the reins.'[105] By 1832 Greville was sure William was 'one of the silliest old gentlemen in his dominions; but I believe he is mad, for yesterday . . . after dinner he made a number of speeches, so ridiculous and nonsensical, beyond all belief but to those who heard them, rambling from one subject to another, repeating the same thing over and over again, and altogether such a mass of confusion, trash and imbecility as made one laugh and blush at the same time'.[106] In 1833 Sir Thomas Hardy expressed the conviction that 'the King would certainly go mad; he is so excitable, *loathing* his Ministers . . . and dying to go to war. He has some of the cunning of madmen, who fawn upon their keepers when looked at by them and grin at them and shake their fists when their backs are turned.'[107]

The monarch's near-madness was a problem for all who had to deal with him. 'He is now and then mad – or very nearly so,' Ellenborough wrote.[108] Even the Prime Minister, Lord Melbourne, was reduced in 1836 to crying out: 'The King is all but crazy.' On 22 May 1837, just before her eighteenth birthday, his niece Princess Victoria of Kent noted that 'the King was in a very odd state'.[109] William himself, like all the sons of George III, 'was haunted by the memory of his father's madness', we are told by a recent biographer.[110] Indeed, as Roger Fulford explains, after the reigns of

George III and George IV it had become natural for people 'to regard madness as almost part of the kingly office'.[111] On hearing of the 'very disgraceful' way the King was treating his senior advisers in 1835, Charles Greville predicted: 'His habitual state of excitement will probably bring on sooner or later the malady of the family.'[112] When one of William's sons shot himself in 1842, contemporaries concluded that he, too, must have been 'tainted with the hereditary malady'.[113]

Physically, too, William IV was considered to be gravely ill and about to go 'the way of both his brothers'.[114] The King had 'gout stones in his fingers' and was frequently unable to hold a pen. Queen Adelaide would bathe his hands in warm water every evening before he settled down to sign state papers.[115] Allen tells us: 'William fell ill in the summer of 1837 with his annual ailment, and could not this time muster his forces to defeat it . . . He could scarcely climb the stairs . . . His condition deteriorated quickly; for the first time in his life he could not eat, he kept fainting, and had trouble with his breathing.'[116] Ziegler informs us that, at his death, William's 'liver was enlarged and hardened, a condition which must certainly have given him much trouble'. In addition, 'his lungs were turgid with blood, the heart valves ossified', and 'the spleen double its normal size'.[117] These findings are remarkably similar to the condition in which George IV's internal organs were discovered when he was dissected.

Charlotte, Princess Royal and Queen of Württemberg (1766–1828)

Throughout her life, George III's eldest daughter Charlotte had a tendency to liver trouble. As early as 1768, when she was two years old, Lady Mary Coke noticed the unusual 'yellow mark' on the princess's cheek. In 1796, not long before her marriage to Prince (later King) Frederick of Württemberg, she fell ill with 'jaundice', the 'yellowness' of which did not 'begin to go off' until the end of the year. After her marriage, her appearance deteriorated alarmingly. Her sisters Elizabeth and Augusta were both shocked at the unrecognizable sibling who met them when they visited her at Stuttgart in 1819 and 1821 respectively, the former writing that 'her person, alas, is sadly changed, for she is certainly very large . . . with a great deal more lower stomach. She . . . certainly does not dress to advantage, for her hair is very thin, and combed flat upon her face, which is three or four times larger than it was.'[118] Augusta's reaction was even more distraught. 'I found my sister very much altered at first; and had I not had the picture previous to seeing Her, I should not have guessed it was her . . . She is very large & bulky. Her face is very broad and fat, which makes Her features appear quite small and distended. But what strikes the most is, that from not wearing the least bit of Corset, Her Stomach and Her Hips are something quite extraordinary.'[119] Charlotte found it difficult to write because her hand was 'much swelled'.[120] She complained of pains in her side, and in 1824 of having been 'unwell the whole winter'.[121]

When, in 1827, she received an invitation from her brother, now George IV, to visit England, she was afraid he would be upset by her enormous bulk and resolved to take no less than thirty baths at a local spa before leaving Württemberg. Even so, she warned that the King would have to send 'a Chair to draw me up in' from the yacht, 'as with my shortness of breath I should be quite knocked up if I was to attempt the going up the accom[m]odation ladder . . . I must do all in my power . . . not [to] alarm you all with one of my Suffocations.'[122] The British medical profession was of the opinion that the old Queen had been 'afflicted for many years past with a dropsy', and that this was 'the cause of her extraordinary size'. On the advice of Sir Astley Cooper, she underwent tapping while in London to siphon off pints of surplus fluid, and, as the Annual Register for 1828 put it, 'there were flattering hopes that the operation would lead ultimately to a perfect cure'.[123] The operation did little good, however, and soon after her arrival in England Charlotte suffered an attack of another ailment altogether, one which might prove to be of significance for our quest: she was afflicted with a feverish inflammation of the skin which the doctors diagnosed as St Anthony's fire.[124] Thereafter her health declined steadily, her eyesight failed, and she died on 6 October 1828 after an apoplectic seizure.[125]

What was wrong with the Queen of Württemberg, the Princess Royal – the grandmother, incidentally, of George V's consort Queen Mary? Given her swollen size, it seems that she was indeed suffering from water retention, i.e. dropsy, on a massive scale, as the English doctors supposed. However, a number of letters in the Royal Archive at Stuttgart from her doctor to her husband the King point to an additional condition involving migraines and sharp 'rheumatic' pains in the side, back, hands and legs which could well have had another cause. On 9 April 1811, Dr Du Vernoy reported that, though the Queen's health was now on the mend, progress was bound to be slow, as 'pains more or less acute' were still occurring at intervals, 'and it is principally at night that the warmth of the bed . . . contributes to their development, thus disturbing her sleep'. The affected foot, he went on, had not got worse, raising hopes that the infected parts would remain confined within certain limits. The doctor ended his letter by explaining that the Queen was 'absolutely in no condition' to write herself.[126]

Some three years later, Du Vernoy reported on a similar 'indisposition the principal character of which is rheumatic'. The Queen suffered from a migraine in mid-October of that year, but otherwise her health at that time appeared to be 'quite tolerable'. On 30 October, however, she was 'attacked by a very strong migraine accompanied by biliousness ['*maux de coeur*'], but without any noticeable alteration of the pulse'. During the day, in addition to her biliousness, the Queen complained of feeling cold. On the following day, the migraine lessened, 'but the Queen's pains became sharper and her pulse more agitated'. At this point in his report, the doctor provides us with precious information on the condition of Queen Charlotte's urine but – tantalizingly – stops just short of describing its colour! 'The urines . . . flowed abundantly, they did not show any abnormal character except that they were more viscous ['*plus épaisses*'] than usual, then separated afterwards to deposit a copious sediment.' Du Vernoy thereupon observes that 'the increase in pain which every sort of movement of the body occasioned proves that it is principally the muscles of the back which are affected'. Though the pulse returned to normal in the course of the day, 'there did not as yet appear to be any noticeable change relative to the Queen's biliousness', nor were her 'rheumatic pains in the back' any the less severe. Her headache became worse again and there was now a swelling in the glands of the neck, but the doctor nevertheless expressed the hope that 'with an appropriate regime, aided by certain remedies', the Queen would slowly recover. Later that day, however, her fever returned, the pains in the back grew worse, the swollen glands in the neck spread on both sides, and she complained of piercing pains in the head.[127]

The evidence on Princess Charlotte is thus inconclusive, and it is difficult for us at this great distance in time to reach a diagnosis. However, given Du Vernoy's record of two separate attacks of great pain in the head, neck and back in 1811 and 1814, which were linked with an unusual cloudiness of the urine, and the appearance of a painful skin inflammation – St Anthony's fire – during her final illness in 1827–8, variegate porphyria (in addition to dropsy) can certainly not be ruled out as the cause of her complaint.

Edward, Duke of Kent (1767–1820)

As Queen Victoria's father, the medical biography of Edward, George III's fourth son, is of special interest to us. Like his elder brothers, the Duke of Kent suffered from 'rheumatism' and chest trouble.[128] In 1787, while in the care of Zimmermann at Hanover, he complained of difficulty in breathing, with the result that the doctor sent him to take the waters.[129] In 1788, at the time of his father's first serious attack, Edward was himself recovering from 'a violent rheumatism . . . which nearly deprived me of the total use of both my hands'.[130] Two years later, he wrote to his father of the 'frequent bilious attack from which I have felt the most violent and serious effects', and reported that his doctor had warned him that if he remained in Gibraltar for another summer he might be subject to 'the most fatal attacks of a complaint, the severity of which is, I believe, not unknown to your Majesty'.[130] Edward often complained of 'violent bilious attacks' and once of 'a very violent rheumatism [which] settled in my head for several days'.[132] His correspondence also provides strong evidence of a skin condition consistent with variegate porphyria: in spring 1800 he confided to his brother George that for the past six weeks he had been unable to wear anything but loose trousers on account of 'a troublesome humour which, after shewing itself in several parts of my body, at length settled in my legs; indeed at this moment one of my eyes is nearly closed from the same cause'.[133] Though the evidence is sparse, it is nevertheless strong and persuasive – and crucial to our thesis that the porphyria gene was passed on by Edward's daughter to later generations.

The duke died suddenly at Sidmouth on 23 January 1820, just a week before his father's death. The mysterious condition from which he suffered was carefully chronicled by his wife Victoire, in a lengthy letter which she wrote to her mother at the end of February. She recalled how Edward had not taken care of himself in the cold house they had rented, with the result that his catarrh developed into a 'terrible illness'. On Friday, 7 January, he began to complain of a severe headache and of cold feet. Within days he was running a high fever and sleeping badly, with vivid dreams and a violent cough, yet still refusing to take the medicine prescribed by Dr Wilson. On the Tuesday he was so hot and delirious and complained of such severe headaches and chest pains that leeches were applied to his head, yet the night was worse than ever – he vomited and had a fainting fit. The daily blood-letting from the head and elsewhere, which on one occasion lasted for no less than four hours, only made him weaker, but the doctors were adamant that this was the only way to prevent an inflammation. 'His head ached so very badly, and unfortunately he began to spit out a little blood!' Victoire recorded. A week after the onset of the illness, 'he complained of a very violent pain in the right side'. He was unable to keep down his food. 'The melancholy fact is that His Royal Highness is now sinking fast, and is not likely to survive many hours,' General Wetherall reported on 22 January.[134] His pulse was so fast that Baron Stockmar predicted his end by midnight; in fact he died at ten o'clock the following morning.[135]

The nature of the Duke of Kent's final illness becomes clearer from the post-mortem examination which was carried out by Samuel Lascombe, the senior physician at the Devon and Exeter Hospital, and which we referred to in Chapter 2. Lascombe registered that the internal organs – the stomach, intestines, liver, gall bladder and spleen – all appeared to be healthy, but that the left lung was 'of a deep red colour', and 'the Cavity of the Chest of the right side contained ten ounces of a Semipurulent fluid, with numerous and large portions of coagulable lymph floating in it'. Moreover 'the left Cavity contained four ounces of a red coloured fluid, in appearance [similar] to venous blood before coagulation', and a further 'two ounces of bloody fluid were in the Pericardium'.

When Lascombe cut into the lungs, that of the right side was found to be 'in a complete state of suppuration, or abscess, it being entirely gorged with pus or matter' – clearly the immediate cause of death – whereas the left lung was 'very much inflamed and charged with blood'. The heart itself was of a pale colour and flabby. On cutting into the stomach, he found the internal lining to his surprise to be 'studded with circular red spots, easily removable by the nail of a finger'. Similar red spots were also to be seen on the internal coat of the small intestines and at the beginning of the larger one. The right kidney was slightly inflamed, but the left one sound, as was the bladder. The blood vessels of the pia mater, or immediate covering of the brain, were 'turgid', Lascombe recorded, but otherwise the brain appeared sound.[136] The immediate cause of the duke's death, it seems clear, was pneumonia, but again this does not account for the numerous unusual symptoms – which included skin rashes, bilious attacks and severe rheumatic pains – from which he suffered throughout his life.

Princess Augusta (1768–1840)

Like several of her brothers and sisters, George III's second daughter, Augusta, who never married, suffered all her life from mysterious 'cramps' and 'spasms'. Her doctor, John Turton, perhaps despairing of helping her with less severe remedies, once urged her to 'boil herself in the warm bath'.[137] In 1815 she was unable to attend a dinner at Carlton House owing to a bilious attack.[138] On a visit to Brighton in early 1835, her sister Elizabeth recorded that Augusta had been 'confined for above a fortnight with a fit of gout, which she has borne most patiently and [with] great good humour'.[139] Otherwise, little is recorded of the medical condition of this unfortunate princess until the late summer of 1840 when, at the age of seventy-two, she lay dying of what Halford described as 'an incurable disease' and a 'formidable complaint', meaning, one imagines, cancer of the bowel. 'The moment must come when a mortification will take place', he informed Lord Melbourne on 27 August, 'but no sagacity can discover . . . when that moment is to arrive. The Princess suffers severe attacks of pain every now and then, but the remedy provided against such visitations generally succeeds in a short time, in subduing them.'[140] By mid-September 1840 Augusta was close to death, suffering 'severe paroxysms of pain occasionally' and showing daily evidence of 'fixt mischief in the tract of the intestine'. She was released from her torment on 22 September.[141]

Elizabeth, Landgravine of Hesse-Homburg (1770–1840)

Princess Elizabeth, George III's third daughter, was a fat and sickly child, and her life was constantly considered to be in danger. The letters and diaries of the time contain frequent references to her many illnesses. When she was fifteen, she had a severe attack variously described as 'an inflammation of the lungs' or 'whooping-cough' which gave rise to alarm, not least because it was accompanied by the mysterious 'very strong . . . spasms' – cramp-like pains that were to plague her throughout her life. After several weeks of illness in Elizabeth, Mrs Mary Delany could record that she had had 'a very severe return of her spasms', and Queen Charlotte, after visiting her daughter on 4 January 1786, could write, more in hope than with conviction, that Elizabeth's 'spasms still continue, but I flatter myself the intervals are longer'.[142] Mrs Papendiek records the significant information that these spasm attacks coincided with the appearance of 'a scrofulous abscess on her left side'.[143] In the midst of their anxiety, 'on account of the dangerous situation of the Pss. Elizabeth', friends at court could at least take comfort from the knowledge that 'the spasms have not affected her head'.[144] Elizabeth was blooded by the doctors twelve times in as many days, losing seventy-five ounces of blood according to the King, who 'seemed quite filled with concern for her danger and sufferings'.[145] The young princess's pains continued until February, when they abated as mysteriously as they had set in – only to return in the late summer. On 2 September 1786, the King himself informed Dr Hurd, the Bishop of Worcester: 'We have had some alarm in consequence of a spasmodic attack on the breast of Elizabeth which occasioned some inflammation, but by the skill of Sir George Baker she is now perfectly recovered.'[146] It was not until after Christmas, however, that the princess was to be 'perfectly restored to health' and even obtained Baker's permission to dance.[147]

The year 1787 brought little improvement in Elizabeth's condition, one lady at court describing her as 'so extremely delicate in her constitution, and so sweet and patient in submitting to her destiny'. By the time of the King's birthday on 4 June she was still only convalescent, after months of being confined to her room 'ever since her dangerous illness', and she could hardly bear the sound of the band playing in honour of her father, so hypersensitive was her hearing.[148] Her illnesses at this time were so frequent and so severe that she was assigned a residence at Kew as a sort of personal sick bay.[149] Everyone lived in fear lest any excitement might occasion 'a return of her spasms'.[150]

As she grew older, she became prone to 'hysterick fits', as her mother called them,[151] and Elizabeth herself admitted that one such seizure was 'of that kind to give me *serious alarm*, and I own fairly I look forward to what I had always thought with horror of, a sudden death'.[152] In the following year, she was once more seized with a long illness which brought her close to death and robbed her of her looks.[153]

In 1818, when she was approaching forty-eight, Elizabeth was finally able to marry Frederick VI, Landgrave of Hesse-Homburg, a diminutive principality in the hills overlooking Frankfurt. Ten years later, shortly after her husband's death, she 'nearly lost' the use of both legs and was henceforth virtually lame for the rest of her life, being able to walk only painfully and slowly with the aid of iron callipers.[154] She suffered painfully, too, from 'rheumatism'. Writing to her companion Louisa Swinburne in 1832, she explained that, 'tho' not ill, I have so dreadful a Rheumatism in my back that I cannot at this moment *move*'.[155] Only a few weeks later, the widowed Landgravine reports: 'I have had one of my severe billious spasms in my hip, so that I only got up for the evening. I shall begin some remedies which my friend, Sir Henry Halford, has sent me, and which I shall take with great gratitude this night, I am easier in a degree, but very like the old nurse in "Romeo and Juliet", – oh my arm, and oh my back.'[156] On Christmas Day, she was still in pain but hopeful of a speedy recovery, telling Miss Swinburne: 'I hope to be out again but I have been very lame; I put myself on the gruel system and with Sir Henry Halford's medicine I am getting easy.'[157]

For a number of years, Elizabeth was able to make the journey to Hanover, where her brother Adolphus was Viceroy, but she found the rooms there insufferably overheated and longed to escape into the open air. To Swinburne she complained: 'The room where I found myself was so *hot* that I was *half dead*.'[158] The stuffy rooms at Hanover continued to plague her well into the spring. 'I took a drive to-day to get some air, for the great heat of the rooms kill me [*sic*] and I require bracing,' she recorded.[159] Not just in Hanover but in other places, too, she felt the (in her view) overheated rooms to be a torment.[160] Thus in the Taunus Mountains she complained in July 1838: 'The heat is so great I am near dead.'[161] 'I am nearly knocked up with the heat, even *here* I am absolutely *subdued*,' she wrote from her *Schloss* in Bad Homburg.[162] Even in Brighton in January 1835 she complained of the 'extreme heat of the rooms' in the Royal Pavilion.[163]

In the last years of her life, Elizabeth was troubled by rheumatism and lameness, by pains in the chest and abdomen and by bilious attacks. Getting up in the morning was for her a lengthy and difficult procedure, as she told Louisa in 1833. 'I blush to think how often I am late of a morning, which is not like me, but my poor legs require time.' Only her 'bathes' seemed to provide some relief.[164] In 1834 she was confined to her bed for several weeks 'with a most tremendous cough and various pains and aches, which my excellent good Stucklitz thought very seriously of at first; but he is now aware that my constitution is a most wonderful one'.[165] In the heat of that summer she found it almost impossible to eat, as it made her 'bilious' – 'but I keep it all right by applying to Sir Henry Halford's box of *bonbons*; they do me much good'. Visiting Adolphus in Hanover in 1837 for the last time, she complained that 'the snow makes me very rheumatic, and I dare not go out . . . To-day I am lame, having the rheumatism in my left leg, so that ill as I now generally walk, it is worse.'[167] Back in Bad Homburg that summer, she looked forward to taking the waters at Wiesbaden, admitting that she enjoyed 'everything but walking, which is totally out of my power, and getting up off my chair when I have been long seated', which gave her 'great pain'.[168] 'My legs have been so very painful and weak,' she now complained in an uncharacteristic show of despondency.[169] Her stay at Wiesbaden had not been a success 'as I went when it was far too hot for me', and when she found herself facing another cure there in 1838, she exclaimed: 'It annoys me, as I meant to have got well *here* [at Homburg], but the uncertainty of the weather has made me so great a sufferer with Rheumatism that I must consider my health.'[170]

Shortly thereafter, in September 1838, another distressing symptom emerged: Elizabeth was afflicted with a painfully swollen face. To Louisa Swinburne she confided: 'I have so bad a *swelled face* I am not shewable . . . I hope in a few days to see you, at present it is out of the question for I am a perfect monster . . . I am too stupid to say more for I am in such pain with my face.'[171]

Throughout 1839, her last year, the Landgravine was ill with abdominal pain.[172] Her legs were particularly bad in May, but she quickly recovered. The old pain in her side returned, but in her letters to her sister Augusta she was so cheerful that the latter was unable to regard it as 'a disease likely to terminate her precious life'.[173] Returning to Frankfurt on 5 November 1839, she took three days to complete a letter to Augusta which ended in the words '*now I am useless*'.[174] On 9 January 1840 Elizabeth was seized by a state of agitation which gave way to unconsciousness. She died on the evening of the following day.[175]

Much pious nonsense has been written about the cause of her suffering and death. As her most recent biographer has stated, the underlying cause of the many illnesses which plagued her all her life – pneumonia, whooping cough, skin inflammation, pain in the lymph nodes, spasms and severe rheumatism in the back, sides and legs – was almost certainly porphyria inherited from her father.[176]

Ernest, Duke of Cumberland (1771–1851)

When Dr William Cookson visited the Duke of Cumberland at Carlton House, he found him in 'a very nervous state', supposedly because of the large quantities of laudanum which he took. Cookson told the diarist Joseph Farington: 'He suffers much pain and is much afflicted with spasms.'[177] Otherwise, little seems to be recorded on the medical history of George III's fifth son.

Augustus, Duke of Sussex (1773–1843)

Prince Augustus, the sixth son, on the other hand, was 'so delicate from his birth, that the air of England was found too severe for his system', and in fact he hardly spent any time there at all.[178] In 1788, when he was only fifteen and in the care of Zimmermann at

Hanover, he was seized by 'fearful paroxysms' which puzzled the doctors so much that they made detailed notes on his condition. The young prince was afflicted with spasmodic constriction in the chest producing a reddish-brown discoloration of the face which resembled asthma except that it was accompanied by extreme pain. Simultaneously Augustus suffered from giddiness, severe headache, insomnia, nocturnal excitement, restlessness, anxiety and listlessness. At times the paroxysms were so violent that the doctors feared the patient might suffocate. Their most telling observation was that the prince's urine 'repeatedly changed' its colour in the course of the illness, being at times 'very pale, at others deeply coloured'; during acute attacks it was 'deep amber' or 'reddish', but in remission 'the colour returned to normal'.[179]

In reporting the illness to George III, Zimmermann was at pains to stress that, though their cause was a mystery, the attacks did closely resemble those which had afflicted the Duke of York from 1783 onwards. He and the other three doctors in attendance, he said with remarkable perspicacity, could only conclude that Augustus had 'a peculiar disposition to paroxysms of a violent kind, but in what this disposition consists we are unable to determine . . . It has come to our knowledge that several members of the Royal Family and in particular His Royal Highness the Duke of York and Prince Edward [the Duke of Kent] are subject to the same paroxysms and this arouses our suspicion of a hereditary predisposition.'[180]

Augustus had many more such attacks. Until 1817 his chief complaint was asthma, which prevented him from sleeping more than 'one night out of six'.[181] As he was unable to lie down, an enormous invalid chair was constructed to accommodate him on his restless nights.[182] Even in this period, however, he had bouts of illness of a different kind. In August 1811 Mrs Jordan wrote to the Duke of Clarence: 'I was extremely shocked to hear of the Duke of Sussex's illness, but still it was a consolation to me to perceive by the papers that the danger did not proceed from his old complaint.'[183] Then, in 1817, after tormenting him all his life, his asthma completely left him, but for the remainder of his life he wore a black skullcap, being convinced that if he left it off the asthma would return.[184] There were times when his brothers feared that his 'intellect' might be 'deranged'.[185]

On 12 April 1843, at the age of seventy, Duke Augustus 'was attacked with erysipelas, and for some days went on favourably; but on the 19th a relapse occurred', and he died later that day.[186] All his life, the Duke of Sussex had a strong sense of being a medical curiosity and often said that if only the doctors could open his head they would discover some anomaly.[187] In his will he asked that his body be opened and examined in the interests of science, as he was sure there was a 'peculiarity in my conformation'. He found the thought consoling, he said, that 'even after death, my bodily frame may advance that which I always desired during my life – the good of my fellow men'.[188]

When the post-mortem examination was carried out, Augustus's *head* was found to be free from disease, but in several other respects the autopsy revealed a condition astonishingly similar to that of King George IV on his death: the mucus membrane lining the throat and windpipe was 'of a dark colour in consequence of its muscles being unusually turgid with blood'; the heart and arteries were ossified; the liver 'in a state of disease presenting a granular appearance throughout its whole substance', and 'in the lower bowel there were some internal haemorrhoids'. However, the lungs, which had given Augustus such trouble in the early part of his life, showed no marks of illness.[189] As we noted earlier, the retrospective diagnosis of variegate porphyria in Augustus of Sussex was one of the most convincing to be achieved by Macalpine, Hunter and Rimington.[190]

Adolphus, Duke of Cambridge (1774–1850)

The Duke of Cambridge spent most of his life up to 1837 as Viceroy in Hanover, being sent to England by his doctors only from time to time to take sea-bathing at Brighton for his gout.[191] In 1833 his sister Elizabeth reported that her brother had been suffering from 'a sort of confined gout which has attacked the nerves, but he is better'.[192] The interesting phrase 'confined gout' was also used by the duke's doctors at Hanover.[193]

Princess Mary, Duchess of Gloucester (1776–1857)

George III's fourth daughter Mary, like her younger sister Sophia and quite unlike her three elder sisters, was slender and delicate.

The family correspondence is so full of references to her 'cramps' and 'spasms' that historians have despaired of using such evidence to identify any specific illness.[194] She was ill for many months in 1788, and from then until her final illness the doctors described her complaint in terms of 'spasms'.[195] After nursing both her sister Amelia on her deathbed and her father during his descent into darkness in 1810, Mary herself fell ill with headaches, insomnia, fever and 'some nervous symptoms' which made her 'unequal to bear light and noise, or conversation'.[196] In 1840 she was said to be 'timid about her health, in which she is totally unlike the rest of her family', and one of her sisters feared that her constitution contained 'the seeds of dropsy'.[197]

Mary, who in 1816 married her first cousin William Frederick, the Duke of Gloucester, was also prone to eccentric and irrational behaviour, as at the christening of Queen Victoria's daughter Louise in 1848, when the young mother wrote of her: 'The poor Duchess of Gloster is again in one of her nervous states, and gave us a dreadful fright . . . by quite forgetting where she was, and coming and kneeling at my feet in the midst of the service. Imagine our horror!'[198] It is only fair to point out that by this time Princess Mary was well into her eighties.

Princess Sophia (1777–1848)

Princess Sophia was also extremely delicate from birth, her poor health being attributed at first to her abrupt weaning, when her wetnurse left to attend to her own mother.[199] In her teens she suffered from a mysterious illness which involved trouble with what she called her 'swallow'. A year later, in 1793, her hands trembled so much she was barely able to write.[200] She is frequently described in the correspondence of the time as being 'far from well' and 'in a most delicate state'.[201] Another 'long illness' lasting one and a half years is recorded for 1813–14,[202] but in her case it hardly seems worth attempting to separate periods of illness from periods of good health, as she seems to have suffered all the time. She grew ever more ethereal, sad and withdrawn, and in 1818 the Princess Royal wrote of her younger sister: 'It grieves me to hear that poor dear Sophia is so seriously ill . . . Her health has so long been delicate, that we must ever look on her as a Hot House plant which requires every care to prevent its being destroyed.'[203] Her 'nerves' were said to be sensitive, and she was subject to 'low spirits' and insomnia.[204] She was short-sighted and went blind – like her father – in 1838, the only one of his children to do so.[205] Her hearing also became very poor, and in addition she 'could not move from her seat without being carried'.[206] Towards the end of her life she is said to have cut a 'pathetic, sightless figure', being 'old, blind, and stricken'.[207]

Like her sister Mary's, Sophia's life was so plagued by 'cramps' and 'spasms' and recurrent attacks of 'pain in her limbs or side' that one observer referred to her illness simply as 'her usual spasmodic complaint'.[208] In 1809, after witnessing violent quarrels between her brothers, the attacks were particularly severe, her sister Mary complaining to the Prince of Wales: 'Our dear Sophy . . . was taken with one of her worst spasms yesterday . . . All that past [*sic*] in her room last Monday was more than her delicate little frame could stand, therefore I own I expected this attack would follow.'[209] In fact, her 'spasms' were so common that people began to remark on their absence rather than their presence, as when a relative wrote on the death of George III: 'Sophy still without spasm, but I fear we shall not put it off much longer.'[210] Her siblings learnt to expect a 'spasm' after every excitement, and were relieved when the attacks turned out to be on the mild side. 'Thank God that our dearest Sophy has so well got over her last spasm, and has not suffered from paying you a visit, which must have agitated her,' the Queen of Württemberg wrote on 2 April 1828.[211] Surprisingly, in view of her delicate constitution, Sophia reached the age of seventy, outliving all her sisters except Mary and all her brothers except Ernest and Adolphus.

Princess Amelia (1783–1810)

In 1798, at the age of fifteen, the King's youngest daughter Amelia began to suffer from 'tuberculosis of the knee', her increasing ill-health turning her into an invalid and making any kind of regular education impossible.[212] Her sister Mary wrote that she was 'quite confined to the couch and suffering so much pain'.[213] Even at this stage, Amelia, like almost all of her sisters, had to be 'painfully lifted from her seat'.[214] However, the pain in her 'poor knee' eventually disappeared and did not return for another ten years, and in that interval she was able to ride, walk and even dance.[215]

Amelia also suffered from a 'very delicate state of Nerves' and complained of hypersensitivity to noise, once wishing that the wind would lessen as it '*hurts the Drumsticks of my Ears*', as she put it.[216] There was also a strange 'Noise in her throat' which lessened from time to time but always returned.[217] Shortly after arriving at Weymouth in 1801, at the age of eighteen, Amelia confided to the Queen that she was suffering from 'Bile and a caught attack of St Anthony's fire' in the face, an early sign of the condition which the doctors were to regard as a contributory cause of her death nine years later.[218] Not long after this first attack of a feverish skin inflammation, she was 'confined with those Boils', as her mother later reminded her.[219]

In their vain efforts to cure her 'erysipelas' and her pains, Christopher Hibbert tells us, the doctors 'bled her, purged her and blistered her; applied leeches to her skin and quills beneath it, immersed her in hot sea-water baths, prescribed beef-tea, calomel and Madeira; poured emetics and laudanum down her throat accompanied by a variety of powders, medicines, restoratives and stimulants'.[220] In 1806, they thought it necessary to insert a 'seaton' – a surgical drainage tube – in Amelia's chest in the hope of relieving the pain in her side, but all it did was to increase her agony, not least because the resultant inflammation of the open wound was treated with caustic.[221]

Less than two years later, Amelia began to suffer from a mysterious complaint from which her sister Elizabeth, the Landgravine, tried to protect herself by taking great quantities of snuff and draping camphor bags around her body – a reaction, one imagines, to an unsightly skin disease. Amelia placed herself in the care of Dr Pope, a Quaker physician from Staines, which inevitably caused ructions with the Court doctors, particularly Halford and Baillie. But, as Amelia explained to her brother George, Halford was too much of a courtier for her liking, and Baillie, though very skilful, had an unpleasant manner. That 'dear honest old Pope', on the other hand, was her 'best friend . . . for I know I am his only object & where he thinks my good concerned he goes strait [*sic*] forward without heeding any one . . . I am sure Pope understands me better than any one else.'[222] Pope diagnosed her illness, interestingly, as 'inflammation of the membrane of the liver', but the remedies he prescribed were no more effective than those of his courtly rivals. On his orders, the princess was to take a 'warm bath every other night, 5 drops of antimonial wine twice a day, some elm-bark tea, to sweeten the blood', and a little sudorific powder at night to cause sweating. Later Pope prescribed large doses of calomel, and again sent her to Weymouth in the summer of 1809, where she had to protect her eyes from the glare of the sea by means of a green curtain covering the window of the bathing machine.[223] As Sophia wrote after visiting her there, 'this obstinate pain in the side yields to nothing, and what she has to go through nearly breaks my heart'.[224] Amelia was unable to climb the seven steps of the pier or to cross the room without fainting or falling into fits of coughing, and even speaking exhausted her.[225]

Instead of getting better at Weymouth, Amelia became gravely ill, with vomiting and terrible shooting pains in the right side; she was unable to eat or sleep.[226] She was still hypersensitive to sound, had an intractable cough and severe pains in the head. Soon her nerves began to give way 'with the length of the illness'.[227] On her slow journey back to Windsor in 1810, her twenty-seventh year, Amelia was reported to be 'very faint, and in great pain with her side'.[228]

The doctors who were called in to examine her at Windsor were puzzled by Amelia's condition – they referred to it as a 'disturbed state of the nervous system which may be expected after so severe an attack'[229] – and at a loss to know how to treat it, other than by giving her laudanum and laxatives. She slept for only two or three hours a night, coughed a great deal, vomited frequently, was hysterical and restless, complained of constipation and headaches and 'much of the hot pain in the side', and had a racing pulse (but no temperature) which fluctuated around the hundred-mark. 'These varieties depend upon the instability of her constitution, and are very common in nervous Habits,' Dr Baillie explained.[230]

The doctors fed her on a diet of beef tea, mutton broth, arrowroot, panada of chicken, grapes, cherries, oranges, nectarines, strawberries and pineapple, and gave her barley water, ginger wine, brandy, beer, cider and Madeira to drink. Someone stayed with the princess throughout every night, and one of the doctors reported in writing to the King at six o'clock every morning.[231] Amelia herself complained on 9 May 1810 of cold and 'oppression upon my chest' which was aggravating the pain in her side, and thought that the new 'strong' medicine the doctors had given her did not agree with her stomach.[232] On 10 May, Halford reported that Amelia was again complaining of 'pain and tightness across the chest', which alarmed him since 'the extinction of inflammation there had afforded us the best ground of hope of improvement in Her Royal Highness's symptoms lately'. Though anxious to 'take immediate measures' for the removal of this 'new evil', all the doctors could think of doing was to take away 'a small quantity of blood . . . from the neighbourhood of the chest'. But Halford's fond hopes certainly did not materialize that 'this timely recourse to the evacuation will effectually prevent a continuance of that inflammatory condition of the interior of the breast which has been so productive of distress in the earlier period of the Princess's illness'.[233] A week later, he was obliged to report to the King that his daughter continued to suffer 'the same distressful state of constant retching and exhaustion' as before, and two days after that he came close to admitting that he was losing hope of being able to save her life. Her nights were very restless, he said, and both the retching and the princess's 'expression of general uneasiness and distress [were] frequent'. She was clearly getting weaker, Halford told the King, and he could not find 'that any one of the symptoms by which the Princess has been so heavily borne down lately have disappear'd – they are all to be found distressing in their turn – and Her Royal Highness has less power to bear up against them'.[234]

There were, from time to time, signs of a slight improvement. On 23 May Baillie was able to inform the King that Amelia had spent a better night, even though she had 'taken no opium whatever', and that she had been able to keep down four teaspoonfuls of beef tea! 'Her Highness certainly swallows better', he added, and the 'thick white . . . crust is shedding from her Tongue'.[235] Three days later Halford reported with satisfaction that the patient's pulse was 'stronger this morning than it has been during this late most severe attack'.[236] In her overall condition, however, there was no improvement, and at the end of May 1810, Sir Henry had to admit that 'the Princess does not complain less of the pain of the side, and of that internal heat, which Her Royal Highness has been in the habit of finding relieved by a more active state of the bowels'.[237] Throughout the illness, Dr Pope was less sanguine and more open about the princess's suffering than Baillie or Halford, but when her headaches became worse in early June, all he could recommend was the cupping glasses – which brought some relief to the head, though 'the pain in her side remains as usual'.[238]

As the months wore on, Amelia, still unable to swallow or keep down her food and drink, became weaker and weaker, and the pain in her side got worse. On 5 October, Halford informed the King that 'The Princess Amelia's complaint prevail'd with more violence than ever at the beginning of the night – and still continues much as it was yesterday evening.'[239] She now had worrying fits of faintness, and in addition the medical reports to the King speak of her 'feverish irritation' and 'rather more heat upon the skin'.[240] By mid-October her doctors reported that the 'pain and tensionness of the head seem to have been somewhat relieved by the bleeding from the nose in the course of the night', that she was sleeping at most one hour each night, eating and drinking virtually nothing at all, and suffering daily from a 'succession of the attacks of faintness and languor'.[241] She became ever more feeble, and almost faded away. On 29 October she had a very restless night with sickness and vomiting, and her pulse rose to an alarming 116 beats per minute. She died on 2 November 1810.[242]

Her eldest sister wrote of her: 'Poor dear Amelia has had a long and dreadful illness . . . I never saw any body more carefull to disguise Her sufferings for fear of vexing others; and truly it is most vexing to see Her so long in such a sad state of Health.'[243] Miss Knight, who attended her at Windsor, recorded that

day by day she sank more and more under her great sufferings. Though pale and emaciated, she still retained her beauty. She wished to live, but was thoroughly resigned when she found there was no hope of her remaining long upon earth . . . I saw her a few days before her death, when, taking off her glove, she showed me her hand – it was perfectly transparent. She was particularly fond of music, but latterly could not bear the sound of a pianoforte even in another room.'[244]

Amelia's sister Mary reported that she was, on top of her other symptoms, suffering once again from 'slight erysipelas about the head and eyes'.[245] In September 1810, Mary told the Prince of Wales that 'the Eruption he saw the beginning of in her face had increased every day since and had run nearly all over the body'.[246]

What did the doctors make of her illness? Amelia herself summarized their mystified diagnosis when she wrote that they were of the opinion 'that the principal disease was an Inflammation which had taken place in the back part of the right side, and had caused considerable swelling in that part. From its origin being in the neighbourhood of the Liver they think it probable it may have been disordered in its functions and perhaps suffered a degree of superficial inflammation.'[247]

More recent royal biographers have come to a different view. Dorothy Margaret Stuart, for example, writes: 'The medical bulletins of the Princess's last year are so full of sickroom details as to leave little doubt that she died of tuberculosis complicated by erysipelas.'[248] But that is a verdict which is also open to challenge. It is difficult to see what the diagnosis of consumption is based on, other than the dubious opinion that the pain in Amelia's legs when she was a child was caused by 'tuberculosis of the knee', that there was a strange noise in her throat, and that she had a persistent cough during her final illness. The surgical drainage tube which in 1806 was placed in her side was intended to ease her pain, not to cure consumption. The striking fact, surely, is that the fearful symptoms from which Amelia suffered throughout her life – lameness, spasms, the shooting pains in her side, hypersensitivity to light and sound, skin inflammation and boils – are astonishingly similar to those which afflicted all the daughters of George III, and indeed most of his sons as well. They cannot all have died from 'tuberculosis complicated by erysipelas'.

Conclusion

Our brief survey of the medical history of George III's thirteen surviving children has produced a startling result. When we set out on our search through the historical record for symptoms consistent with porphyria, we were expecting to find such symptoms either in about half of the King's offspring – indicating that George did indeed have this dominantly transmitted genetic disorder – or else that none of them presented such symptoms, showing either that George III's agony was of a different nature, or that he did not transmit his illness to his progeny. What we have discovered is that all, or very nearly all, of his children suffered severely from porphyria-like symptoms such as spasms, colic and cramps, sharp headaches, lameness and brachial weakness, pain in the chest, back and side, biliousness, vomiting and constipation, breathlessness, irregularity of the pulse, inflammation and fragility of the skin, mental disturbance and, in one or two cases, discoloured urine. Only Adolphus, the Duke of Cambridge, failed to display such symptoms, but the medical information available to us on him is so thin that the absence of evidence should not be equated with absence of the illness.

It is not only the historian looking back over two centuries who is struck by the similarity of the strange and terrible symptoms afflicting the children of George III, however; they themselves, together with their doctors, were fully aware both that they suffered from some kind of constitutional abnormality, and that that abnormality was shared by the entire family. We have seen how the Duke of Sussex was sure there was a 'peculiarity in my conformation', and how George IV had the acute sense that all his symptoms were caused by his '*very nervous* and . . . *delicate* fibre'. The latter likened his own symptoms to those suffered by his brother Frederick, and the doctors frequently remarked on the similarity of the mysterious attacks endured by the royal dukes: Zimmermann explicitly likened the symptoms he noted in the young Duke of Sussex to those he had witnessed in the Duke of York and heard about on the medical grapevine in the Duke of Kent, and thirty-five years later Sir Henry Halford compared the violent paroxysms suffered by George IV during his final illness with similar attacks visited upon his brothers William and Augustus in earlier years. What is more, as the Duke of Kent's letter to his father of 1790 makes clear, there was widespread recognition among his offspring that the disorder afflicting them all, whatever its nature might be, was the same as that endured by King George III.

But the most telling symptom is that noted by Zimmermann and the other Hanoverian doctors treating the fifteen-year-old Duke of Sussex in 1788. Their observation that the Prince's urine 'repeatedly changed' its colour in the course of the attack from 'deep amber' or 'reddish' back to 'very pale' in remission is such an accurate description of the most characteristic single symptom of porphyria as to leave little room for doubt that Augustus had inherited that disorder. Apart from the passing reference by Du Vernoy to the dense or opaque character of the Queen of Württemberg's urine during a painful attack in 1814, and Zimmermann's observation that the Duke of Sussex's symptoms (he does not specify which ones) were remarkably similar to those endured by the Duke of York some years earlier, this is the only description we currently have of orange or red urine in any of the children of George III. However, now that we have established beyond reasonable doubt that most of his children suffered from the same disorder, it would seem to follow in logic that, if Augustus had porphyria, then that must have been the cause of the suffering of his siblings, too.

We can deploy a similar argument to try to determine the *variety* of porphyria inherited and passed on by George III. In more than half of the cases we have examined – George IV, Frederick, Charlotte, Edward, Elizabeth, Augustus and Amelia – we were able to register strong evidence of an inflammation of the skin, referred to in the medical terminology of the time as 'erysipelas', 'anasarca' or 'St Anthony's fire'. We suggest that doctors in the late eighteenth and early nineteenth centuries used these terms interchangeably to denote a feverish swelling and reddening of the skin in general, and that when they used the name 'erysipelas' they did not mean by it the specific infection, caused by the dangerous *Streptococcus* bacterium, which is known by the name 'erysipelas' today. The very frequency with which this symptom showed itself throughout the lives and in particular during the final illnesses of George III's children over seven decades would in itself seem to rule out streptococcal infection as its cause. We are dealing instead, as Croker rightly pointed out in 1834, with a '*family* complaint' which we may now tentatively identify as porphyria of the variegate kind.

CHAPTER 5

The 'Hereditary Malady':
The 'Peculiarities' of Queen Victoria

The Q[ueen] is so excitable that the P[rince Consort] live[s]
in perpetual terror of bringing on the hereditary malady.
Charles Greville, 12 December 1858

These nerves are a species of madness, and against them it
is hopeless to contend.
Sir Henry Ponsonby on Queen Victoria, 5 October 1871

In her unfinished biography of George III's granddaughter
Victoria, Cecil Daphne Woodham Smith, while accepting that both
George III and George IV had porphyria, is insistent that the illness
did not affect the British Royal Family after 1837. 'There is no
evidence whatsoever to suggest that Queen Victoria suffered from
porphyria or passed it on to any of her children,' she categorically
states.[1] This belief has led historians to abandon their search for
signs of the disease in subsequent generations. In the following
chapters of this book, however, we shall demonstrate that an
overwhelming amount of evidence exists to indicate that Queen
Victoria's eldest child Vicky had the porphyria gene and passed it
on to her eldest daughter, Charlotte, and she in turn to her
daughter, Feodora. The conclusion seems inescapable, then, that the
Queen must herself have carried the gene, though clearly she did not
suffer much from the symptoms, since otherwise the countless
historians who have investigated her life in such detail would have
come across evidence of the illness many decades ago. Nevertheless,
given that she passed the gene on to at least one of her nine
children, it is worth reviewing her own medical history in a fresh
light.

Modern biographies of Victoria, and not least Woodham Smith's own sensitive portrait, provide us with many fascinating clues about the 'peculiarities' of her system (as her personal physician termed them) which suggest that the disease might not have been entirely dormant even in her. Almost all of her biographers note, for instance, that Victoria – like her Aunt Elizabeth – revelled in cold draughts and felt uncomfortable in warm rooms and sunshine. At seventeen, she lamented that a hot July was 'quite dreadful to me, *who love cold*, & am always poorly & stupefied in hot weather'.[2] She was 'broiled and exhausted and done up' by the heat of summer and 'suffered severely from headaches . . . on account of the terrible heat', she wrote in 1858; she longed to escape from London and the 'dreadful' smell of the Thames.[3] On a July evening in Windsor she complained that it was 'so terribly hot I can hardly sit still or hold my pen'.[4] Similar complaints abound in her later correspondence.[5] In 1887, when she had been on the throne for fifty years, she insisted on having a large block of ice placed at the centre of her dinner table even on cool evenings so as to lower the temperature further.[6] Though her hands were ugly, swollen and red, she found it uncomfortable to wear gloves.[7] She insisted that she was having her new dresses made larger not because she was getting fatter but because she could not bear to wear anything tight.[8]

There were other 'peculiarities', too, which will strike us as familiar. When she was just fourteen, Princess Victoria complained of biliousness, of feeling sick, of being 'prostrated' by severe headaches, and of having backache, sore eyes and frequent colds.[9] In the following spring she records being 'indisposed' and confined to her room for a whole month, and we know from other sources that she was in poor health – again she felt sick and had constant pains in her back – and suffering from emotional tension.[10] In the autumn of 1835, her diary is full of complaints of 'dreadful headaches', backache, nausea, loss of appetite and immense fatigue.[11] At Ramsgate in October of that year she fell dangerously ill with a mounting fever and a pulse of 130. She was delirious at times and had to keep to her room for five weeks. Throughout her long life she remembered 'Ramsgate in 1835' as the most serious illness she had ever endured.[12] Dr James Clark, who attended her, described the illness as a 'bilious fever', whereas Victoria herself came to believe that it had been typhoid. (Many years later, when

Prince Albert was dying of typhoid, the Queen recalled that his symptoms were 'much what I had at Ramsgate, only that I was much worse and was not well attended to'.) On Clark's orders she took quinine draughts, but she could eat little and walk only a few steps. Whatever her illness was, she grew thin, lost a lot of hair and complained – unusually – of having ice-cold feet. By February she had recovered sufficiently to resume her lessons.[13]

Not long after her accession to the throne, just after her eighteenth birthday, Victoria lamented that she felt 'poorly' and 'faint', 'sick and miserable' and was suffering – once again – from 'nausea'.[14] On 10 July 1838, perhaps still exhausted from the strain of her coronation, the young Queen developed a rash on her hands which then spread to her neck. Alarmed, not least because he had seen similar symptoms in Victoria's uncles and aunts, Lord Melbourne, the Prime Minister, warned her 'on no account to scratch it'.[15] Later that year he noticed that she was looking 'rather yellow' and was often 'cross and low', though on occasions she would delight in bouts of frenetic enjoyment. Melbourne warned her against overeating, which he considered to be the family failing and the cause of her 'sick headaches' and fits of irritation. He urged her to walk more, since otherwise (like so many of her relatives) she would lose the use of her legs, but Victoria retorted that she disliked walking, as it made her feel tired and sick and caused her feet to swell.[16] She complained that her conflicts with Lord Palmerston made her physically ill, and told her doctor that reading Palmerston's dispatches before dinner made her bilious.[17]

In the prime of her life, Victoria had serious problems with her 'nerves'. In the days before her marriage to her cousin Albert, she was 'very nervous and feverish, so much so that they fancied she was going to have the measles'.[18] She frequently complained of 'sick headaches' and 'shocking nervous headaches', particularly after she and Albert had quarrelled, which they often did, even though they were famously close.[19] Soon rumours abounded of the young Queen's 'restlessness, excitement, and nervousness'; in early 1844 it was even reported that 'the Queen's mind is not in a right state'.[20] 'She is continually in tears and nothing but the extraordinary good sense of Albert, and the boundless influence he has over her, keeps her feelings under due restraint,' Greville noted in June 1848.[21]

Victoria's first two pregnancies depressed her and wrecked her nerves, she claimed, for '*a whole year*'.[22] For the 'first 2 years of my marriage', she said, she had 'aches – and sufferings and miseries and plagues'.[23] After the birth of Prince Leopold, her eighth child, in 1853, Victoria underwent a series of hysterical attacks – Melbourne called her 'choleric' – culminating in 'distressing' quarrels with Albert, who began to fear for her mental and physical health.[24] 'I have been lately suffering a great deal from nervousness and am therefore not capable of writing so connectedly as usual,' she confided to her friend Princess Augusta of Prussia, the later Empress, in 1854.[25] Over the next few years these nervous attacks were such a regular feature of the Queen's personality that periods of tranquillity and 'self-control' lasting four weeks became a matter for congratulation. 'I am trying to keep out of your way until your better feelings have returned and you have regained control of yourself,' Prince Albert told her on 5 November 1856.[26] In December 1858, Baron Stockmar actually confided to the Earl of Clarendon that he believed Albert to be 'completely cowed' by Victoria, who was 'so excitable that the P[rince] lived in perpetual terror of bringing on the hereditary malady' which had afflicted her grandfather George III, 'and dreaded saying or doing anything which might have a tendency to produce this effect'.[27] Woodham Smith vehemently disputes the accuracy of this assertion, but she herself prints several of Albert's letters showing the Prince Consort close to despair and vowing to avoid all further differences of opinion with Victoria so as not to aggravate her bad temper.[28] Stockmar's interpretation also receives corroboration from the diary of Sir James Clark, who recorded in 1856 that he had never seen the Queen so exhausted, nervous and debilitated, and that he feared for her mental health. 'Regarding the Queen's mind, unless she is kept quiet and still amused, the time will come when she will be in danger,' he wrote in alarm, and continued: 'Much depends on the Prince's management . . . If I could impress him with what I consider necessary I should almost consider the Queen safe.'[29] As Elizabeth Longford has written, Stockmar's insight throws new light on 'the Prince's strange technique for dealing with the Queen's upsets – his refusal to let her "have it out", his resort to notes, his periodic reports as if on the condition of a patient . . . He saw, through the eyes of Stockmar, not a perfectly sane though angry

Victoria, but the mad ghost of George III.'[30]

In their final years together, Victoria and Albert grew increasingly concerned over the wayward behaviour of their eldest son, the Prince of Wales, whose outbursts of childish rage Stockmar also interpreted as a reappearance of George III's madness.[31] In 1858 the Queen experienced a 'sharp attack of neuralgia' as a result of her worries, and rumours again began to circulate about her mental stability.[32] To her eldest daughter she wrote that she had 'horrid neuralgic pains' which 'flowed' about her face. 'I am not in a very fit state ... with my nervous pains,' she admitted.[33] 'My poor face is still not well,' we read days later. 'Though free from real pain (there is a great tenderness) through the day. It has come on each day just for dinner though perhaps less severely than yesterday; the nights are good – but it pulls me, and I can only get out for a short time with double veils and much wrapped as the wind is so cold. I fear it may be long in going off.'[34] The death of Victoria's mother in March 1861 set off a nervous breakdown in the Queen – the depth of her grief was quite inordinate, and she was unable to bear loud noises, particularly the sound of the Prince of Wales quarrelling with her other children.[35] As she wrote to Queen Augusta of Prussia, now her daughter Vicky's mother-in-law: 'I am deeply stricken, and so far have found no consolation! I am not actually ill, but my nerves are terribly upset and I can only bear the most complete quiet.'[36] To Vicky herself she confided: 'My head is so very bad – so fearfully sensitive; I can't bear the least noise or talking in the next room even ... [Bertie's] voice made me so nervous I could hardly bear it. Altogether I never felt in such a state of nerves for noise or sound.'[37] Several weeks later she was no better, telling her daughter: 'My nerves are still very bad, I suffer very much from my head and from that dreadful sensitiveness.'[38] In addition to the pain in her head and her sensitivity to noise, the Queen complained of 'getting bewildered and confused, which is tiresome and trying'. Any new face around her upset her, she said. 'I am dreadfully nervous just now ... Every new person I see – makes me so fearfully nervous.'[39] Several months after her mother's death, the Queen was writing: 'My spirits are very bad, my nerves terribly weak – and there is a heavy weight which weighs upon me and makes everything seem weary work! ... I am so dull and listless still, and London air and noise don't improve one.'[40] She spoke of her 'great depression' and recorded that she had taken 'quite a dislike to music!' as it hurt her head.[41]

Again, whispers abounded concerning the state of her mind. Vicky reported from Germany that there were 'monstrous reports' circulating there to the effect that 'all the doctors of Europe' had gathered to attend the Queen; and Prince Albert did what he could to keep such 'horrid vile rumours' from her.[42] The Earl of Clarendon wrote of the Queen's 'morbid melancholy' and believed that her mind was 'trembling in the balance'. He told the Duchess of Manchester that Robert Ferguson, one of Victoria's accoucheurs, had a 'private opinion about her mind (founded on his attendance upon her years ago when she was in a strange state) [which was] far from satisfactory'.[43] Even so, Victoria's depression after her mother's death was a mild affair compared with the endless mourning which set in with the death of Prince Albert in December 1861.

As her consort fell ill, Victoria too became seriously unwell 'with a violent, sick headache and retching!'[44] After his death she went into a state of nervous lethargy from which she found it impossible to escape. Once more, rumours spread that she had inherited her grandfather's ailment and was becoming mentally unhinged.[45] She shut herself away to a quite worrying extent. 'I do not appear in society because neither my health nor my nerves could bear it, as I find I need the greatest quiet,' she told the Queen of Prussia.[46] 'I feel really very weak and ill.'[47] She lost weight and was barely able to walk. She suffered from severe neuralgic headaches and pains, and was hypersensitive to sound and heat. She was convinced that the pressure of her responsibilities, coming on top of her unbearable grief, would drive her insane.[48] 'I feel more and more disinclined to take any interest in any thing,' she wrote to Vicky in April 1863. 'I am so uninterested because of tiredness and of total exhaustion. I am so dreadfully overworked, that I really can only compare myself to a hunted hare! I am dead beat, and then come headaches, and such forgetfulness and bewilderment, with such yearnings and wild longings for Papa – and accumulations of work which are so annoying and distressing, and I can never get to do what I wish.'[49] Travelling became a 'misery' for her, since she was 'so weak, so shaken and exhausted'.[50] Her life, she wrote, 'cannot last much longer as my increasing weakness and shattered nerves are dragging me down . . .'. She felt 'weak and shaken . . . with my poor vitality wasting gradually away!'[51]

To her eldest daughter she confided on 14 June 1862: 'I am so terribly nervously affected now; my pulse gets so high, it is constantly between 90 and 100 instead of being 74! This wears me terribly. It exhausts me so and I am so weak, and then my poor memory fails me terribly.'[52] In January 1863 she was still suffering from her nervous debility, writing to her daughter: 'You never will believe how unwell and how weak and nervous I am, but any talking or excitement is far too much for me. I must constantly dine alone.' Even now, the sound of her son's voice was 'quite too much for my very shattered nerves'.[53] On 24 May 1863, her forty-fourth birthday, the Queen still felt 'poorly' and complained of a 'violent headache, sickness and great prostration'.[54] More than half a year later she was blaming her deafness on her 'nerves', too, and lamenting that all the hard and unassisted work expected of her 'irritates, excites and exhausts my poor, shaken nerves' which were 'much worse of late again'.[55] She was, she said in February 1864, 'so unwell' and 'quite shattered' from worry and anxiety.[56] In March of that year her condition seemed to be worse, and she confided to Vicky: 'I am very poorly; very weak and exhausted . . . My weakness, nervousness and trembling has so greatly increased.'[57] This general nervous disability coincided with painful neuralgia. As the Queen wrote in April 1864, she had been seriously ill for several days with neuralgia. 'I never was in greater agonies, continuously', and although she was better now, she added, she was still 'much shaken and not well yet'.[58]

Victoria's condition did not improve in the following years. In fact, as late as May 1869 she was insisting that it was getting worse each year.[59] Her political duties, social events, even family gatherings were almost too much for her. In 1865, she explained to her eldest daughter that she would not be able to have her and her family to stay for Christmas on the grounds that her 'poor nerves' were completely 'shattered'.[60] Two years later, she suffered from a disgust for food and very bad headaches that lasted for several days.[61] She was 'broken down in body and spirits', she said, and felt 'as though my head were of china'; she found talking to people unbearable as it caused her 'such positive suffering'.[62] Standing made her feet 'swell so'.[63] More than six years after Prince Albert's death, the Queen found large social gatherings intolerable. She would leave her guests after a brief period and would be 'in a tremble and quite exhausted' afterwards. Life in the capital was especially irksome to her. 'The noise of London, and driving in the streets tires my head and nerves very much,' she complained in 1868. 'The fearful noise in the streets, when I try to get any fresh air, the constant interruption from morning to night and the dreadful atmosphere (we have a dense yellow fog this morning) makes me quite ill, and affects my nerves very much.'[64]

Full of sympathy, her daughter wrote to her:

> I do hope your visit to London will go off well and that the heat and the unwonted exertion will not be too much for you and give you one of your bad headaches. I am indeed distressed to hear that the blood so easily gets to your head and that your feet swell. I fear you are already approaching a stage in your health, which is said to be the most trying and unpleasant in a woman's life, and at which the strongest constitutions suffer as well as the most delicate . . . I shall be fearing you will be in so much discomfort of body which must always affect the nerves and spirits and make the mind more sensitive and less up to exertion.[65]

Vicky was able to put herself in her mother's shoes precisely because she could identify with her symptoms. 'Your description of what you feel like is exactly how I felt in the month of March,' she told her in July 1868. 'The very rustling of a person's gown used to irritate me, and more than one person talking in the room made me feel as if I was going wild. I was ready to cry if I heard anyone speak for a few minutes together, and talking myself made a lump come in my throat! All this is so completely gone now that I have only the recollection left, but that is enough to make me sympathize with you.'[66] That summer Sir William Jenner, the Queen's physician, strongly recommended that she go to Switzerland 'as it might do my nerves good'.[67]

What was the matter with Queen Victoria? As we have seen, there were those who feared that she was teetering on the brink of insanity. Clarendon records how in June 1862 at Windsor the Queen's mood suddenly changed from being warm and welcoming to a state of great agitation during which she tapped her forehead and repeated the words: 'My reason, my reason.' He concluded that a serious political crisis would drive her mad, and warned Lord Derby, the Leader of the Opposition, to this effect. Rumours circulating in aristocratic circles and eventually in the press that she was insane and believed her husband to be still alive were only fed further by ill-considered efforts to deny them.[68] As her seclusion continued from year to year, demands for her abdication, indeed for a change in the British system of government, became ever more persistent. Under Gladstone's first ministry, the 'royalty question' again moved close to the top of the political agenda.

The Queen's physician, Sir William Jenner, regularly reported that she was nervous and suffering from headaches, neuralgia and strain, 'and very ill from the heat and worry', but others – including Gladstone and the Cabinet, her private secretary and several of her own children – were less charitable, attributing her seclusion to simple malingering.[69] In the summer of 1871, however, she was struck down by a genuine, long and severe illness – 'the Queen really was very unwell', Sir Henry Ponsonby recalled – involving a sore throat with a choking sensation, a very painful arm and 'violent spasms'.[70] Her servants had to do everything for her, including feeding her and helping her to blow her nose. A suggestion that her children be sent for was dismissed with the argument that that would have 'killed her at once!'[71] She was to lose two stones in weight by the time she was able to resume her duties. 'Never felt so ill since typhoid at Ramsgate in 35,' she recorded in her diary on 22 August.[72] Looking back on the summer of 1871, Victoria stated that her recollections were 'most painful to me – for I did feel so ill'.[73] As soon as one abscess on her arm subsided, another appeared, and Jenner wrote, mystified, that 'he dont clearly know what it is'. The arm refused to respond to treatment. The Queen's 'rheumatism' spread to her leg.

Jenner, who confided to Ponsonby that at one stage he thought the Queen might have no more than twenty-four hours to live, obtained her permission to send for the surgeon Joseph Lister, who lanced the abscess and prescribed a carbolic spray of his own invention which would 'destroy all organic germs'. Even then, however, she suffered for several weeks more from 'spasms', 'flying rheumatic pains' and 'gout' almost everywhere – hands, arms, knees, ankles, feet, side and shoulder – so that she was irritable and unable to walk: John Brown, her ghillie, had to lift her from the couch to the bed as the maids were not strong enough to carry her.[74] Months went by before she began to feel better, 'though I am not strong – and often have rheumatic pains – but nothing thank God! to prevent my walking or going out in all weathers'.[75] As before, rumours arose even in ministerial circles that the Queen was to some extent 'insane', and the only comfort Lord Halifax, the Minister-in-Attendance, could draw from the situation was that such 'small evidences of insanity' would not increase since 'she has always been much the same in these matters'.[76] In October, Jenner told Ponsonby that the Queen's seclusion was the result of her 'nervousness'; even her high colour at dinner, which made her *look* well, was due to 'nerves'. 'But these nerves are a species of madness, and against them it is hopeless to contend,' he added, tantalizingly.[77]

As she got older, her 'nerves' seemed to improve somewhat, but bouts of 'rheumatism' continued to plague her.[78] On 2 March 1873 she had 'a violent neuralgic attack in my face which I have not had for a long time', she wrote to her daughter in Berlin, 'but I have been overworked and worried and overdone for the last three weeks and it was brought to a climax in London the other day. I am free from pain today but very tired.'[79] In February 1874 the Queen was 'quite sick and headachy' after a visit to an exhibition of Landseer's pictures, and had a 'dreadful headache' and 'sickness' again after a troop review in April.[80] In November 1879 she had a 'bad, feverish, bilious derangement', which she blamed on her failure to drink Carlsbad water as she had always done in previous years.[81]

A succession of painful rheumatic attacks were provoked by a fall on the stairs at Windsor in March 1883. For many days she was unable to walk, and when, shortly thereafter, she received the news of John Brown's death, unable even to stand. Writing to Ponsonby shortly after Brown's death, she complained: 'The Queen can't walk the least & the shock she has sustained has made her very weak – so that she can't stand.'[82] In June she was still not much better, writing from Windsor that, although her leg was on the mend, 'I feel weak and exhausted and dreadfully sad on returning here. I could not well have little Feo here as I am unfit for anything and require quiet as much as possible.'[83]

For many months a French masseuse kneaded her every limb

backwards and forwards and rolled her up in flannel, but even a year after her fall the Queen was still very stiff and lame.[84] 'I am still very cripply – I can't stand except for a few minutes,' she wrote in January 1884. 'I can walk for a short while out of doors – and go upstairs alone if I have a good rail to take hold of – but my own servant must always lead me downstairs and support me in getting in and out of the carriage.'[85] One year later again, in January 1885, she felt stronger and was more optimistic. 'My health is better, and I can walk and stand much better, but I fear I shall never walk for any great length of time again,' she wrote.[86]

The death of General Gordon at Khartoum on 26 January 1885 affected the Queen deeply. 'The worry ab[t] this affair of the Soudan has quite upset the Queen & she is not very well today,' Victoria informed Ponsonby. 'She had been feeling much less nervous but this behaviour of her Gov[t] & the mistrust she has of their conduct & concealment has brought back her nervous existing feeling of exhaustion which she suffered from so much latterly.'[87] Nevertheless, it is stretching things a little far to suggest, as has been done, that Victoria's feverish attack of neuralgia in September 1885 was caused by this humiliating setback at Khartoum eight months earlier. The attack began with headaches, great tiredness and a troublesome cough caught, she believed, from her grandchildren, but it was serious enough for Jenner to fear that it might lead to another nervous breakdown.[88]

An unusual – and far from flattering – portrait of the Queen at about this time is contained in the diaries of the German diplomat Friedrich von Holstein, who recorded in May 1884, after Victoria's visit to Darmstadt for the wedding of her youngest daughter Beatrice to Prince 'Liko' Battenberg:

> I have heard some remarkable details of the way the Queen of England alarmed and tyrannized over her family at Darmstadt. A quarter of an hour before dinner, without fail, she would say which of the royal personages was to dine with her. The rest of them ate elsewhere. She completely ignored the attendants of the various princes and princesses. Our Crown Prince simply did not dare to present to the Queen those of his adjutants who had not already been presented. In the end the Crown Princess made up her mind to do so. The ceremony can hardly have been a pleasure. The Queen

did not even raise her eyes, and there was no question of addressing even a single word to them. Somebody told me . . . that the Crown Princess was petrified in Queen Victoria's presence. Whenever the Queen withdrew, the effect was 'like an ascension to heaven', those left behind stared after her, transfigured. During the whole of her stay in Darmstadt the Crown Princess is said to have been summoned to dine with her mother only twice. I asked whether perhaps the secret of the Queen's authority lay in her personality. On the contrary, he said she was an undersized creature, almost as broad as she was long, who looked like a cook, had a bluish-red face and was more or less mentally deranged.[89]

As her Golden Jubilee drew closer, Victoria's rheumatism, lameness and backache became so painful that the massages had to be resumed.[90] She also suffered from severe attacks of 'sciatica' that kept her from sleeping.[91] 'I can't stand hardly at all any more and hot dinners and standing about after dinner and much talking are impossibilities,' she wrote in 1887.[92] As her eldest daughter, who suffered from the same kind of back pain, commiserated: 'I am so distressed to hear that you have sciatica! I well know how horrid it is! . . . It is so troublesome to cure & get rid of, as the muscle & nerve affected are so deep in the leg & embrocations etc. do not reach them!'[93] In the following winter the Queen's other leg began to cause her trouble: the result, she thought, of a sprain. 'My legs have been very troublesome this winter,' she wrote to her daughter in 1890. 'I slipped just about two and a half months ago in my tub and saved myself from falling by catching hold of a sofa and in doing so I must have strained my sound left leg, though I was not aware of it at the time and since that, off and on, rheumatism got into it and makes me very lame.'[94] By October 1890 she was well enough to dance the quadrille at Balmoral, but the lameness returned in the subsequent years.[95]

In 1894, at the time of Gladstone's resignation, she complained that her rheumatic leg was giving her continuous pain.[96] Thereafter, very gradually, she slipped into the helplessness of old age, being confined to her chair and almost unable to see. She had slight aphasia and suffered badly from insomnia, but this was hardly surprising in view of her great age and all the personal and political setbacks that she had to endure.[97] She died at Osborne House in the arms of her eldest grandson, the Kaiser, and surrounded by many of her children and grandchildren, on 22 January 1901. A few months later Vicky was dead, too.

Viewed purely in its own right, our brief sketch of Queen Victoria's medical history does not amount to a powerful case in favour of the view that she had inherited her grandfather's distressing condition. What our account does show, however, is that Victoria was far from well, and the symptoms of both mental and physical disability from which she suffered all her life were undeniably similar to those endured by so many of her aunts and uncles. It is only when we turn to explore the painful constitution of her eldest child Vicky, the German Crown Princess and (all too briefly) German Empress, that the case for diagnosing Queen Victoria's 'peculiarities' as porphyria symptoms becomes convincing.

CHAPTER 6

Vicky

You are so much the strongest of the family excepting
Bertie. You could do more than anyone I know.
Queen Victoria to her daughter Vicky, 1 July 1885.

In 1858 Vicky married Crown Prince Friedrich Wilhelm (Fritz)
of Prussia, just a decade before Bismarck forged a militaristic and
semi-absolutist Prussia into the core of the new German Reich. If
her father-in-law, King Wilhelm I, had abdicated in 1862, as he was
on the point of doing, instead of summoning Otto von Bismarck to
become prime minister, then Queen Victoria's eldest daughter
would have become Queen of Prussia at a time when the House of
Deputies was overwhelmingly dominated by liberals and demo-
crats, and a wholly different Germany – one unified largely by
consent, and boasting a parliamentary monarchy on the British
model – would have arisen. Even after unification, if the old
Emperor had died, say, at eighty in 1877, there would still have
been a strong chance for Vicky and her husband Fritz, once they
had inherited the powerful Prusso-German throne and dismissed
Bismarck, to have led the country towards parliamentary institutions and a close alliance with Britain; instead, Kaiser Wilhelm I
lived on until March 1888, by which time Fritz was dying of cancer
of the larynx. It was not Vicky and Fritz, but their vainglorious and
impulsive son Wilhelm II, *the* Kaiser, who was to take the helm
when the old Emperor died, with disastrous results.

The bright hopes which attached themselves to the marriage of
Fritz and Vicky faded and soured not just because of Wilhelm I's
longevity and tenacious *Junker* reaction, however. The decades of
impotent waiting, political ostracization and frustrated idealism

118

had a severe effect on Fritz's nerves, and by the late 1870s he was depressed and chronically lacking in self-confidence. And to make matters worse Vicky, easily the cleverer and stronger-willed of the two, was suffering from a mysterious ailment which constantly laid her low and may at times even have affected her judgement. The symptoms of her unnamed illness, which all of her biographers have so far ignored, are carefully recorded in her letters to her husband, in her own correspondence with her mother and in the twenty-five-year diary which Fritz painstakingly kept from 1858 to 1882.

From the first, Queen Victoria's first-born child was frail and edgy. She had digestive troubles, was often sick and lost weight easily. To fortify her she was given asses' milk, arrowroot, chicken broth and calomel, and simultaneously subjected to purgatives – 'doses', 'powders' and 'lavements', as they were called. Her father accused James Clark to his face of 'poisoning her with calomel' and of starving her. 'Take the child away and do as you like and if she dies you will have it on your conscience,' he thundered in a letter to the Queen.[1] Looking back, the Queen blamed Vicky's unhappy childhood on her own nervousness. 'You had not good nerves as a child and young girl', she wrote to her in 1874, 'which is natural as I always was very nervous, an inheritance of my family, and which I am sorry to say from hard work and early and many trials, anxieties and sorrows have certainly become greatly worse and are very bad now.'[2]

As Vicky's marriage to the Prussian Crown Prince drew near, her mother, who admitted to a lack of intimacy with her eldest daughter at this time, nevertheless indicated an awareness of Vicky's ambivalent feelings as the young princess prepared to leave her beloved England. 'Vicky was not quite well on the journey and during the few days here,' the Queen wrote. 'Her stomach was a little out of order, chiefly as a result of the agitation of the dear 26th [Prince Albert's birthday], and of leaving dear, beautiful Osborne, where she has now spent her last happy summer as an innocent child in the happy group of children.'[3]

For the remainder of her life, the intelligent and politically ambitious English princess on whom German liberals pinned such great hopes was racked with bouts of pain. In June 1858, not long after arriving in Potsdam, Vicky had to spend several days in bed with severe headaches, nausea and toothache, not in one tooth but in 'several on one side', though some of these symptoms might have been due to her pregnancy, for she was expecting Wilhelm, the future Kaiser, at the end of January.[4] From late October through to Christmas 1858, she was unwell with a 'cold' and ordered by the doctors to stay indoors.[5] One year later – this time she was pregnant with Charlotte – she was again too ill to go out, and in fact had a fainting fit.[6] In June 1860, she suffered a violent attack of colic, and in November such a terrible headache that she had to go to bed.[7]

In May 1861 it was 'violent lumbago' which forced her to take to her bed.[8] Interestingly, from our point of view, this attack of lower back pain was followed by an unsightly rash in the face. As Vicky told her mother on 4 June: 'My face is quite swollen and red on one side and hurts me so much as if I had had a bad bruise.'[9] She had another attack lasting two weeks that winter, this time with unbearable pain in the 'nerves of the head' and especially in the ears and the left eye socket, and once again the attack was accompanied by an ugly rash thought to have been brought on by quinine. Neither the leeches nor the medicines the doctors gave her brought any improvement.[10] Vicky complained that the attack had left her with 'dreadful fatigue' and that she was 'quite laid up', and Queen Victoria – who again sensed that there was a family pattern at work – admonished her doctor to give her 'strengthening and nourishing things – as you belong to our family who are so easily lowered'.[11]

In the summer of 1862, Vicky suffered 'violent pains in the left side & back'.[12] On 14 June she wrote to her mother:

> I have many torments to go through at present – neuralgia in my left side and left shoulder which I have had for more than a week, and which keeps me in perpetual pain. Then those dreadful nights when I can hardly sleep at all and do nothing but turn and toss, bathed in perspiration and sometimes almost choked. It is really dreadful and makes me feel so knocked up all day long. Then a great deal of mental anxiety about our unfortunate affairs . . .[13]

Just like her mother and her Great-Aunt Elizabeth, she found the heat of a summer's day quite insufferable, complaining in July 1862 in a letter from Potsdam: 'The heat is something awful today. I am in a state which I can not describe – almost suffocated, and everybody else is enjoying so much, and wonders that I find it warm.'[14] On a trip to Malta later that year the Crown Princess blamed her giddiness on the warm Saharan wind, writing: 'I do not feel at all well, so dreadfully giddy – every thing dances before my eyes, the sirocco wind is really most trying, more so than the heat of the atmosphere alone.'[15] In the following year, in Lithuania, she reported feeling 'quite ill', having lost her appetite and her ability to sleep, and suffering from a sore throat and a 'whitlow' on her thumb.[16]

If she was uncomfortable in the summer, the cold Berlin winters were hardly any better. 'I do not feel well and am off my sleep and appetite,' she told her mother, and added: 'This climate does not agree with me in the winter; there is something irritating and exciting in the air without being bracing.'[17] When Wilhelm I complained to Queen Victoria that her daughter was not fulfilling her social obligations at the Prussian court, the Queen promised that Vicky would do her best in future, but asked the monarch and Queen Augusta to bear in mind that her daughter could 'not really stand very hot rooms and late hours well'.[18] Only weeks after this exchange, Vicky reported that she had attended Augusta's soirée at the Berlin court, but that it had been 'so stiflingly hot and so late that I had a violent headache all day yesterday in consequence'.[19] She caught colds easily, some of them beginning with a feverish attack which then went to her head and made her feel miserable.[20]

Other symptoms, too, will strike us as familiar: in early 1863, when workmen were doing repairs to her palace, Vicky complained that the 'perpetual noise' had given her a 'racking headache'.[21] In 1864, she suffered for weeks with another of her feverish colds and a cough which the doctors treated with leeches, mustard poultices, liniments and hot baths, but all to no avail: they eventually sent her to Switzerland for the sake of her health.[22]

The following years – the years in which Bismarck fought his three wars of unification against Denmark, Austria and France respectively – were similarly overshadowed for the Crown Princess by pain and nervous disorders. On 7 October 1864 her husband recorded that she was 'feverish from nervous mood swings', ten days later that she was suffering very badly from terrible migraine, and at Christmas that she had a 'ghastly headache'.[23] The year 1865 began with earache and ended with unbearable headaches which caused her to vomit.[24] In January 1866 she was struck down by an attack involving a high fever, heart palpitations and a pulse of 128, at other times that year it was migraine, lumbago or 'rheumatic headaches' that laid her low.[25] In August, while Fritz was on the battlefield fighting the Austrians, Vicky wrote that she had 'tormenting abdominal pains' which became so severe in the night that her physician, August Wegner, prescribed 'a linseed flour poultice with opium' and several things to swallow; they did her little good, she said, but she was at least relieved to know that it was not cholera.[26] More often than not such attacks were the result of stress, brought on by rows with her domestic staff or meetings with Queen Augusta – in 1866 she admitted that each time she saw her mother-in-law 'I have been quite ill after – my knees shaking and my pulse gallopping'.[27] 'I am suffering again from a hysterical nervous pressure in my throat,' she reported to her husband after a quarrel with Emma Hobbs, the young Prince Wilhelm's English nurse.[28] The seriousness of her attacks can be measured by the fact that in November 1867, after several days of palpitations and headaches, Vicky was forced to abandon a visit to her beloved Windsor.[29] There were even times when she feared that she might lose her mind.[30]

Not long after the cancellation of her visit, a major episode occurred in the medical history of the Crown Princess which is diagnostically of great significance. While she and her sister Alice were staying with their uncle Ernst of Saxe-Coburg at Gotha in 1868, Vicky suffered an acute attack of 'most severe neuralgic headache!' As she herself described it to her husband:

I have been in the most excruciating pain all day long. The nerve pain above my eye has never been so intense as it was this time – I could only cry & moan while it lasted . . . At around 5 o'clock this morning the piercing pain began raging again. All external treatments prescribed by Uncle Ernst's doctor, Dr Hassenstein, were to no avail, & I did not want to resort to quinine because of the rash it gives me – but I cannot go on like *this* any longer. I thus sent a telegram to Dr Gream to inquire whether he would advise quinine in my condition. His reply was *yes*, so I shall take it in any case. In all *other* respects I am not in the least unwell – my stomach is in order . . . Only I am so wrecked & down as if I'd been seriously ill . . . I attribute my neuralgia to a journey I made on a cold stormy day, when the wind was blowing violently & bitingly in our faces – and to the unaccustomed gaslight in the theatre. – In Berlin I always spent the evenings in the half-light in my library, & now my eyes were very sensitive & the gaslight and the intense peering at the stage have irritated the nerves.[31]

As she had feared, within hours of her taking quinine, Vicky's face turned 'fire-red'.[32] As she explained in a letter to her husband:

I was supposed to leave here tomorrow – but the quinine has given me such a nettle rash that I shall have to postpone my journey, as I am unable even to leave my room. My face has swelled to a dark red sphere, and my skin is taut and itches & burns in a way that is as hard to describe as it is to bear. There is only a hint of eyes, nose & mouth, & I look such a fright that I ask forgiveness of everyone for having to lay eyes on such a sight! It's a pitiful condition to be in – but hopefully it won't last long. The neuralgic pains have ceased . . . It's a good job you can't see me – I think you'd hold your sides with laughter, for I myself am forced to laugh when I look in the mirror & see, instead of my face, this fire-red shapeless mass.[33]

Two days later she reported that the swelling was 'still so severe that I can only look straight ahead, as if through a narrow chink – for my eyelids are so swollen that my eyes are almost *completely* shut, making it impossible to look up or down. My ears are so swollen that I can hardly hear, & I have to keep my mouth wide open because my nose is so swollen that I can only breathe through it with great difficulty. The tautness of my skin, the burning heat & the itching are almost intolerable.'[34] In her distress it was something of a consolation for her to hear from Dr Hassenstein that workers in the quinine factories often suffered from the same severe nettle rash, 'so one can see that my constitution is not the only one which has an idiosyncratic reaction to this stuff'. She was thankful that, though the attack was a severe one, it had affected her only externally and had not been accompanied by a fever or gastric problems.[35] This relatively optimistic mood gave way to one of exasperation, however, for after nearly two weeks her face was still 'fire-red' and the nettle rash worse than ever. 'My eyelids, ears &

hands are swollen', she complained, sighing that 'the itching is *practically* unbearable'.[36]

Another diagnostically significant peculiarity of her affliction was the coming and going of her unsightly rash. As she remarked in a letter to her mother:

> Is it not strange that my nettle rash comes out again every day? From one o'clock in the middle of the day until after I go to bed, so that of an afternoon I am obliged to hide myself, I am such an awful object, and it is so uncomfortable. In the morning there is not a trace to be seen. Do what I will – go out or stay indoors – eat or not eat – try medicines etc., washes and salves, nothing is of the least use – and the weather hot or cold makes no difference whatever. It is too provoking.[37]

When finally the rash did begin to abate, Vicky came down with 'colic' attacks, which worried her since she was pregnant again.[38]

At the beginning of this savage attack of 1868, Vicky, who had evidently tried quinine before and knew she was allergic to it, had stoically asserted that 'in spite of everything, I could not have done without the quinine, for there *is* no other sure means of curing these raging, gruelling nerve pains'.[39] After the crisis of that spring, she never again took quinine and accepted that there was probably no cure for her suffering. But why did she react so badly to an apparently harmless substance? Was hers a case of general quinine poisoning, the symptoms of which can include porphyria-like conditions such as exanthema – a scarlet skin rash with eruptions? Or can we deduce from her dramatic reaction to the medicine that she was suffering from porphyria? At first sight the former explanation seems the more likely, since quinine is not listed among the numerous substances which porphyria sufferers are nowadays counselled to avoid. However, we need to remember that quinine was only produced synthetically after the First World War. Until then, it was extracted from the bark of the chincona tree, and its purity or impurity depended very much on the skill and care of the workers entrusted with its production. The bark of the chincona tree harbours a number of other alkaloids, apart from quinine, such as cinchonine, cinchonidine and quininide. Once the drug has been obtained, it has to be mixed with other substances before it can be taken. In the nineteenth century it could be infused with lime water, lemon juice or magnesium oxide, acidulated with aromatic sulphuric acid or macerated in alcohol. Substances such as camphorated opium, dried orange peel, saffron and snakeroot were often added, as was glycerin. One compendium of the time lists no fewer than forty formulas for elixirs containing quinine.[40] We do not know where Vicky's quinine came from, nor what dosage she was given. Nor do we have any information on what additives her medicine contained; the one thing we can be certain of is that the potion she was given would not have passed the rigid pharmaceutical controls in place today. Whatever substances her 'quinine' preparation contained, we have firm proof of a link between the prescription of impure drugs in use in the early part of the twentieth century and the onset of porphyria attacks. Several such cases are referred to in Jan Waldenström's pioneering articles of the 1950s which first established the true nature of the porphyria disorders.[41]

The attacks of colic which the Crown Princess experienced in May 1868 returned with a vengeance in the August of that year, striking her at night and lasting for several days. 'The last few days have been quite too much for me,' she wrote to her mother on 19 August, 'I have had cholics and Diarrhea & feel quite wretched; the heat is really intolerable, & the nights are as bad as the days.'[42] In April 1869, Vicky's 'neuralgia' was again so painful that 'morphium injections' became necessary.[43] A year later, she suffered '*such* violent pain in my side that I couldn't get a wink of sleep & was truly at my wit's end'.[44] Her skin rash returned in early 1870, and the description she provides in her correspondence with her mother is again diagnostically revealing: 'What a state my skin is in I am quite ashamed of – and can hardly show myself I am such a figure. My forehead, nose and chin are covered with large red blotches and so chapped and stiff that it is very uncomfortable and yet I never was out in the coldest weather.'[45]

During the dramatic events that transformed Europe in the next few months – the German victories against the French armies, the establishment of a powerful German empire under Kaiser Wilhelm I, the annexation of Alsace and Lorraine – Vicky, now heiress to the imperial title as well as the Prussian crown, was almost helpless with pain. As the great battles raged, she was suffering from headaches and stomach complaints brought on, she believed, by thunderstorms.[46] In January 1871, as the new Reich was being proclaimed at Versailles, she complained of 'neuralgia in the head' and 'agonising rheumatic pains'. A little later it was 'a dreadful sore throat with inflammation', followed by 'acute neuralgic pains' that plagued her for many days.[47] On New Year's Day 1872 Vicky wrote to her mother complaining of 'great pain . . . from neuralgia in my face, my right cheek and ear'. She had been to the Emperor's palace twice that day, 'which was so fearfully hot that I had not a dry thread upon me and then coming out into the cold air, has brought this on', she explained.[48] This attack was followed by alarming pains in her back and legs. 'I felt very unwell and knocked up yesterday, still I went to the Opera Ball for an hour, – in spite of a pain in my back and limbs wh. quite frightened me,' she confided to her mother.[49]

For much of March and April 1873, as her husband's diary records, Vicky again suffered from a 'violent sick headache', 'rheumatic headaches', 'severe nervous headaches', 'pain near the right ear', and 'horrible neuralgia'. As her eyes were inflamed she was ordered to wear blue-tinted glasses.[50] On 24 March she wrote to Queen Victoria: 'The last few days have been so horribly fatiguing, and the exposure to suffocating heat in the rooms and violent draughts on going in and out of the houses has been such that I am very unwell. The blood goes so frightfully to my head from the fatigue, heat, noise, bustle etc. – and having a cold besides gives me a dreadful rheumatic headache so that I can hardly move my head – a swelled face, sore throat and pain in my limbs!'[51] The attack got much worse in the next weeks, with Vicky writing on 6 April that she was 'next to insensible with the frantic violence of neuralgia in my eye. I cannot describe what I have suffered these last three days. I have been nearly mad. I took arsenic without any effect, tried hydrate of chlorate in order to make me sleep – I did not sleep and was only very sick – I tried carbolic acid, and rubbing acoustic salve [a soothing ointment] over my head but all to no purpose. Today I am able to stand on my legs.'[52] It was to this attack that Queen Victoria was referring when she wrote to the Empress Augusta: 'Vicky's convulsive pains disquiet me very much, for they prove that she is not as strong and well as she should be.'[53]

After a journey to St Petersburg in 1874, Vicky reported from the Hermitage: 'I meant to have written yesterday evening but I really was so knocked up and my head ached so with the dreadful shaking of the railway train that I was unable to collect my thoughts sufficiently.'[54] That October, she had an attack of 'violent neuralgia worse than anything in the last 3 years'. It was accompanied by 'headache and dizziness, as well as nausea'.[55] Just a few weeks later, Fritz recorded that his wife had 'gall-colic with vomiting . . . although without fever'[56]

In 1875, while Angeli was painting her portrait, another attack of 'very acute neuralgia' ensued, although this time the pain was 'distributed more throughout the body'.[57] This bout, which Vicky described as 'this most violent and with me uncontrollable neuralgia', sparked an interesting correspondence between the two Victorias on the subject of which preparations might ease their pain, indicating once again that they recognized their symptoms to stem from a complaint common to both of them. The Queen asked whether Vicky had ever tried 'the application of aconite', a poisonous alkaline derived from monkshood or wolfsbane, which in modern medicine is used only as a last resort. Queen Victoria also recommended 'a new application which never affects the skin, oleate of morphia –', which 'should be rubbed in, in small quantities but for some time'. She offered to send Vicky some if she had difficulty in obtaining the oil in Berlin.[58] The Crown Princess replied that all the painkilling preparations she had tried merely brought on her skin rash. 'I do not know the oil of morphine, but have a salve of morphine which I suppose answers the same purpose, aconite, bella donna, and veratrine salves have all been tried. Aconite irritates instead of soothing. Even smelling salts I cannot use as everything a little sharp seems to set it on. The only thing I take inwardly is bromide of potassium but I do not perceive that it has any effect.'[59] Hardly had she written these pessimistic words when her 'violent nervous headaches' returned to torment her for no less than six weeks that winter.[60] 'I have had dreadful neuralgia again!' she told her mother on 29 December 1875. 'What shall I do, when the carneval begins, I am sure I shall be knocked up altogether.'[61]

In early 1876, the pain came to affect her upper limbs and her back. 'I have had rheumatics in my hand and arm – the *right* one,' she informed her eldest son.[62] Only a few weeks later it was 'sciatica pains' that she complained of, writing to Wilhelm on 27 March: 'I have not been well ever since your Grandpapa's Birthday [22 March], the dreadful fatigues of the Ball added to those of the day, had upset me so completely, that I had "*Ischias Schmerz*" [sciatica pain] from the long standing!'[63] By the summer she was describing her back pain as lumbago, explaining to her son: 'I have had a terrible attack of "lumbago", which was dreadful pain, – the tears ran down my cheeks with the pain each time I attempted to move, it is only a very little better, and the nights are wretched as I cannot turn round!'[64] As if this agony were not torment enough, the attack was accompanied by a serious inflammation of her right eye and a return of her 'nettle rash'. 'I have had a terribly bad eye & suffered very much indeed!' she wrote, adding: 'I had to go about with a bandage, & I feel quite ill from all the pain I have suffered with it.'[65] In mid-June she had a violent attack of fever which lifted as suddenly as it had come.[66] The 'racking headache' returned in November and tortured her for more than three weeks.[67] Next, it was the 'lumbago' and the 'rheumatic pains in the side' that laid her low.[68]

In July 1877 the family travelled to the Belgian coast for a holiday in the sun, where Vicky's 'neuralgia', already severe before they left Potsdam, became acute. Among the guests bathing at Ostende was Professor Robert Ferdinand Wilms, who prescribed a medicine which gradually alleviated the pain. Unfortunately the Crown Prince's cryptic notes do not tell us what the wonder drug was, but whatever it was it brought no permanent relief, for the week-long headaches, the neuralgic pains and the eye infections continued at intervals for the rest of her life.[69]

When her youngest son Waldemar died of diphtheria in 1879 – she had already lost her beloved little Sigismund in 1866 – Vicky was understandably inconsolable. She suffered from hormonal irregularities, giddiness, neuralgia, rheumatism and depression accompanied by feelings of suffocation and perpetual noise in the head.[70] Looking back on Waldemar's death several years later, Vicky admitted that ever since that traumatic event her nerves had been in pieces. 'My hand shakes, my heart knocks loudly, & my entire organism seems to become agitated & disordered as soon as anything upsets me!! And then sleep & appetite are gone!'[72]

When the Crown Princess's agony failed to abate (in May 1879 her husband recorded 'violent rheumatism . . . reaching down as far as her foot'),[72] the doctors ordered her to take a long rest in Pegli – the first of many lengthy sojourns in Italy. To everyone's dismay, though she was able to enjoy bathing in the sea and does not appear to have suffered from being in the sun, the nine months Vicky spent on the Italian Riviera brought not the slightest improvement in her condition. She continued to suffer from 'dreadful neuralgia', and her husband expressed his 'bitter disappointment' that 'neither the Riviera nor the Roman baths seemed to function as painkillers'.[73] Vicky had two wisdom teeth extracted in a vain effort to alleviate the pain in her head.[74] After visiting her in Italy in March 1880, Fritz wrote in despair to Ernst von Stockmar:

> My poor wife has been suffering from dreadful neuralgia for days now, which this time is unbelievably violent, forcing us to galvanize the sensitive head nerves. We cannot deny that the pain has taken on a different nature since yesterday, but as a rule it begins at 4 o'clock in the morning and lasts until 11 at night ... without letting up. You can imagine what kind of shape her head is in, especially as her stomach also strongly feels the effects of the agonizing pain.[75]

The Crown Princess returned to Berlin thinking that her long rest in the south had healed her, but within weeks the 'rheumatic' pains in her neck, shoulder and right arm had returned, as had the 'neuralgia' in her head and eyes and her attacks of 'colic'.[76] Miserably she confessed to her mother that she was 'growing very unsightly', having lost almost all her hair. Her face, she said, was 'full of lines and wrinkles especially round the eyes and mouth'.[77]

The following years were to be overshadowed by her husband's bleak depression as the realization dawned that he would never be able to put into effect the liberal reforms he and his wife had planned. From late 1886 onwards, though they both outwardly denied it, cancer relentlessly destroyed his larynx and finally – in June 1888 – his life. Fritz's mortal illness must not blind us to the fact, however, that Vicky's own medical history in these years amounted to an almost unrelieved catalogue of pain. Though there were periods of remission, the contemporary record is riddled with references to her neuralgic, rheumatic and colic attacks and to the pain in her head, eyes, arms, legs and feet. In March 1882, for example, she suffered 'indescribably from an inflamed retina and tear duct with raging headache and eye pain' which prevented her from sleeping, 'despite chloral'.[78] As the Crown Prince noted in his diary: 'V[icky] 3 hours sleep with chloral, acute neuralgic pain during the day; in the evening 3 boils opened up, pain lessened, also through applying pressure with my hand.' However, the 'torturous' pain in both eyes and the purulent boils continued for another month.[79] In April 1883 Vicky apologized for the incoherence of a letter she had written to her mother, pleading that she was 'half wild with a neuralgia in my forehead and eye the consequence of a violent influenza'. This was an attack which lasted till well into the month of May.[80]

As her husband's final agony began, Vicky put on a brave face, but behind the smiling public mask she too was frequently in pain. Thus in March 1887 she suffered from 'neuralgia for 5 days' and spent whatever time she could lying down in her own room.[81] In the following month she admitted to her mother: 'I am tormented a good deal with Rheumatism – in the neck, back & right arm. I have had it now for 3 weeks & it gets worse instead of better!' Several weeks passed and the pains in the arm and right side were as bad as ever, particularly at night, despite daily massages.[82] At the end of 1887 she claimed that, though she was again ill with 'neuralgia', her attack was 'not as violent or with fever as I have at Berlin'.[83] In May 1888, with her husband (now the Emperor) dying and all the cares of the world resting on her shoulders, she was struck down again by her 'horrid neuralgia' which made her feel so 'wretched'. As she informed her mother, 'the neuralgia was so frightful & accompanied with such shivering & retching that I had to go to bed & remain there for half the day. Such a *bore* when there is so much to do, but I felt *so* ill that I could not keep on my feet any longer. It is quite like the ague.' The following day she was not better in the slightest, sighing in torment and frustration: 'I am again obliged to go to bed with the violence of the pain.'[84]

After the terrible end of her husband and the trauma of widowhood, it will not surprise us to learn that the 'rheumatic' pains were never absent for long. Five weeks after Fritz's death she wrote to Queen Victoria: 'I suffer again of rheumatism in my neck & collar bone, & cannot turn in bed, it has *never* been so bad! – besides feeling weak & tired & my nerves much unstrung.'[85] A

130

month later, she reported to her mother: 'I am feeling *so low* – & so shaky – yesterday the rheumatism was much better, today it is worse again.'[86] In the following summer the inflammation of the eyes and the pain returned – 'I suffered from the most racking neuralgia all day,' she wrote from Bad Homburg in May 1889. That July, she told her mother that she had 'the most frightful cramps in my thigh; I do not know what to do with pain at night, & it comes without warning and hurts all the next day.' Diagnostically significant is the fact that these attacks of neuralgia and cramp were accompanied by a skin rash. 'My nettle rash is unabated, in spite of all I have tried against it,' she reported to Windsor.[87] In autumn 1889 she wrote (from the steamer taking her from Venice to Athens for her daughter Sophie's wedding to the Crown Prince of Greece) that, although the journey had so far gone well, 'the carriages shook and rattled fearfully, wh. with my neuralgia was not pleasant'.[88]

Powerless to intervene, the Empress Frederick, as Vicky now called herself, looked on in dismay as her autocratic son and his narrow-minded, haughty wife made one blunder after another. The bouts of extreme pain which had afflicted her ever since she had arrived in Berlin thirty years earlier continued to torment her every few months. Thus in April 1890, shortly after Wilhelm had dismissed Bismarck, she complained in a letter to her mother: 'I have had such neuralgia in my right arm.'[89] In October of that year, she suffered an attack of 'lumbago & rheumatism in my knee' and had to put herself to bed. She described the attack as 'something of the same kind as last year – at this time! Violent sickness & Diarrhea, pain in my limbs & head – shivering etc.'[90] By December she was attributing her discomfort to the menopause, writing to her mother of 'the sudden dreadful flushes & perspirations that come over me, – and the very little sleep I get at night.'[91]

While on a visit to London in the spring of 1891, Vicky made an intriguing observation which sheds light not only on her own condition but also on that of her elder brother, the future Edward VII, suggesting that he might have had occasional attacks similar to her own. Writing to her mother from Buckingham Palace on 24 March, she reported that the Prince of Wales was severely ill with influenza-like symptoms, weakness and savage back pain.

Dearest Bertie came to pay me a visit, but I was quite unhappy to

see him looking *so* ill! – *so* pale, such black rings round his eyes, so
languid – & with no voice! – He has no more feverishness & says
he is much better, but that he has not been so ill since his typhoid
fever; certainly, he *looks* so! . . . He has *no* cold in his head, but
seems to have a kind of influenza! . . . I am so distressed for him.
These are the sorts of attacks I used to have at Berlin, & take *weeks*
to recover from.[92]

That summer, she confided to her mother that she was having
'such bad nights; such palpitations & giddiness and the blood to my
head, & such perspirations – & my nerves are so easily upset!' If
people remarked that she looked well, she said, that was only
because she was very sunburnt from being out in the open air.[93]
Two weeks later she had 'such an attack of sickness & diarrhea'
that she was 'hardly able to hold up my head!'[94] At about this same
time another distressing symptom appeared – a painful rash in the
gullet. 'My mouth & throat are still so painful that I can only
swallow *liquids*,' she informed her second daughter Victoria who
was now married to Prince Adolf of Schaumburg-Lippe. 'The rash
is all down the "*Speise Röhre*" – wh. we call in english by the Greek
name of "Asophagus",' she explained.[95] Toothache, pains in the
ribs and back, a racking cough and 'stomach catarrh' troubled her
again throughout February 1892.[96]

The attacks continued to occur, though perhaps less frequently
than before, right up to the time she herself was diagnosed as
having cancer in late 1898.[97] Thus in 1894, Vicky commiserated
with her mother's chronic rheumatism, recurrent headaches and the
difficulty she had in walking, but added that she herself was also in
pain. 'My head & neck & shoulder are still very painful and give
me no rest at night!'[98] In January 1896 she reported to Windsor: 'I
have inflamed eyes (an "*Augen Catarrh*") and neuralgia in my head
wh. is wretched.'[99]

The Empress Frederick died in Schloss Friedrichshof, which she had
built for herself in the Taunus Mountains, on 5 August 1901, just
half a year after her mother had passed away at Osborne in the
Kaiser's arms. The rich historical record – in particular the diary
kept by her husband and her thrice-weekly intimate correspondence
with her mother, a fellow-sufferer – enables us to establish with

remarkable precision both the pattern of Vicky's illness and the nature of her symptoms. Throughout her life, from her marriage to Fritz in January 1858 to the onset of her cancer in December 1898, the Princess Royal of Great Britain and Ireland, George III's great-granddaughter, was struck down by excruciating pain in the head, neck, arms, shoulders, back, side, abdomen, legs and feet. She described the pain variously as 'rheumatism', 'neuralgia', 'colic', 'lumbago' or 'sciatica'. Such attacks occurred several times each year and could last for anything between a few days and six or seven weeks. Often, they were accompanied by dark red blotches, a nettle rash or blisters on the skin, and by biliousness, giddiness and vomiting. Not infrequently she experienced a sort of malarial fever, with hot and cold flushes and sweating. Sometimes, in addition, her eyes were inflamed. On occasions she had difficulty in swallowing. Vicky made several half-hearted attempts to explain her pain in terms of external causes – the heat, the cold, the hot wind, thunderstorms, bright lights, overcrowded rooms – but she herself had to admit that at best such factors acted merely as triggers setting off an inner mechanism she did not understand.

To us, there seems little doubt as to the nature of her distressing condition, particularly as her correspondence with Queen Victoria contains several strong hints that the two women sensed they were both suffering from the same family disorder. True, the one symptom that would put the retrospective diagnosis of variegate porphyria in Queen Victoria's eldest daughter virtually beyond dispute – dark-coloured urine – is missing from the record of Vicky's medical history. It is not missing from that of *her* eldest daughter.

CHAPTER 7

'Charlotte the Brat'

Urine dark red.
Princess Charlotte to her physician, 7 April 1906

Charlotte, Princess of Prussia, Kaiser Wilhelm II's eldest sister, was Queen Victoria's granddaughter and therefore a great-great-granddaughter of George III. Born in 1860 and surviving until after the First World War, she occupies a crucial position in our search for the porphyria mutation in the descendants of the Hanoverians. Though her death on 1 October 1919 came before Waldenström's pioneering work which identified porphyria as the product of a dominant genetic mutation, towards the end of her life scientists were establishing that symptoms such as hers were the result of inborn errors of metabolism.

From the early 1890s, Charlotte was in the care of one of the greatest physicians of her generation, Ernst Schweninger (1850–1924), who was also Bismarck's doctor. Schweninger, realizing that her unusual condition was incurable but not wholly unmanageable, convinced Charlotte that an operation would be useless and eventually placed her in the hands of his pupil Georg Groddeck (1866–1934), whose clinic became a refuge for her when her suffering became unbearable. It is largely thanks to Charlotte's own correspondence with Schweninger that we are able to reconstruct her medical history in detail. In addition, her family correspondence, and in particular her intimate letters (written in English) to Baroness Ellen von Heldburg, the half-British third wife of her father-in-law, the venerable Duke Georg II of Saxe-Meiningen, provides us with yet more information about her illness and enables us to arrive at a retrospective diagnosis as surely as we

134

can without actual access to the patient herself. Beyond that, as will become apparent in a later chapter, we hope that Princess Charlotte will act as our conduit from the rather murky world of the historical past through to the bright clinical certainties of present-day genetics.

For the early years of Charlotte's life, it is of course not her own correspondence but the concerned letters of her parents, Crown Princess Vicky and her husband Fritz, that are our best source. These letters reveal how, from the age of two and three onwards, little 'Ditta' – her nickname was derived from her brother's attempts to call her 'dear sister' – caused much anxiety on account of her 'dangerous disposition'. 'Alas, she is an unsatisfactory child, poor little thing,' the Crown Princess wrote to Queen Victoria about her own eldest daughter.[1] Shortly before her fourth birthday, Charlotte is described by her mother as 'very sensitive and nervous' and 'easily upset' but 'definitely not very bright'.[2] Her tutor and her governess exclaimed that they had never encountered such a troublesome young pupil.[3] 'Stupidity is not a sin', Vicky sighed in resignation, in anticipation of the difficulties that lay ahead, 'but it renders education a hard and difficult task.'[4] In 1863, when the princess was just three, her mother complained of her hyperactive nature, writing to the Queen: 'Her little mind seems almost too active for her body – she is so nervous & sensitive and so quick. Her sleep is not so sound as it should be – and she is so very thin.'[5] Charlotte without her clothes on, her mother remarked, was 'an object for studies in anatomy, nothing but skin and bones'.[6]

Even at this stage, there were problems with the child's digestion. 'While we were in Italy', the worried young mother reported to Windsor, 'I fear Mrs Merrifield was not quite attentive enough to her – and did not cut up her food fine enough – so that her digestion got completely deranged – and upon that by some carelessness or other she caught a violent cold wh. threw itself on her stomach and liver – and since then she has never been altogether right and gives a gt. deal of trouble.'[7]

However, it was her violent tantrums that caused her parents the gravest concern in these early years. Shortly before Charlotte's second birthday, when such tantrums might be considered normal, Vicky noted in alarm: 'Ditta has such outbreaks of rage and stubbornness that she screams blue murder.'[8] Four years later, she wrote again in exasperation: 'Today, Ditta had a tantrum – the worst she's had in a long time, rolling around on the floor, flailing and screaming blue murder.'[9]

When she reached fourteen, Charlotte's disposition seemed briefly to improve. As her mother informed Queen Victoria in May 1874, 'She is gentle and amiable and willing to do all she is told, and much nicer towards the brothers and sisters . . . Clever she is not – and never will be; she has few or no interests – no taste for learning or reading, for art or for natural history, so it is no use to expect these things of her . . . If she only grows up a nice and good girl – and in time becomes trustworthy and conscientious that is all I can expect. Her temper is very even and good now!' However, the condition of Charlotte's nose, which had been blocked for several years, and more generally her tiny size, caused her parents and doctors some puzzlement and concern. The Crown Princess reported to Windsor: 'She grows so little that you would think she was nine or ten, has not an atom of figure, or waist, and shows no sign of her health beginning to change . . . Charlotte is in everything – health, looks and understanding like a child of ten!'[10]

When she did eventually reach puberty, her mother considered her clumsy and almost misshapen, with an unusually long neck and waist, 'immense' arms and breasts, and very short legs. She was what the Germans call a *Sitzriese* – a giant when seated but short when standing. Her gait was awkward and ungainly, since she tended to 'trundle' along with her elbows stuck out.[11] A trait now reappeared which had worried Vicky in Charlotte as a tiny girl: her propensity for cheeky flirtatiousness, malicious gossip and mindless troublemaking. Then she had referred to her as a 'little coquette'.[12] Now, when she was only sixteen, Charlotte chose to marry her cousin Bernhard, the heir to the tiny Thuringian duchy of Saxe-Meiningen, and as the wedding day drew near, Vicky confided to her husband:

I cannot tell you how it saddens and troubles me to think of Charlotte! – That pretty exterior – & the empty inside, those dangerous character traits! Everyone is initially enthralled, & yet those who know her better know how she *really* is – and can have neither love nor trust nor respect! It is too sad. There is nothing to be done, it is just a fact, & one can only hope that time & life will serve as teachers to her, & that the good Bernhard will *protect & guide* her. Then at least her wicked qualities will not be able to cause any harm.[13]

Charlotte's father entirely concurred and confessed that he was just as depressed at the thought of the ominous future that lay ahead.[14] Their sense of foreboding was only confirmed by Charlotte's capricious and mischievous behaviour after her marriage, so much so that on 9 September 1879 the Crown Princess confided darkly to her own mother:

> The one that causes me *most* anxiety is – *Charlotte*. In later years you will perhaps understand me, – – perhaps much may change in her, though I fear where most people only see her pretty face – and are taken with her amicable exterior. – She *has* the wish to be amicable & make herself pleasant, but the poor Child can never be a help mate or a resource to any one. I admit it is not her fault. Nature has made her so – and education *cannot* do *all*! Education cannot give either capabilities of the mind nor a thoroughly good *kind warm heart*! – This *is* a *great* trial . . . She is *very* independent, and very obstinate, so one cannot influence or direct her, as one wd. wish.'[15]

Such forebodings were realized when Charlotte grew to adulthood. Looking back on her daughter's childhood in 1888, Vicky admitted that 'this poor child has always caused us more concern than happiness, she was indescribably difficult to educate, & unfortunately nature has given her a difficult & unhappy character with many qualities that are dangerous for herself as well as for others! . . . She has ruined her strong and blooming good health through her stupidity – & because she has not seen the point of living sensibly & hygienically & refuses to accept good advice.'[16]

When Charlotte was in her early twenties, her mother became alarmed by her chlorotic appearance – she was sure her daughter's greenish pallor was a symptom of anaemia.[17] In 1885, when she was twenty-four, we find an initial but very powerful hint that the cause of Charlotte's pallor and disturbing behaviour might lie in her physical constitution. On 2 January of that year, in what is for our enquiry a key document, the Crown Princess wrote to her sister-in-law, the Duchess of Connaught:

> Charlotte is slowly improving at Cannes under the clever care of

Dr Franks! She had a thorough malaria poisoning, & consequent anemia to a high degree, – and it is *very* difficult to get her round. Every one of the organs were starved – & the *Blutbildung war eine falsche geworden* [the formation of her blood had become a false one]. – But I am quite satisfied as to her treatment & hope she will recover altogether. – She cannot walk yet – and only leaves her Bed at 12 in the day! But the neuralgia, fainting and nausea have left her, wh. is a great deal gained![18]

Abnormal constitution of the blood with severe anaemia, 'malarial' feverishness, neuralgia, biliousness, fainting fits and semi-paralysis of the legs – it reads like a textbook list of the symptoms of porphyria, and this several decades before the disorder was clinically identified.

When her brother inherited the Prusso-German throne in June 1888, Charlotte, resentful at being marginalized by the chromosomal accident of gender and an age difference of only nineteen months, became a figure of some notoriety in the court society of imperial Berlin. Smoking heavily, her dark hair piled high on top of her head with a fringe falling over her eyebrows, her diminutive figure balanced precariously on high-heeled shoes and her waist laced into a corset of breathtaking tightness, she was the heart and soul of a fast set of aristocrats, foreign diplomats and young court officials who amused themselves by mocking the strait-laced low-church morality of the Kaiser's dowdy wife Auguste Viktoria, known as Dona. Ditta loved to shock her brother by turning up unexpectedly in foreign capitals during his state visits.[19] 'Charlotte *must* go everywhere, and put herself *en evidence* – she *never* can keep quiet, and is always gadding about,' her mother complained.[20]

The princess used her inside knowledge of her brother's intentions to spite her family, friends and rivals alike. Her own mother considered her to be '*dangerous* in the extreme' and openly expressed the fear that Charlotte's 'untruthfulness' might hurt her. 'I am really quite *afraid*!', she admitted to Queen Victoria, and went on to explain: 'I am always rather alarmed at all the nonsense, mischief & gossip she carries about, wh. one believes, not knowing what confusion she always makes. There is a great deal of harm done in that way, perhaps even unintentionally.'[21] Naturally the gossip and hurtful jokes of the Kaiser's eldest sister were 'passed from mouth to mouth and whispered and passed on' in the claustrophobic world of Berlin high society.[22] 'She knew things, though not as many as she gave you to believe,' the Queen of Romania recalled of Charlotte many years later.[23] Her brother Henry nicknamed her 'Charley the Pretender' on account of her insistence on making herself interesting as the bearer of the latest gossip, and she signed herself 'Charlotte the Brat' in her correspondence with her English cousins.[24]

The Hereditary Princess of Saxe-Meiningen barely bothered to conceal her numerous love affairs.[25] She took the greatest pleasure in match-making and in generally making mischief in the sexual arena, and the rumours which circulated in Berlin to the effect that she and some of her friends were behind the obscene anonymous letters which poisoned the life of so many high-ranking people at Court in the early years of Wilhelm II's reign are by no means implausible.[26] Soon, however, the jolly japes and malicious mischief-making had to stop.

In the early 1890s worries about Charlotte's health began to resurface – the result, it seemed, of 'fits of violent excitement'.[27] Vicky urged her other daughters to eat plenty of wholesome food, since otherwise their blood would get 'poor' and their circulation low, and 'you will have constant neuralgia!' If they failed to keep the constitution strong, she warned, they would become 'out of health as Charlotte was for years'.[28] In 1893, Charlotte 'quite suddenly' became 'so very thin', and the doctors ordered her 'off South' to recover.[29] Her mother despaired of her appearance and unfortunate lifestyle. 'Charlotte is under the influence of "nicotine" wh. is a poisonous substance,' she told her second daughter Victoria.[30]

Just a few months later, suffering from painful legs, swollen knees, rheumatism, almost daily headaches, nervous problems, insomnia and an inexplicable blood disorder, the Kaiser's eldest sister sought the help of the celebrated Professor Ernst Schweninger. In August 1894, her husband, the Hereditary Prince Bernhard of Saxe-Meiningen, registered Schweninger's surprise at discovering her to be severely anaemic.[31] Charlotte herself wrote to Baroness Heldburg after her first examination by the great doctor:

Schweninger was amazed at my Anemie & broken down nerves, &

yet praised me for my energy I had proved so far, & my quiet regular simple way of living & trying daily to walk. The other troubles are nearly cured, such a blessing, now the headaches, consequence of so little blood, & sleeplessness, are to be cured by eating eggs, salt in quantities, drinking salt water, bathing of a morning in the sea, of an evening hot, & his 'Rumpf – & Beinbewegungen [trunk and leg exercises]' & lyings up. I know well – more one can't do.[32]

Two years later, another symptom emerged which was to pain the princess for the rest of her life: what she rather touchingly called her 'dentical torments'.[33] She had to undergo a series of operations on her teeth and gums to combat abscesses and an inflammation of the roots which MacFarlane, her Scottish dentist, identified as Knochenhautentzündung – alveolar periostitis.[34] In 1902, when the condition got worse, her doctors and dentists diagnosed the problem as 'a form of scurvy' – except that no amount of dietary change or medicine brought any improvement. Her gums consisted, Charlotte said, of 'lumps of crimson, or strings of white flesh' which looked so 'disgusting' that she had to refrain from laughing and to cover her mouth with a thick veil whenever she went out.[35] Charlotte was clear that this condition, too, resulted from her unfortunate general constitution and had nothing to do with her teeth as such. As she told Ellen Heldburg after a visit to MacFarlane, the 'excruciating pains that nearly drove me mad . . . do *not* come from my *teeth*, which are *perfectly* in order, but abscesses, also *on* my body, all over the gums: else I *should* have mine out'.[36] As late as 1917, after seeing a German dentist, she was firm in maintaining that 'there is *nothing* wrong with my teeth; they have only become loose on account of the dreadful swellings'.[37]

Charlotte was emotionally and physically ill and in pain for weeks or even months at a time, but then mysteriously well again. Schweninger, on examining her in May 1896, was alarmed at the state she was in but professed himself confident that, with rest and good air, 'I should soon pick up & be myself again!'[38] However, only a few weeks after this optimistic prognosis, Charlotte had to admit in a letter to him that she had swellings in the limbs, hands and hips. She begged Schweninger for advice on how to deal with these afflictions and the accompanying sudden increase in weight, since the 'diet and hot baths' he had prescribed 'didn't help in the least to counter the swelling of my stupid limbs; the worst swelling was in my hands & hips', she informed him.[39] 'Tomorrow Schweninger comes, that means fresh life & help,' she told her confidante Ellen Heldburg that winter.[40] He arranged for a female assistant to massage her legs three times a day. 'I get pinched & wrenched & beat about,' she wrote, but she soon began to feel and look better.[41] A year later she reported that an attack of mycodermitis (athlete's foot) had given her a 'nasty foot' for which she was having treatment.[42] In 1898 she was thrilled by the new craze of cycling – but shortly thereafter, in October, she suffered 'the total collapse of my nerves' – which left her without sleep and crying without cause.[43]

Schweninger's presence in itself often made her feel better, but his visits were always too short and his remedies of little help in the longer term. 'I don't feel well ... & my nerves are in a stupid condition,' the princess wrote to Ellen in December 1898. 'Schweninger is not satisfied with me: but mentally he has already done me *so* much good, if only I could keep him longer than 1 day.'[44] 'Schweninger 3 weeks ago was shocked at me; but I am better now,' she confided to the same friend six months later.[45] A year later again it was the same story: 'Have been so poorly for days', she told her motherly friend, but 'Schweninger was luckily here (to see to me).'[46] There was little even he could do for her, however, and only a few weeks after this particular visit Charlotte wrote to him complaining again of 'a great deal of pain that refuses to let up. My abdomen often swells, too, and the most distressing thing is my digestive trouble with spasmodic pains. But in spite of the tiredness and listlessness I do ride ... and look well, or so I am told.'[47] Schweninger was obliged to visit her again in September 'to patch up my idiotic nerves!'[48] At the end of 1900 she had to give up riding because the pain from 'rheumatism' and an 'inflammation of a tendon and its sheath' was too severe. She also complained that her 'idiotic nerves [were] giving way', the result, she believed, of 'old age creeping on gradually'.[49]

In October 1901, on one of her many visits to King Carol of Romania, she reported stoically: 'Giddyness, headaches & bad nights, must be borne, & hope much from the pleasant, fatherly quiet sympathetic ways of the loved King.' After a further week at

Sinaja, however, she admitted to feeling 'low & depressed', and to be suffering still from 'headaches & bad nights'.[50] As soon as she returned to Breslau, where her husband was now the Commanding General, she arranged for another visit from Schweninger.[51] She also discussed her case on several occasions with Dr Reinhold Franz, Baroness Heldburg's brother.[52] 'When yr. Brother comes give him my special love,' she wrote to Ellen. 'I wish he would remain for Xmas, so that I could have some nice medical chats with him.'[53] Charlotte was also an avid reader of the medical journals, in the vain hope of finding a diagnosis or a cure for her affliction.[54]

From about this time – she was now in her early forties – Charlotte's condition deteriorated even further, a development which Schweninger attributed to the menopause and the drastic hormonal swings that the change of life brought with it, whereas Bernhard, her husband, was convinced that it had been the waters of Franzensbad, a spa in Bohemia, that had 'ruined her for life'.[55] 'I have been poorly & had stupid fainting fits, & other disagreeable-nesses,' Charlotte informed Ellen Heldburg on 17 June 1902. 'Schweninger believes certain age changes are beginning & the cause of my inconveniences & bad nerves: a nice look out!! added on to all other bothers.'[56] 'My left cheek, glands & side of my head are swollen,' she sighed in despair in November of that year.[57] Symptoms – sickeningly familiar to us by now – regularly appeared which put the true cause of her agony beyond reasonable doubt: unbearable 'wandering' abdominal pain, abscesses, boils and itchy oedematose inflammation of the gums and skin, swellings in various places, headaches, fainting fits and biliousness, lameness and chronic constipation. In a despairing letter of 26 June 1903 to Schweninger the princess sighed: 'Time has been too hard on me & I cannot manage to recover. My nerves are in shreds, although my appearance does not show it. But a terrible headache on one side & dizziness on the left side *so* depress me, & completely irregular [period] malaise, with a rash & itching.'[58] She would not envy Schweninger, whom she nicknamed her 'Master' and her 'little Devil', she said bitterly, in his efforts to control her 'simply dreadful . . . vomiting!!'[59]

Throughout 1904, Charlotte complained of swollen legs, of severe pain in the back (almost wholly on the left side), and of

George III, by Allan Ramsay.

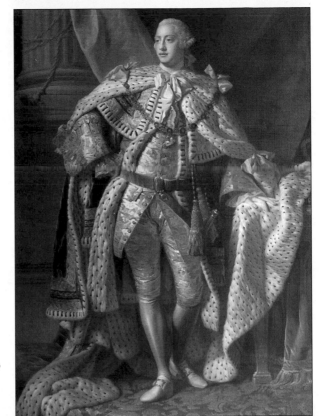

The thirteen children of
George III and Queen Charlotte,
detail from *Queen Charlotte*,
by Benjamin West.

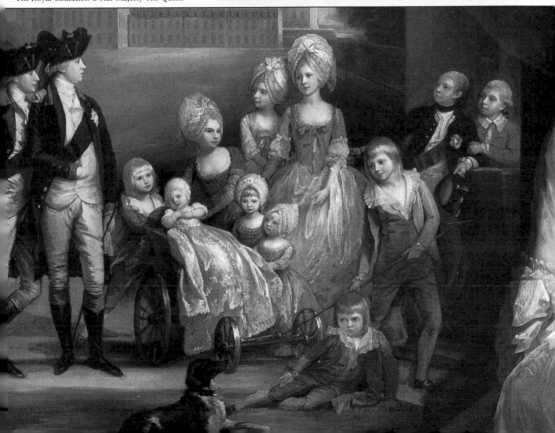

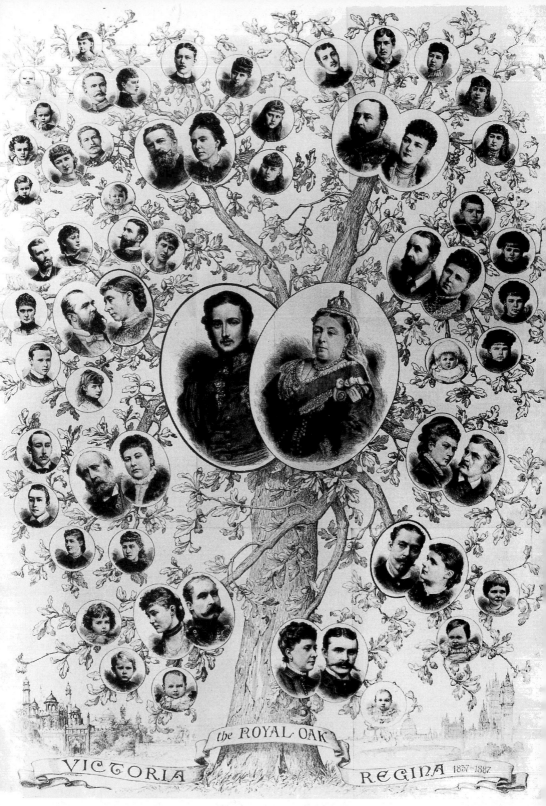

Family tree of Queen Victoria, printed in the *Illustrated London News* in celebration of the 1887 Jubilee. Illustrated London News

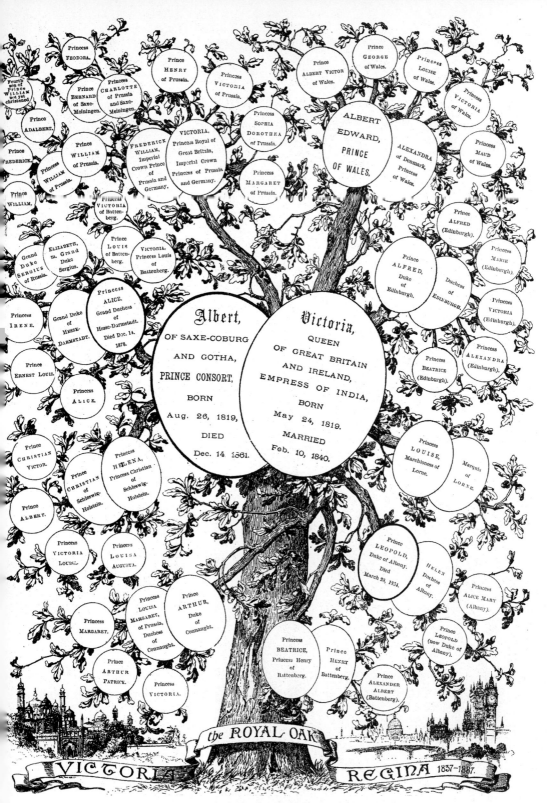

Key to the family tree opposite, from the *Illustrated London News*.

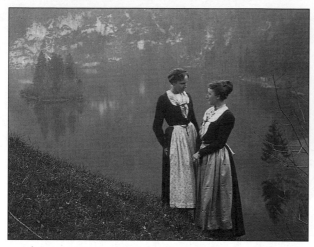

Princess Adelaide (patient A, *right*) and Princess Feodora (Feo II, *left*) on the shore of Lake Königsee in the Bavarian Alps.

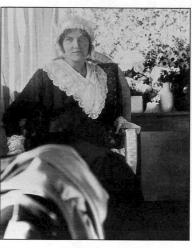

Princess Adelaide (patient A) in her sickbed.

Thüringisches Staatsarchiv, Meiningen

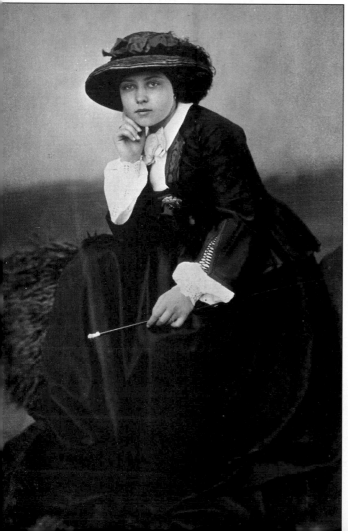

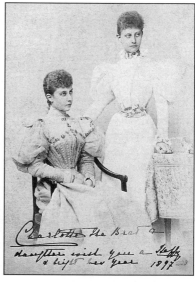

'Charlotte the brat'. Signed photograph of Princess Charlotte (*seated*) with her only daughter, Princess Feodora (Feo I).

The Royal Archives © Her Majesty The Queen

Princess Victoria (Vicky), eldest daughter of Queen Victoria, photographed at Osborne House in 1855.

The Royal Archives © Her Majesty The Queen

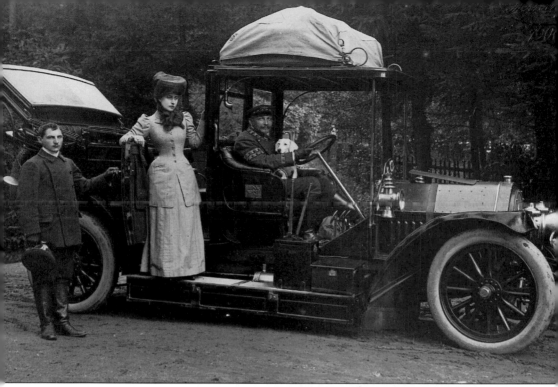

Princess Charlotte with her beloved car, 'Angel'. Thüringisches Staatsarchiv, Meiningen

Portrait photograph of Princess Feodora (Feo I), taken in 1891.

The Royal Archives © Her Majesty The Queen

Princess Feodora (Feo I) with her husband, Prince Heinrich XXX of Reuss. The Royal Archives © Her Majesty The Queen

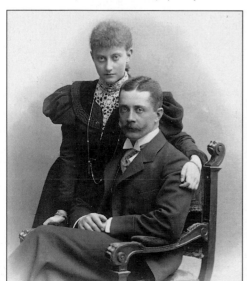

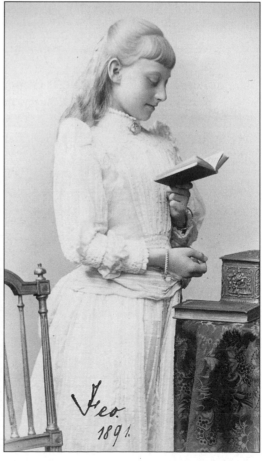

Feo.
1891.

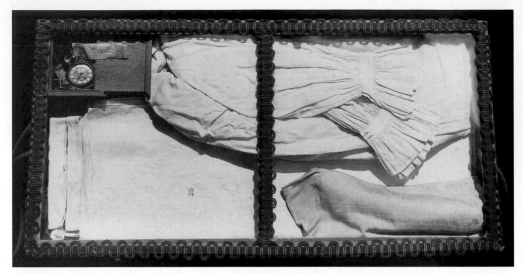

The relics of Charles I, kept on the Ashburnham Estate since his execution at Whitehall on 30 January 1649. The display case contained a shirt, undergarments, a stained sheet, and a lock of hair. A distinctive royal emblem (CR) was embroidered onto the sheet. © Photograph Judges Postcards Ltd, Hastings

The authors at the grave of Princess Feodora and her husband Prince Heinrich XXX of Reuss in Kowary, Poland (August 1996).

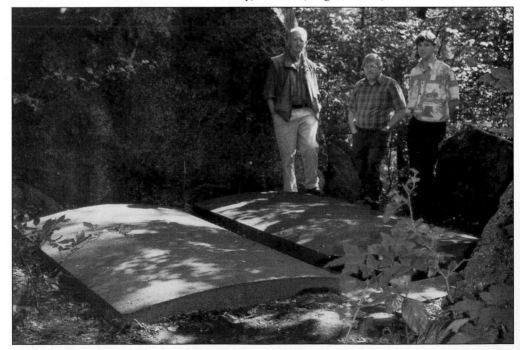

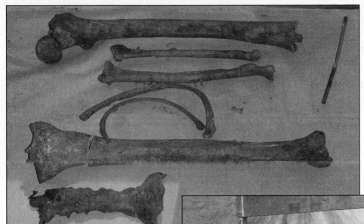

Bones recovered from the graves of Princess Feodora and her husband.

Opening the grave of Princess Charlotte in July 1997, at Schloss Altenstein, Germany. The stone slab weighed over three tons.

Remains of the flag that had been draped over Princess Charlotte's coffin. Carrying the emblem of the cross of the Teutonic Knights, it is a regimental banner from the 1870–71 Franco-Prussian war.

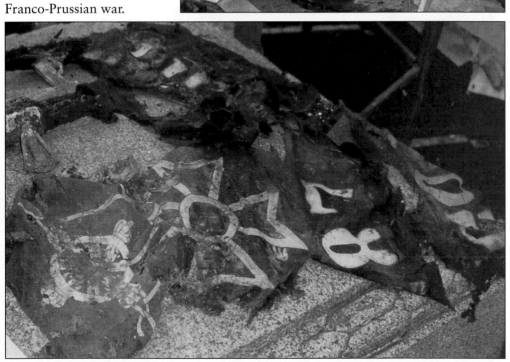

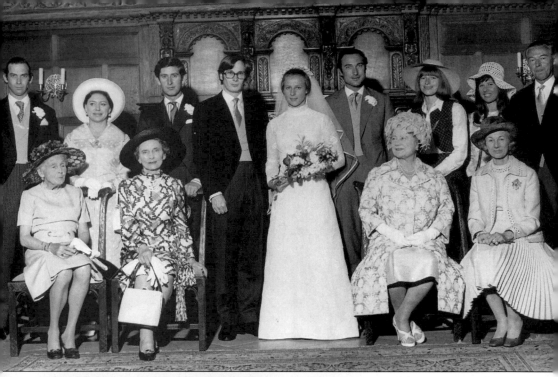

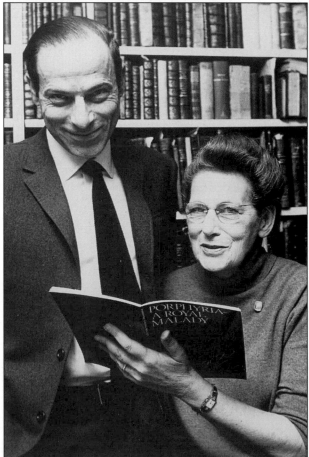

The wedding party at the marriage in July 1972 of Prince Richard of Gloucester. The party includes Prince Charles and Princess Margaret. William of Gloucester is standing to the right of the bride. The photograph was taken just six weeks before his death.

Tom Hustler/Camera Press

Dr Ida Macalpine and her son Dr Richard Hunter, taken in 1968 after the publication of the British Medical Association booklet 'Porphyria – a royal malady'. The Press Association giddiness and severe constipation.[60] In late October, she and her husband checked into the Hotel Regina at Baden-Baden for six weeks to be 'inspected' and treated by Georg Groddeck for the first time. Although he was later to become a convinced (if rather unorthodox) Freudian,[61] Groddeck identified the root cause of the princess's suffering as physiological and in line with Schweninger's teaching prescribed massages twice a day, together with hot baths and a liquid diet to combat constipation.[62] The massages were 'abominably' painful – she felt 'bruised & sore all over', Charlotte reported[63] – but appeared to do some good, especially in conjunction with a strict diet and hot leg and hip baths. The diagnoses Groddeck provided now and later – 'totally false circulation', leading to a damming-up of the blood (*'Blutstauungen'*) in some parts of the body and an absence of blood in others – were fanciful but by no means without value. 'The *"Blutstauungen"* in my lower!! back part & womb are great & cause all the trouble & lameness, the other surrounding parts being bloodless, of course are swollen; my B.T . . . is the worst', forcing her to lie on her tummy, Charlotte explained to her friend Ellen soon after Groddeck's first 'inspection'. 'Sitting 20 minutes in hot water at night, until I perspire, seems very good, but all in all I feel naturally *"zerschlagen"* [broken].'[64]

In spite of her horror of Groddeck's massages, by the following spring a further stay at Baden-Baden had become 'highly necessary'. As she reported to her confidante in telegraphic style shortly after her arrival there on 2 May 1905, her cure had begun immediately to deal with all her 'swellings & *"Schlackungen"* [quakings] which have increased on left side only. Giddyness & pains same cause: twice a day treatment & very strict diät & hot leg & hip baths: day filled.'[65] From now on, her twice-yearly visits to Groddeck became an agony she needed to endure in order to secure even the minimum of relief. In September 1906, she informed Ellen with just the faintest trace of hope: 'The massage has begun mightily in new places & head too, which is more painful than I can describe; [but] riding has decidedly improved the leg.'[66]

In addition to her regular visits to Baden-Baden, from 1905 onwards Charlotte and her husband spent the winter months in Cannes, not suspecting that the stronger Mediterranean sunlight might actually exacerbate her problems; in December 1908 they bought the beautiful villa La Forêt there from Prince Serge Galitzin.[67]

It is tragic to witness the disenchantment that followed upon the hope and joy of the early visits to this magical part of the world. Leaving Baden in the pouring rain in her car (nicknamed 'Angel') in October 1905, the princess exulted at the 'blue sea & sky' and felt certain that the Mediterranean brightness would 'soon pick me up again'. It was, she wrote, 'quite a dream to be here, Summer weather after eternal wet dark & damp. Lying at open window, sun pouring in . . .'[68] Not long after arriving at Cannes, Charlotte suffered one of her severest attacks to date. In despairing letters to Schweninger she complained of 'swollen joints & acute pain, at times in the back, at times in the legs & arms: then, for hours at a time, none at all. But moaning, wailing, poor appearance, even worse moods & constipation – these are neither pleasant nor easy to bear.' She had nothing but contempt for her French doctors, who despised Schweninger (as she told him) and prescribed her Vichy water and embrocations. Contemptuously dismissing their diagnoses – 'I think it is neither gout nor rheumatism!!!' – Charlotte (curiously, after all that she had gone through) considered her attack to be influenza and looked forward to being treated by Schweninger and Groddeck – the latter being due to visit her in Cannes in the near future.[69] A week later she reported having been forced to take aspirin 'because I truly could *no longer bear* the *excruciating* pains in my eye sockets, nose & forehead. I always have to take 1 capsule every 7 hours. For I cannot see *a thing* for the pain.' Schweninger having colluded in the diagnosis of influenza, Charlotte thanked him for the reassurance that this spurious support had brought her. 'Am so relieved that you consider our illness to be infl with all the torture it brings with it; I refused to accept the idea of gout or rheumatism, despite the opinions of the doctors.' Once again, she complained of constipation and lack of appetite. Most revealing of all, from a diagnostic point of view: for the first time in her correspondence, tucked away in brackets at the end of this letter to her 'Master', we read the tell-tale words: 'Urine dark red'.[70]

Returning to Cannes in the autumn of 1906, Charlotte was once more full of hope that 'this wonderful, sunny land' would bring relief 'both in body & soul', but again the reverse was the case, and soon it was an insufferably itchy skin rash that became the predominant problem. In a letter to Schweninger she pleaded: '*13 full days of strong [menstrual] plagues (like never before) have succeeded in bringing me down: am lying down or sitting outdoors here: and beg you for advice on . . . alleviating my swelling. Since the 4ᵗʰ I have been drinking as little as possible and eating fruit, but things will not get better, & *this* itching!! – on the upper part of my body with a rash is enough to drive me mad: cold warm gives momentary relief.'[71] Shortly after writing this letter Charlotte had to spend several days in bed 'with dizziness and fainting spells' during which she 'saw only stars against a black background'. She continued to be plagued by her 'rash & itching, with abdominal pains', she told Schweninger.[72] None of the remedies he or Groddeck recommended brought release from her torment, however, and on Christmas Eve 1906 she again complained of feeling 'constantly nauseous' and that her 'dizziness & itching' were getting worse.[73]

In the following spring, the Kaiser's sister was again admitted to Groddeck's clinic and was soon able to report to her Master: 'Dear Groddeck came in early today and treated the bad spots, *quite* excruciating: but he hopes that massage twice daily & hot compresses in the morning and evening will cure them by the 15ᵗʰ. I can only compare it to being *flayed*.'[74] To illustrate her agony she sent Groddeck a postcard depicting the flagellation of a naked woman by monks in a crypt, with the inscription '*Ich heisse Schinder* – my name is Torment'.[75] Returning to the clinic in the autumn, she was full of hope that the massages would relieve her pain. 'I can observe the improvement brought about by Groddeck's fingers', she reported to Schweninger, 'but my thighs are exceedingly painful, as is a new bout of alveolar periostitis, which still refuses to abate.'[76] As usual, her optimism was misplaced, and within days of praising Groddeck's 'miracle massage' she was forced to ask Schweninger for a tranquillizer as her

> old pains have returned with full force, accompanied by such intense nausea that I am very nearly unconscious. The burning, shooting pains extend up into the left side of my abdomen; something new must be happening, & therefore my coming to see you is urgently necessary: self-massage & hot-water bottles

bring relief from the pains for brief moments; from one hour to the next I think my plagues have come, but it turns out to be nothing. The urine is slightly cloudy, the constipation comes and goes . . . It really is *too* stupid . . . The redness between the breasts & the itching all over my body have flared up again in full force.[77]

'These are dreadful days which I am going through,' she complained in a letter from Meiningen after receiving Schweninger's reply three days later. 'It is possible that the unpleasant itching, the red blotches, the nausea & the sharp pains lasting for hours at a time are only the side effects of my plagues which keep announcing themselves . . . but never actually arrive.' She was grateful for some painkilling drops – morphine – that Schweninger had sent her.[78] A visit to the Master's clinic outside Munich in November 1907 only brought more pain and a confirmation of Groddeck's diagnosis: 'Cold better, *no* influenza but treatments have been "tearfully" painful,' she reported to Ellen Heldburg. 'The whole thing caused by "*Stauungen*" [damming] & change of life.'[79]

At the end of 1907, back in Cannes, Charlotte reported that, though the pains had temporarily abated, her itching had become worse and the colour of her urine was now 'changeable'.[80] Just a few days later, however, she told Schweninger that 'spasmodic labour pains & heavy bleeding with hefty pain in or *above* the left buttock [have] set in, so that my left leg has gone numb'. She was forced to spend her entire time lying on hot-water bottles as the only way to cope with the pain.[81] In the winter sun things rapidly went from bad to worse, and on 7 January 1908 she wrote: 'The day before yesterday I had a lovely attack in the kidneys!!! After 3 hours of torture, 60 drops [of morphine] finally brought relief & sleep . . . Since then, my rash has grown much worse & is almost unbearable in the evenings due to the itching. The buttocks too are now sore. It's time that my Master came to console & help me. The weather is ideally beautiful: brilliant warm sunshine,' she added in her innocence.[82]

Her suffering was now virtually continuous, without the remissions she had enjoyed earlier. Her 'disorders & pains' were 'atrocious & so dismaying', she wrote. 'I have been in bed again with strong plagues which, even though over and done with, culminated in regular labour pains which spread up to the breast, which is purple. Pains, little abscesses, constipation, then sudden loosening & orange urine are among the more amusing of my additional symptoms.'[83] The only thing that had helped her through this 'nasty attack', she admitted to her friend Ellen, had been Schweninger's 'soothing' drops.[84] 'Everything is as it was before', she wrote to Schweninger in despair in February 1908,

> with the difference that the middle plagues are even more painful than the real thing, with biliousness & pain against which only your drops are of any help; for 3 days the urine was bad again; I shall now have to hold on bravely until the beloved thumbs gently touch the affected parts. The labour pains, which occur frequently, are so short & violent that they take my breath away. Urine changeable, constipation brilliant. The sun continues shining brightly . . .[85]

After eight more days of intense suffering, during which her only comfort was morphine and the thought that she would be seeing Schweninger in late March, she complained again of 'labour pain-like' spasms with 'pains on my left side' and 'itching in the evenings', both of which were 'almost unbearable'.[86]

Though she lived in hope that some new medicine or other remedy might yet release her from her martyrdom,[87] the princess's condition deteriorated alarmingly in Cannes in the spring of 1908. Still tending to link her abdominal pain to the menstrual cycle, she reported to Schweninger that for two weeks now she had been waiting for her 'stupid, labour pain-like plagues' to materialize. On a visit to Monte Carlo she had been unable to attend any of the dinners arranged in her honour but had spent the time either in bed or in the bath. She had tried to quench her terrible thirst with a new mineral water given to her by the Queen of Italy, she sheepishly confessed to her doctor, and claimed that this had helped to alleviate 'the itching & rash, & the abscesses', and that even her urine was 'lighter, better & much less painful since then'; her constipation, on the other hand, was as bad as ever, and she was getting fatter.[88] Two weeks later she had to admit that nothing had changed, and that if anything she was worse than before. 'The devil take fistulas, suppuration, abscesses & pain,' she cried in frustration. Her pains were more intense than ever, and were starting to affect the right side as well. 'My mental depression & my frequently crying alone because everything is always going wrong, as well as my anger, can only be cured by *you*,' she told Schweninger.[89] Just a week later we read: 'My pains are *not to be endured!* and are now accompanied by new symptoms . . .'[90] Her condition was so bad – in addition to everything else she was now quite lame again – that it was agreed that she should leave Cannes for Munich and enter Dr Hauffe's sanatorium at Ebenhausen, where Schweninger could visit her daily.[91]

From the sanatorium she wrote to Baroness Heldburg on 8 May 1908: 'My prison life I'm now getting accustomed to, but the first days I howled.' Her treatment, consisting of a 'beastly' diet, massages, hot showers and lying on hot-water bottles, had had one good effect already, she reported: 'The horrid itching & rash have *gone*; else I can't speak of any improvement yet, after 8 days; what has been so long coming cannot be got over in a short time, but I'm convinced it's the right thing; & Schweninger's daily kind visits, gentlest treatment "*u. mir Muth zusprechend*" [and his words of encouragement] are a comfort.'[92] Within weeks, miraculously, she seemed all but cured, and could hardly believe the feeling of well-being she tasted. 'I can but wish *you* felt as well as *I do*,' she wrote in triumph to Ellen. 'I can *never* thank Schweninger & Hauffe for restoring me so; sometimes I think it's a dream, my pains having left me.'[93] In July the terrible pains in her teeth and gums returned, 'but otherwise I am free from pain & can cope with *all* the duties daily life brings with it, it's fabulous!'.[94] Her daughter Feodora refused to believe that she was cured. 'Does she really look her old self?' she demanded to know. 'No more so ghastly white & ghostlike & thin? I only hope she will remain so, but doubt it.'[95]

Sadly, by late August 1908, the all-too-familiar symptoms began to reappear. 'I'm fairly well, but need seeing to at Ebenhausen,' she reported from Bayreuth, followed – after her visit to the sanatorium – by the disappointing news: 'I had a touch of my old pains & Schweninger as well as Hauffe found a small swelling again on the left side: so I'm put down for another 10 days on liquids, hot bottles & hot hip baths; they are certain to help; but luckily no return of anything else.'[96] All too soon she was having to admit that her old pains, her 'plagues' and 'labour pains', her dizziness and biliousness – all the symptoms of a serious porphyria attack – had returned.[97] By October her skin rash was also back to torment her, all over her body, in spite of zinc ointment.[98] 'The itching on my neck is unbearable, and on the breasts, too, which are sore in various places,' she informed Schweninger who, on examining her at Ebenhausen in November, established that the *'right* kidney & womb [were] not right'.[99]

The annual winter visit to the French Riviera brought on a further worsening of Charlotte's condition. Bitterly she wrote from Cannes on Christmas Day 1908: 'Sometimes I cannot get up because of the pain (above the buttocks!); hot-water bottles offer some relief; & if I can walk a little things are better.'[100] 'My left side is now without a doubt the most painful,' we read in a letter to Schweninger of 7 January 1909, and a week later we learn: 'Pain, constipation (for up to 7 days), urine very changeable in quantity & colour, rash & itching are on the increase, and in addition little ulcers everywhere, the mouth, nose & 6 on the buttocks!! Very attractive. I feel like a little volcano that keeps erupting. A plague (very late) has been on its way for a long time!!'[101] To the belated period she attributed 'perpetual contractions & pains, with nausea & cold sweat: The itching is intensifying, particularly at the nape of the neck.'[102]

In February she complained of having to spend several days in bed with 'dreadful shooting pains, just like 2 years ago. Once again I endured ghastly suffering & at night ran about in my room moaning & crying. But hot baths, compresses, [hot-water] bottles did the necessary work, & now I am up and about, wrapped in brown paper, if a bit wobbly... Very amusing!'[103] Later that month she reported that 'for days I have been dragging myself around with the familiar pain in my left side ... the night was so awful, with swollen joints, that I had to stay in bed today lying on hot-water bottles.'[104] At the end of March she likened her suffering to 'a belt of nails (around my hips & tummy), it pricks & torments me, and takes my breath away; perhaps there's a missing plague on its way, for my thighs are paralysed & swollen'.[105]

Unable to bear the pain and discomfort any longer, Charlotte left Cannes for Baden-Baden to be treated by Groddeck. The imaginative 'soul searcher' now compared her abdominal pains to a wandering stone, and the princess incorporated this analogy into her letters to Schweninger and Ellen Heldburg. His painful massages were designed to rid her of her 'stone', which they both liked to think of as a 'savage beast' that was refusing to be tamed.[106] As she told the baroness soon after her arrival: 'The wicked *Nierenstein* [kidney stone] caused agonies with *Koliken* [colics] lying high up & hidden deep; now he has achieved in bringing it down low & hope to be rid of it shortly. The swellings have quite gone & am able to walk several times a day in this lovely place, like one huge flowering garden.'[107] As always, such optimism was unfounded, and before very long Charlotte's husband was obliged to inform Schweninger that her pains, which were 'a consequence of the kidney stones', were as strong as ever, and that 'not a day passes without her having to suffer, more or less. But we are convinced', he added, 'that your skill will be able to release her from these pains in time.'[108]

October 1909 found Charlotte back in Groddeck's hands at Baden-Baden. She had, she explained, 'been bad & in such pain' on account of her 'stone' that she had been forced to seek his help.[109] 'Groddeck is gradually managing to get me back on my feet', she wrote a week after her arrival, 'although progress is slow: the stone-beast is now low down. But the *pain*!! when he grabs it, pokes it & sticks his knee into it!!! Urine is bloody again, but there's much more of it and it flows easily; bowel movements very irregular.'[110]

In addition to the 'bad colour' of her urine, she was 'sleeping miserably on account of toothache & swollen cheek inside & out', she said.[111] The attack was so severe that she could not manage without morphine. To Schweninger she wrote:

I have been suffering from *such* raging pain in my teeth and nerves over the last 3 days that Groddeck stopped the massage treatment and allowed 2 injections. The night from 1st to 2nd I screamed & ranted so much for 5 hours that at 3 a.m. Schliep was called in; after a strong injection the drug finally took effect an hour later. Head, teeth, every corner of my mouth, & now my hips are afflicted with these raging pains. Since noon today the attacks have abated somewhat, but I have become cowardly & am completely exhausted from ranting and raving during the night, waking everybody up. Groddeck is touchingly patient with me. His iodine tincture did little good. The stone is low down & well-behaved: perhaps *it* is the cause of all this. For MacFarlane's examination has shown that the teeth are *all* in good shape.[112]

Still without a clue as to the true cause of her illness, the princess looked forward to the winter sunshine at Cannes, although she accepted that it would 'not get rid of my pains'.[113] 'Weather simply divine & warm & much in the garden & roasting in sun,' she wrote in innocent joy in January 1910.[114] Not surprisingly, soon after arriving in the south of France, her condition worsened once more. 'Teeth painful, the stone too, the rash now even on the bottom, unbearable,' she told Schweninger. 'The sun here shines every day & renders nature a delight ... I shall try to let its rays shine on those parts of me that itch. My rash has got worse, in addition ... a swollen foot, extravasated oedema & a swollen knee. I hobble about like an old, lame sparrow that must prop up its leg at night; what a stupid beast I am!!'[115] She was delighted with Groddeck's visit in January, who was convinced that 'the stone was wandering about again'. The cocaine preparation he had prescribed was having a beneficial effect on the activity of her kidneys and bladder, Charlotte reported.[116] On 14 January 1910 she was able to tell Heldburg: 'Groddeck's skill has brought me on at last, & after 3 weeks of solitude & laying up I'm beginning to walk slowly on a stick, & pains nearly gone as well as inflammation: my troublesome "*Nierenstein*" [kidney stone] played me a nasty trick of a "collique" attack, but the Dr. has mastered this finally too.'[117] Shortly after Groddeck's departure, she was a 'wreck' again, lying on hot-water bottles suffering from 'a weak plague with swellings, vomiting, kidney pains'.[118]

In accordance with the pattern of life that she had been forced to adopt several years before, at the end of April 1910 Charlotte had herself driven in her 'Angel' from Cannes to Frankfurt for 'dentical sittings' with MacFarlane and from there on to Baden-Baden.[119] In misery she wrote to Ellen on 6 May 1910: 'Since my arrival I'm layed [sic] up, horrible achings & pains from inflamed nerves specially between ribs, & *Ischias* [sciatica] too ... But today I'm better & hobbled in my room & hope in a week's time to be human up & dressed again; but it's been beastly.'[120] To Schweninger she admitted that the pains she had had, though diminishing now under Groddeck's 'tortures', were as savage as those she had suffered in Cannes two years earlier, and that her legs and kidneys were still completely inactive.[124] As always, the painful treatment Groddeck meted out did do her some good, and soon she was able to tell

Schweninger: 'The legs still don't want to move much, but in other respects you will see a huge improvement.'[122] She found the heat of that summer insufferable, complaining that she was sweating the whole time, even at night, and enduring her first 'plague' in four months 'with unbelievable labour pains' and swollen legs and feet. 'I can only report that I am in pain and constipated,' she informed Schweninger in July.[123] At the end of that month she 'collapsed physically!, vomiting often', and was 'still a wreck with violent cramp-like labour pains which press terribly on the bladder'.[124]

Before leaving for Cannes that winter, Charlotte needed to see MacFarlane in Frankfurt, as she was 'in such pain from a horrid abscess' in her mouth. She described her swollen face as a 'hideosity', but it had returned to its normal shape by the time she reached the shores of the Mediterranean in December 1910.[125] The abscesses continued to torment her in Cannes, however, and in addition her rash and the wandering 'stone' caused her much pain. 'For days swollen & excruciating pain from 2 abscesses in my mouth (1 is not enough) . . . Glands and tonsils are so swollen; the nights (with rash) are *such* a joy!! & on top of this hot flushes and sweating spells!'[126] In February she complained once again of an abscess in her mouth, of painful tonsils, and that she was 'swollen to the shoulder blade'.[127]

Despite her dreadful suffering, the Kaiser's eldest sister bravely determined to attend the coronation of her cousin George V in June 1911, but not before visiting first Schweninger in Munich 'for a few days, to get put in order for London', and then MacFarlane in Frankfurt. Her recent cure at Baden-Baden had done her 'much good', she told her friend Ellen, and Schweninger was keen 'to see the good results'.[128] From Frankfurt she wrote that she was in the dentist's chair three times a day with abscesses and a 'black tongue', as well as suffering from abscesses on her buttocks which made sitting difficult.[129]

The visit to Britain in the summer of 1911, just three years before the outbreak of war, delighted her in many respects. 'What I've seen, learnt to admire, heard & witnessed, I can't describe,' Charlotte wrote from Sandringham on 25 July. 'There is no place in the world like England, & if possible I'm more English than ever . . . Have made several trips with my Sailor Brother [Prince Heinrich of Prussia] & other friends, running down to various lovely country houses. Seen hospitals, Pierpoint Morgans marvellous private collections, seen Drs., states- and tradesmen, politicians & colonial gifted men . . .'[130] But she found the heat of that English summer overwhelming: her joints, feet, hands and eyes swelled up, and she was confined to bed for several days with 'violent pains' and a 'face swollen beyond recognition', unable to eat or speak on account of swollen tonsils, glands and gums.[131]

On returning to Germany, and suffering from constipation and 'acute pains in the side', she lost no time in visiting Baden-Baden, from where she reported on 4 October that she was 'finally feeling better', and that Groddeck had 'done a good job; only his genius and skill could even come close to those of our Master! . . . The stone has shifted & I can now breathe again, although sleep still eludes me.'[132] But as always the relief was short-lived, and in December she was complaining to Schweninger from Cannes that she was hardly able to enjoy the 'radiant sun' as she could get no further than the garden, and spent 'more time *in* bed than out; the dreadful sciatica, which has settled in my back and kidneys, has me firmly in its grip'.[133]

Charlotte's life continued along this pattern until the outbreak of war in 1914. Groddeck's massages of her 'kidney stone' brought relief from time to time,[134] but otherwise she was in almost constant pain in her swollen legs and feet, her kidneys and hips, writing: 'I am completely lame, so swollen are my foot, leg and hip . . . it's too stupid, and then this heat & hot flushes & sweating (I am so embarrassed by the sudden reddening). Oh! This damned change of life.'[135] She complained of the pain her 'stone' was causing her, as well as lamenting that her 'rash, bad foot, swollen leg' were plaguing her greatly.[136]

With the outbreak of war, her husband, who was now the reigning Duke of Saxe-Meiningen, put Charlotte in charge of his miniscule principality while he himself went to the front, but she was hardly in a position, physically or mentally, to run the country, and the news that Duke Bernhard was resuming his powers was greeted with relief and even joy.[137] Trips to the Mediterranean were of course out of the question now, but otherwise her illness and its treatment continued much as before the war. She complained of kidney pains, digestive and intestinal disorders, constipation, toothache, boils and oedema, and bemoaned the fact that the skin on her face had become 'wrinkled, peeling and itchy . . . and looks simply awful'.[138] All she could do was to 'hobble around the room on sticks for short periods', she told Schweninger in December 1917, adding that as a result her feet and legs had become 'quite atrophied & thin'.[139] At the beginning of 1919, after the collapse of the German Reich and the abdication of both her brother and her husband, she complained of a 'very painful infection of the colon' and of 'cramp-like digestive pains' which were affecting her heart.[140] She was forced to spend much time in bed, although unable to sleep. 'Unfortunately last night was very trying; I tossed & turned in pain until 4 a.m., doing trunk exercises, applying compresses, massage, nothing helped.' The pain was especially devastating when she tried to walk, as she informed Schweninger; she asked him to commend her 'steadfastness' in managing to get through *'without medicine or morphine'*.[141] She died on 1 October 1919 at Baden-Baden, with Georg Groddeck at her side. Her tiny body was transported across revolution-torn Germany, to be buried at Schloss Altenstein in the forests of Thuringia.

Princess Charlotte's detailed self-portrayal in her letters to Schweninger and Ellen Heldburg leaves little room for doubt that she suffered from variegate porphyria, for what else could the cause of her excruciatingly painful condition have been? In terms of the historical evidence alone, hers is our strongest case.

CHAPTER 8

Feodora, Our Last Princess

Tactless as usual, [Heinrich Reuss] named the illness
straight out, [asking] why I would not say so, [since] all
the world knew it.

*Charlotte, Hereditary Princess of Saxe-Meiningen,
to Ellen Baroness Heldburg, 5 December 1900*

On 26 August 1945, in the cataclysm that visited Germany at the
end of the Second World War, one of Queen Victoria's great-
granddaughters, Princess Feodora of Reuss, for many years an
inmate of the Sanatorium Buchwald-Hohenwiese south of the
Silesian city of Hirschberg, entered into a suicide pact with her
companion Meta Schenck, put her head in the oven and gassed
herself. Her grave, a deep vault covered by a heavy stone slab in the
woods less than a mile from the clinic, had been ready since before
the war; her husband, Prince Heinrich XXX of Reuss, had been laid
to rest there back in March 1939.[1] Their ramshackle house of
Neuhoff, near Schmiedeberg, not far from the sanatorium in which
they were both to end their lives, was about to become the south-
western corner of the new People's Republic of Poland. Princess
Feodora, who was Princess Charlotte's only child, died without
issue. With her, the blood line we have been tracing from George III
through the Duke of Kent to Queen Victoria, her daughter Vicky
and *her* daughter Charlotte comes to an end. Feodora is our last
princess.

If Charlotte cut an unattractive and insignificant figure on the
political stage of imperial Berlin, her daughter was positively
obscure. Not a line has been written about her in any history book.
Through an extraordinary stroke of fortune, however, we find that

the matriarchal Baroness Heldburg also acted as mother-confessor to Feo, both in her incessant quarrels with Charlotte and in matters pertaining to her health. Hundreds of Feo's letters to the baroness, which, like those of her mother, were written in English, are preserved in the Thuringian State Archive at Meiningen. Together with Charlotte's own comments on her only child, Feo's self-descriptions in her letters to Heldburg of her torments and her increasingly desperate attempts to find a cure provide us with plentiful evidence suggesting that she had indeed inherited the porphyria gene.

Very much as with her own eldest daughter, Vicky was struck by the diminutive size and the physical and mental peculiarities of her first granddaughter Feo, who was born on 12 May 1879. As a child, Feo would often come to stay with her grandmother, and it was on such occasions that Vicky remarked on the girl's tiny frame and curious looks. 'Little Feo looks more pinched & peaky & thin than ever, with such *old sharp* features, *much* too big for her diminutive body, – and a way of talking like an old woman; she is not a bit like a child & has none of the charm & roundness of youth,' the widowed Empress wrote in 1892, while Charlotte was in Constantinople. A few months later, she complained: 'I find dear little Feo hardly grown, she is very plain just now, especially in profile – a huge mouth & nose & chin – no cheeks, no colour – the body of a child of 5 & a head that might quite well belong to a grown up person!' In 1893, when the twelve-year-old had once again come to stay, Vicky remarked that her 'sharp pinched features are more old looking than ever', and added: 'I do *wish* she could grow – she is the shortest child I ever saw.' It was not only Feo's stature that reminded Vicky of Charlotte, however. Though she was quick to assert that Feo's 'disposition & character' were different from those of her mother, she nevertheless noted that her grand-daughter was 'very fond of telling stories – and hardly ever says *exactly* the truth! I am afraid she will be her Mama over again.' Feo, she observed, was superficial and forgetful, and seemingly incapable of anything approaching deep thought, just like Char-lotte, but she was '*far* easier to manage than her Mama was, – & makes one far less anxious'.[2]

When Feo was ten, the first symptoms appeared of the mysterious illness that would torture her throughout her life. Describing one of her own violent attacks of sickness and diarrhoea with shivering and pain in the limbs, back and head in October 1890, Vicky gave Queen Victoria the telling news: 'I have not seen little Feo yet, as she has had an attack similar to mine!'[3] When she was sixteen, Feo told Ellen Heldburg in one of her first letters to her grandfather's wife that she had been confined to her bed for several days with a 'dreadful cold' which had been accompanied by a 'real *Migräne* & lots of other headaches'.[4]

Meanwhile, Feo's looks improved.[5] Her mother noted that she was 'simply flourishing & looks very well indeed: quite round in the face & good colours'.[6] The Crown Prince of Serbia asked for her hand in marriage, but was turned down on the grounds that 'for *such* a throne she is far too good', and besides, one could not marry into '*such* a family'.[7] In 1897, however, to her mother's intense annoyance, Feo became engaged to Prince Heinrich XXX of the junior line of the Reuss family,[8] a penniless Prussian army officer fifteen years older than herself; they were married in Meiningen in September 1898.[9] Though blighted by childlessness, the marriage was for a time quite a happy one, but almost immediately after it was solemnized, Charlotte broke off relations not only with her son-in-law but with her only daughter. From now until well into the First World War, a campaign of mutual vilification, unprecedented even in the gossip-ridden court society of imperial Berlin, poisoned relations between the two generations, calling into question the mental and emotional health of both mother and daughter – and confronting the historian studying their letters with something of a Cretan paradox.

After their wedding, the young couple settled in Frankfurt-an-der-Oder, where Heinrich – his nickname was 'Haz' – was kept busy by his regimental duties. When they could, they went for long rides together, but otherwise Feo – who was universally known by the English nickname 'Babes' – occupied herself by joining a reading circle and making the occasional visit to the opera and theatre in Berlin. Her great sorrow was her failure to conceive – she cried whenever her period came. She soon began to look worryingly 'tired . . . pale & thin', and wrote to the baroness that she had been in bed for several days and felt 'shaky'.[10] Both her mother and grandmother accused her of not looking after herself but failed to persuade her to lead a more sensible lifestyle.[11] After a visit from the couple in 1899, Charlotte observed: 'Babes I don't find looking well, & he [Heinrich] grown fat heavy lumbering (& to me not sympathetic); she of course is different too, & shifts & shrinks away, whenever I try to influence her, concerning her person & health. It's of no use, so I must keep aloof & let her go her own way.'[12]

Soon the rupture between mother and daughter was almost irreparable. 'Babes is incomprehensible to me!' Charlotte complained. 'Although totally wrapped up in her H. she might at least have a feeling of filial gratitude for *me*, who did so much for her . . . I never was blind about her faults & character, but never thought she would turn round against me.' Soon she was describing Feo as a loud, selfish and self-righteous girl with bad manners, and Heinrich as heartless and conceited.[13]

Rapidly the adjectives used – on both sides – went from bad to worse. 'The lies she has told Papa . . . about me . . . are really disgusting,' Feo wrote about her mother in November.[14] 'She only causes me pain & becomes rude, I can't stand any more. The less I think of them & hear of them the better,' was Charlotte's hurt response.[15] She proceeded to spread 'such absurd and hair-raising stories' about Feo and her husband that the conflict between the two couples rapidly spiralled out of control. By spring 1900 the hapless Prince Bernhard, wholly under Charlotte's sway, was writing of Feo's 'loud mouth' and her 'mendacity and passion for gossip and calumny which she has certainly not inherited from us'.[16] On 3 April 1900, Bernhard gave notice that he would not be able to see Feo and her husband again until Feo had withdrawn her accusation that Charlotte was a liar.[17] Thereafter, communication between them ceased almost entirely. 'She is beyond *my* comprehension,' Charlotte asserted in bewilderment, and then proceeded to exclude her daughter from her home 'for ever'.[18]

It is perhaps no coincidence that this emotional crisis coincided with a recurrence of Feo's earlier illness, one which quite unnerved her. From September 1899 to March 1900, she had a series of severe attacks of what she, in a letter to her grandfather, referred to as 'the old story'.[19] She repeatedly had to take to her bed with influenza-like symptoms accompanied by terrible pains, semi-paralysis of the legs, dizziness and diarrhoea. As she herself described her plight in the seventh week of her illness: 'I had a severe attack of

Influenza which kept me in bed over a week, half paralysed. I could not move a limb excepting my arms; neck, whole back & legs were totally stiff; & the frightful pains are not to be described. For three nights I could not close an eye & only lay there moaning; & when I wanted to turn round Haz had to lift me . . . I still feel weak, & cannot write long, it always makes my back ache afresh.'[20] The 'influenza' struck again in March 1900, this time together with a 'bowel disorder'; the attack kept her in bed for a further three weeks and rendered her 'half idiotic', she said.[21]

In the summer of 1900, Feo paid her grandmother a long visit at Kronberg – her parents heard later that she had told 'fearful lies' to try to wheedle some money out of Vicky[22] – and then visited her great-grandmother, Queen Victoria, at Windsor. Vicky was shocked not only by Feo's 'superficiality' but also by her physical condition, 'thinking her anemic & delicate' and suggesting that she spend six weeks taking the cure in the Trentino.[23] Not long after her return to Frankfurt-an-der-Oder, Feo suffered another 'attack of malaria', for which she took quinine, which brought only temporary relief, however, as she soon had to take to her bed with a 'frightful' migraine.[24] In the following months, too, Feo complained of 'feeling rotten' and of having 'raging headaches' that were like hammers inside her head.[25]

In December 1900, after an unsuccessful attempt at reconciliation, Charlotte described her daughter as 'pale, thin, ugly, all freshness gone, funnily dressed, hair parted on the forehead (like a dairy maid), talking of dancing, acting, Lieutenants, not looking at anything, inquiring after *nobody*!! I could hardly believe this curious, loud personage *had* been *my* Child!! . . . I could *not* cherish motherly feelings any *more* . . . I *cannot* love her! & my heart seemed & felt a stone.' She was appalled by the 'hatred, disdain & flippancy which came out of that Child' and asked: 'How can a Child's mind be so poisoned & totally changed in 2 years by such a stupid man?' Even worse were Charlotte's impressions of her son-in-law, who had 'grown *so* fat, heavy & ugly' and lolled about, looking '*so* done for'. The climax to the meeting came when Reuss, 'tactless as usual, named the illness straight out', asking 'why I would not say so, [since] all the world knew it'.[26] We must assume from the context that this tantalizing passage refers to the illness both Feo and Charlotte were tormented by, but what was the name

159

that Heinrich used to describe it, which he claimed 'all the world' was using, too? The documents are silent on this vital point.

After a number of icy encounters with her daughter in 1901, Charlotte again described her as looking 'pale & thin & old'. Feo's behaviour, too, she said, 'jars to such an extent on my wracked nerves', for she 'jabbers & tells such fibs, doing nothing all day, that I shall be heartily thankful when at last . . . she leaves me. Sad to behold such an utter change & vulgarity & untruthfulness in her.' She was, Charlotte sighed, an 'incredible personage!!!'[27] At this point, the mutual hatred and contempt which mother and daughter felt for one another, coupled with the reputation that both women had as mischief-makers and liars, begins to pose serious problems for the historian who is dependent on the testimony of their letters for establishing their medical condition.

This is most evident in the mysterious interpretation Charlotte placed on yet another attack of 'malaria' – the gravest yet – suffered by her daughter in the winter of 1901–2 and lasting several months. In early January Feo had to enter a clinic at Köstritz, and in mid-February she was still there, feeling 'too dreadfully down from that beastly Malaria'.[28] By the following month, the 'malaria' had turned into a 'Darmentzündung', an infection of the intestines which was not, she assured her confidante, appendicitis. Whatever it was, the illness forced her to lie on her back. It was 'very painful & tiresome', she wrote, and she felt 'quite stiff', but the fever was now at last gone.[29] In April 1902 she returned to her home in Frankfurt-an-der-Oder, still extremely weak, but convinced that the cause of her suffering had been an infected appendix after all. As she wrote to Ellen: 'Your old Babes is a *very* miserable old Babes this time. I never felt so down before in all my life, & it seems as if I shall never pick up again. Four weeks are passed now, since I began with that beastly *Blinddarm* [appendix], & still I go tottering about in a teagown all day, and am more on the sofa than on my beetle-squashers. Well, everybody, not *only* the doctor, says to comfort me that *Blinddarm* always lasts weeks even months.'[30] Not until 16 April did Feo feel a little better, though she realized the need to be extremely careful, especially with her food. 'No bread is allowed, & excepting *Spargel* [asparagus] & *Kartoffelbrei* [mashed potato] no vegetables, & not all meats.' The doctor was coming shortly 'to look at the beastly old *Blinddarm* again', she wrote; he was advising her to get away completely, perhaps to Italy.[31]

Charlotte disagreed with the doctor's diagnosis and believed she knew the true nature of Feo's troubles. On 30 November 1901 she hinted darkly in a letter to the baroness: 'Astonish *me*, her condition does not in the least: *I* know full well what it comes from, but cannot entrust to pen & ink. All her & *his*!! fault, & nothing to be done, except a long treatment both flatly refuse to undergo, as naturally [it would] put *him* in bad light & fault.'[32] Four months later, with Feo still in bed, Charlotte refused to believe the explanation given by Reuss that the cause was appendicitis, for 'the symptoms are *wrong* to *my feelings*'. She was sure, she said, that it was 'an "*internal* inflammation!!!" I have been dreading for years!!!'[33] To her sister Victoria of Schaumburg-Lippe and her 'favourite' brother, Prince Heinrich of Prussia, and then to numerous outsiders, too, Charlotte confided that she was convinced that Feo had venereal disease. As an outraged Feo finally confided to the baroness in 1907, after years of keeping the matter to herself, her own mother had gone around saying 'that I had *not* had appendicitis, that time in Frankfurt-an-der-Oder, but Haz had infected me with a dirty venereal disease through his own bad lifestyle!!!'[34] Charlotte demanded that her daughter allow herself to be examined by Schweninger, and saw in her refusal 'proof' that her suspicions were true. Feo and Reuss, meanwhile, informed several members of the family, including the Kaiser's wife and brother, of Charlotte's incredible behaviour; everyone agreed that until she withdrew her accusations the younger couple could not set foot in the latter's house.[35]

Whatever its cause, Feo's serious illness of 1901–2 lasted for well over a year, with several ups and downs. Towards the end of 1902 she felt she was beginning to recover, writing to Ellen Heldburg: 'I am *so* well & strong like I never was with this mess before.'[36] A month later her husband reported that she was being wheeled regularly into the fresh air, which was doing her good.[37] But four weeks later still she felt 'wretched' again, complaining that her 'head & limbs ache[d] violently' and attributing this setback once again to 'Influenza'.[38] Such attacks became less frequent in 1903, though from time to time she did still suffer from 'beastly migraine' and was compelled to spend several days in bed.[39]

At the end of 1903, her husband was transferred to Flensburg, near the border with Denmark. Feo, now twenty-five years old, was delighted, since the climate there was similar to the weather in England, and since her Uncle Heinrich, the Kaiser's brother, lived near by. They found a small house with a garden which she loved to tend. Here Feo began to feel better for a number of years. She even put on weight. Her letters to the baroness bubbled with happiness and robust well-being. She led an active life marred only by her childlessness, money worries and the surreal conflict with her mother.[40] 'I went for a long walk this morning, along the water,' she wrote in early 1904. 'It was simply lovely, I felt I could scream with joy, the seagulls did it for me. If it goes on like this, & remains so warm, we shall soon ride again . . . I feel *so* well & strong now, like I never have before.' Many similar letters followed throughout 1904 and 1905.[41] In June 1905 she spent four weeks at the sanatorium run by Baroness Heldburg's brother, Dr Frank, at Langenschwalbach, but that was to improve her chances of conceiving, not because she was in pain; when the remedy failed to produce the desired result, she cried out in frustration: 'These everlasting disappointments are too disgusting.'[42]

Though she insisted that she was '*not* ill' and only in need of 'general strengthening', Feo's underlying condition had not changed and continued to be a source of worry even in this relatively happy period.[43] In May 1904, when she herself was exulting in a sense of well-being, her husband informed Heldburg after a consultation with Professor Ludwig Renvers: 'Babes is all right as far as it goes, but she needs to go to some spa or other on account of her anaemia ['*Blutarmut*']. On the other hand I don't really believe that spas can do her condition any good, things like that usually pass with time. Renvers recently stuffed her full of arsenic-and-thorium pills, so that she expanded like a plum pudding, but as soon as she stopped taking them she reverted just as quickly to her thin and pale old self.'[44] As with her mother, 'anaemia' was the term which came to be used within the family to describe her illness.[45]

Not only did Feo's stay at Reinhold Franz's clinic fail in its aim of helping her to have a baby; she complained that the cure had 'turned my inside topsey turvey', so that she could never predict when her period was coming. 'Before Schwalbach it was all in such good order.'[46] She came to blame her sojourn there for the setback she endured over the following months, complaining in March 1906, three-quarters of a year after returning to Flensburg: 'I don't feel well, funny to say, ever since I left Schwalbach I don't feel quite myself, they say here ever since I came back from there I looked pulled, drawn & tired, & that's what I feel like too.'[47] Even so, she decided to return to the sanatorium in another attempt to conceive, particularly as her grandfather the duke agreed to pay.[48]

Though the treatment again failed in its chief aim, for a time Feo's health returned. She bought a new horse and adored her early morning rides with her husband through the beautiful beechwoods full of singing birds.[49] The mysterious and painful influenza-like symptoms were never far away, however, and a cure could not be found, no matter what they tried. Thus in August 1907, on a visit to Meiningen, Feo complained that she was 'dead tonight with heat & fatigue, my head aches like mad, I only hope I shall not have a migraine tomorrow'.[50] From Meiningen she went on to Berchtesgaden in the Bavarian Alps for several weeks, to be treated by a Dr Lacher, who declared that her heart was much better and that she should go for long walks up the hills. 'Which I promptly do. Yesterday evening I had a three hour walk. Tomorrow Lacher wishes to see me once more after all these long walks to see how all behaves.' In spite of feeling so well, however, Feo suffered from toothache and terrible headaches that prevented her from sleeping.[51] In October, just before returning to Flensburg, she was struck down by 'influenza' which made her weak, though she believed that she was 'so very much stronger this year than I *ever* was'.[52]

That summer, the princess took the fateful decision to place herself in the care of Professor Albert Döderlein (1860–1941), director of the Department of Gynaecology at Munich University, in whose private clinic in the Sonnenstrasse she was to undergo the most extraordinary treatment over the next three years. Her main purpose was to try to have a baby – a girl, she hoped, 'Babes No. 2'. As she told Ellen Heldburg in a letter from the clinic on 6 July 1909, 'the torchers [*sic*] I went through these last 3 weeks ought really to be rewarded I think, & to have to go through all that *alone*, without Haz! And yet . . . the more I suffered, the happier I was, as it was *for* Haz, for his future happiness, I should *gladly* have borne more, & the greater the pains, the surer I felt, that Döderlein was getting at the root of all evil, & I nearer my prize.'[53] On releasing her from the clinic to return to Brunswick, where they now lived, Döderlein urged her to avoid all 'malarial areas' and not to travel by train, but 'walking & driving is expressly allowed & wished for from Professor Döderlein', who assured his patient that 'all chances were there now for me to get a Baby', but asked her to return to Munich if she were not expecting within three months.[54]

In addition to trying to conceive, Feo was visiting the clinic in order to get to the root of the pain and lameness from which she had been suffering ever since her attack of 'influenza' in the winter of 1907–8. On her first stay in 1909 she was able to report: 'I am *ever* so much better now, can walk again alone, & feel much stronger too.'[55] When she returned to the Sonnenstrasse in January 1910 for a second attempt, she told the baroness: 'I hope with *all* my heart that Döderlein will put an end to all these pains, & I shall *gladly* go through an operation, if he thinks it necessary.'[56] The professor, however, was more cautious, warning that it would not be possible for him 'to alleviate immediately her very troublesome pains and complaints', for her condition was 'so very unsatisfactory' that the treatment would take several weeks. Döderlein's diagnosis was unexpected, to say the least.

> I attribute the pains suffered by Her Serene Highness to a disorder caused by a congenital narrowing of the uterus and to exceptional sensitivity, so that the smallest occasion or intervention instantly provokes violent and long lasting pain. The attendant disruption of sleep, the reduced ability to take nourishment, the impediment of normal movement then cause further disorders in their turn, with the result that a summation of all these things produces discomfort in the Princess which severely disturbs her sense of well-being but which she tolerates with admirable patience.

Feo was to remain in his clinic until he had solved the problem; she would then have to keep away from all excitement for at least a quarter of a year, the professor pronounced.[57]

In spite of this strange diagnosis, and in spite of the fact that Feo was suffering from 'terrible, dreadful colic and fainting fits',[58] Döderlein went ahead with an attempt to inseminate her artificially which nearly cost her her life. As Feo's aunt Katharina, who lived in Munich, reported in alarm after visiting the clinic on 20 February 1910:

In the course of the artificial insemination D[öderlein] inserted two injections of sperm with great force into the uterus. (Feo said one should normally inject only a small quantity.) Thereupon Feo had horrific pains & a feeling as if she were going to burst. After two hours D. wanted to remove the injected matter from the uterus but to his horror he was unable to find it. It had spread up as far as the oviducts. He had to leave it. Now it began to putrefy up there, – and then the fever started! D. realised that this would lead to festering, that he would have to wait for a climax . . . As the temperature rose to dangerously high levels, he anaesthetised her and cut open the entire uterus (Feo says from top to bottom), the purulence was removed & he scraped the entire organ clean,'

so that the 'catarrh' from which Feo had suffered ever since she was a child, so she said, had now cleared up. Feo had the impression, Katharina went on, that for three days she had been hovering between life and death, but she (Katharina) had the distinct impression that in her solitude Feo was embroidering the story each time she relived it. There were other aspects of the incident which puzzled her too. Feo informed her, for instance, that 'in the high summer she had infected herself (on a toilet), that she had suffered very severely for five weeks from a rash, etc. I must admit that I soon lost the will to ask any more questions, as I had the feeling that I would never get to the bottom of the whole story. Who knows it? Whether Döderlein knows it is very questionable?!'[59]

Feo, accompanied by two nurses from the clinic, was able to return to Brunswick at the end of March, but she was barely able to walk, was 'swollen still', with a 'sticking out tummy & no waist' and unable to bear the slightest pressure. 'I have nearly lost my thinness', she reported six weeks after her operation. 'My goodness what a skeleton I was, one could see every bone in my body, arms & legs were sticks, legs are still so, that is why I can walk so badly.' She had indeed been 'at death's door', she told the baroness. But, far from condemning Döderlein for botching the insemination and endangering her life, Feo was ecstatic in her admiration. 'When today 6 weeks ago, my Professor came in & said he would operate, I could have hugged him, for happiness, only I was immovable with pain. I was not afraid a single moment, only happy, because I knew that would do me good, & Döderlein is so safe & great as

Operateur. Although he made a mistake, & a *great* one, I never was angry with him *one* second, or doubted him, for however great, a Professor is human, & mistakes are human too . . .'[60] In her admiration for Döderlein and indeed all the doctors who treated her, Feo of course did not realize how often the misdiagnosis of porphyria and the consequent false treatment can be fatal.

From that time on, the pain hardly ever left her. 'I believe I *never* shall be my old self again,' she admitted in May 1910. 'Sometimes I am quite disheartened with these everlasting pains. Not a day passes without them coming, & that now soon for a *whole year!*'[61] She spent many hours each day asleep in bed to make up for 'all those sleepless weeks in the clinic', she claimed, and seldom got up before lunch.[62] When she did get up she had to hop up and down the stairs, could only hobble about with a stick, and was able to sit only on an air cushion. A Sister of Mercy came once a day to massage her. Her husband Heinrich grew so concerned at her condition that Döderlein was sent for. 'Haz had grown *so* frightened, that it was more for him than for me that I asked the Professor to come.' Döderlein's 'quiet yet energetic way put an end to all Haz's fear, & in the evening he was gay & whistling, so up went old Babes too'.[63] But soon Feo was hiding her pain from her husband so as not to alarm him.

> Something which Haz does not know . . . is that I have pain almost daily, here & there. Professor Döderlein knows of it & says that it will continue for some time but was nothing to worry about. But I keep it a secret from my darling, because he would only become frightened, & would ask questions, and then I would *have* to tell him the truth. Sometimes it is very hard to hide it from him, when the pain comes suddenly & violently, but so far I have always managed it.[64]

She had written to Döderlein telling him of the constant pains and insisting that, though she 'would wait patiently till the year was up, if then *still* they went on, then I would bully him to death, till he had freed me of them. I simply *won't* go on like this all my life, & should gladly undergo a second operation if necessary.' She felt so helpless and useless in her present condition, she said, 'to be tied down like this, not to be able to twist & turn about my body as I choose, a thing I have never known until now. It's better to be really ill & in violent pain than like this!'[65]

Not until June 1910 was she able to report that she had been '*completely* without pain for a longish period, a *most* pleasant condition & one wholly unknown to me for a whole year'.[66] She was, she said, 'getting on well now, only for going down stairs I need my stick a wee bit still'. The heat had been intolerable over the past two weeks, she added, 'we felt quite ill, & helplessly stupid, incapable to do *anything*, I never felt anything like it'. Feo was delighted to read in the newspaper that Döderlein had been offered the post of director of the Gynaecological Department in the Charité, the famous hospital in Berlin; she hoped he would accept so that he would be nearer at hand.[67] Döderlein, however, stayed in Munich, married the daughter of a Bavarian general and ended his career as head of medical services of Himmler's police force.

Feo was examined again by Döderlein in Munich in September 1910, on her way to Berchtesgaden. She had been unwell with serious pain for five weeks when she saw him, and he ordered her to return to his clinic 'for a few weeks . . . for fango-packs [hot clay poultices] and internal massage'. Döderlein was confident, Feo assured Heldburg, 'that after that cure, I shall be perfectly alright again. I hope so with *all* my heart, but who knows what silly pranks that inside of mine will play again.' She was not afraid, she insisted, and still trusted Döderlein in spite of the mistakes he had made. 'He now knows me *inside and out*, & I don't want to go to another doctor because I don't want to become a guinea pig again!'[68]

For a brief spell in the early months of 1911, the princess, now thirty-one years old, appeared to have recovered her good health. 'Just think how different last & this year,' she remarked on 8 February. 'Tomorrow a year ago was my operation, & this year I shall go to the big court ball.'[69] By the summer, that good spell was just a memory. In May her remorseless pains returned, and she realized she would need to enter Döderlein's clinic, possibly for a second operation. 'I myself was rather miserable the last five weeks,' she reported, 'those horrid pains tormented me again, & showed me that I *must* see Döderlein, & the sooner the better.'[70] The pains got worse while she was staying at Schloss Altenstein that summer. Finally, at the beginning of September, she broke down altogether, and an operation seemed urgently necessary.

When Döderlein cut open Feo's abdomen on 9 September 1911, he found the reproductive organs to be fused together and to the peritoneum in one 'completely unmovable' mass. In his report on the operation he describes the situation that met his eyes in the following words: 'Both ovaries and the oviducts lie conjoined behind and alongside the uterus ... and have degenerated into tumours about the size of a fist. The uterus lies anteverted [i.e. bent forwards] and the lower part of its rear surface is conjoined to the peritoneum by membranes similar to a spider's web.' Once he had separated the two ovarian tumours from the peritoneum, Döderlein established that they were cystically degenerated and suffused with an old haematoma larger than a hen's egg. The Fallopian tubes were in themselves healthy, but their serous covering glued them so tightly to the ovaries that their separation from the latter proved impossible. The right ovary was in such a bad state that it had to be extirpated; but Döderlein was able to remove the affected parts and so save most of the left ovary. Once he had freed the uterus from its web-like membranes he discovered on its rear wall a growth the size of a hazelnut, which he excised. The other abdominal organs – both kidneys, the liver, the gall bladder, the spleen, the stomach and the intestines – proved to be perfectly healthy. There were no signs of old or new infections of the appendix, leading him to conclude that 'the pains previously experienced in this region were probably already being caused by the changes in the ovaries'. As to the cause of the degeneration and fusion, Döderlein concluded that no infection can have been involved. The haematoma in each of the ovaries, on the other hand, suggested an ovulation disorder of long duration. He confidently expected a full recovery.[71]

In fact, Feo's condition after the operation was abysmal. She was ashen-faced, bleeding profusely, in great pain, dangerously weak, listless and without appetite, and barely able to sleep even after morphine injections. Alarmed, Heinrich Reuss, Baroness Heldburg, Professor Döderlein and in the end Feo herself all begged her parents to relent and visit her in the Sonnenstrasse.[72] However, both Charlotte and Bernhard were outraged that the operation had been decided on at all. Bernhard said he was 'greatly alarmed' to hear of Feo's decision, and when she heard of the 'vile operation', as she called it, Charlotte declared herself to be 'grieved & shocked'. 'Those murderous knives are too wicked & dangerous,' she exclaimed. In what was her first letter to her daughter for a decade, she wrote coldly: 'The knife I *abhorr* & you know cannot agree with, & can but be fatal in *every* respect . . . I know neither the Dr nor the Klinik so I am no judge & don't even know to what *purpose* the operation is. You were *ever* a *strong* & *healthy* girl & all your internal organs were in perfect condition & order; so what has suddenly made yr. inside go so wrong, I fail to comprehend or take in.'[73] Her second letter, though a shade warmer, still expressed disbelief that Feo should have chosen to resort to the knife. It was little wonder, she wrote, that Feo's 'splendid constitution' had been 'so cruelly . . . harmed by the operation'. In an interesting comparison with her own illness and the treatment she had received, Charlotte termed her daughter's operation 'an incredible sad fact, which I shall *ever fail* to comprehend, as my dangerous internal diseases were cured & my life saved by such splendid treatment'.[74] As in the case of Vicky's correspondence with Queen Victoria, this exchange between mother and daughter suggests that Charlotte believed Feo to be suffering from the same disorder as herself.

Feo's hypersensitivity and depression did not lift on her return home.[75] 'I am so far quite well again, can walk without a stick', she assured the baroness just before Christmas 1911, but then continued: 'but inwardly I am not my old self, I feel so dreadfully sad & miserable, & it is all I can do not to let my old man notice it . . . They say it's nerves, *you* know how I hate that word, & yet I know that *this* time it is true. It was *not* true last year, because there I really *was* ill.'[76] Not only was she depressed, her violent pains returned and often caused her to stay in bed.[77] Not until February, nearly six months after the operation, was Feo able to report the recovery of her old strength. 'Now I am better in every respect, & feel myself that I am getting on,' she wrote. 'I sleep like a top now, nearly 12 hours . . . That does wonders; I feel my old strength & will coming back, & that makes the spirits rise too.' The doctor had assured her that with all this sleep her 'nerves' would soon be in good order again.[78]

Unexpectedly, in February 1912 Reuss was posted to Kassel, which was so close to Meiningen that he feared Feo was bound to see more of her mother.[79] By April 1912, she was suffering badly from stomach cramps. As she told Heldburg on 18 May, 'Since many weeks now & again I get such horrid internal cramps, I thought they would pass, but they don't, & always drag me down again so. Then "something else" [her period] behaves so curiously, too, & so we have asked Döderlein to come. If it is necessary to go through a treatment, *no* operation I feel sure, I shall go [to Munich] then. It *may* be it is all only nerves, but the pains after the cramps tell me no.' Feo was anxious that her mother should not hear of her new symptoms, since she had complete faith in Döderlein, and her mother's harsh judgement upset her. 'She sticks to Schweninger, I to Döderlein,' she declared defiantly, again hinting that there were two approaches to managing the same complaint.[80]

When he examined her on Whitsunday 1912, Döderlein found Feo to be in good condition internally but ordered her to take a long holiday in Tarasp in the Lower Engadine, a village noted for its mineral baths.[81] As Feo reported the results of the consultation to the baroness, 'Döderlein was so far satisfied with my interieure & the *Narben* [scars], but said that my whole condition now were [*sic*] shattered nerves, & that he wished me to go to Tarasp in July for four weeks, to have the good *Höhenluft* [mountain air], it's 1300 meters high, & to take the *Kohlensauere Bäder* [carbonic baths] there. Haz is to go with me, Döderlein expressly wishes it, as he says *every* disagreeable excitement of *any* kind harms me.' After Tarasp she was to go to Berchtesgaden for an after-cure rest.[82]

Reuss begged Feo not to tell her mother of Döderlein's advice, but she felt she had to. 'Of course she was angry', she reported, '& said he would ruin me, that he had done so already, & that Tarasp was the worst thing for me. But *I* feel *sure* it is right what Döderlein says, & that it will do me good ... I only wish I could passifie Mama, she can make one *quite* ill with *one* word ...'[83] When Charlotte saw her daughter immediately after Döderlein's visit, she was alarmed both by Feo's appearance and by what she declared to be the doctor's mistaken advice. 'Saw Babes for a half of an hour: shocked at her looks!' she told Baroness Heldburg in exasperation. 'Döderlein had been with her Sunday, found her *well*!!!! if you please! Forbidden her to write etc.!!! & she is to go to Tarasp in July! Slightest exertion finishes her out [*sic*], always layed [*sic*] up. Can't do anything as she won't listen; hopeless case.'[84]

In actual fact, the Alpine air and the long walks Feo was able to take in the Engadine did do her good. She was happy and felt her strength returning, and her husband was relieved to see the back, as he put it, of the 'eternally vibrating bundle of nerves' that she had become for the past 'dreadful year'. 'Döderlein was therefore right to send her here,' the prince concluded. In the mountains around Tarasp, Heinrich and Feo Reuss determined to settle at Neuhoff, their ramshackle house near Schmiedeberg that Heinrich had inherited, since it now seemed clear that mountain air and peace and quiet was all she really required.[85] Soon after her return to Kassel, Feo wrote to Ellen full of optimism: 'Well here your old Babes sits, well & strong again, quite her old wicked self, jolly & happy, full of fun & *ah* so happy! To be able to do *all* again, to have one's head & nerves again in the right place, is an unutterable joy . . .'[86]

Then, in October 1912, while passing through Munich on her way to Berchtesgaden again, she suffered a 'complete breakdown' with 'terrible pains & a fever', which Döderlein diagnosed as a 'uterine colic, resulting from excitement'. For the fourth time she found herself in the Sonnenstrasse, but this time Döderlein declared that there was nothing physically wrong with her: she was suffering merely from emotional strain.[87] 'I am gravely concerned about Feo's condition and can't begin to imagine what is going to happen,' her husband confessed in alarm to the baroness. 'For the past 12 days the same symptoms have recurred time and time again: In the evenings horrible pains & a rise in temperature, bad nights & an inability to walk. Döderlein assures me with complete certainty that there is no organic illness involved & that her condition is a purely nervous one. That is something I fail to understand.'[88] After six weeks in the clinic Feo seemed cured, apart from the occasional attack of diarrhoea, with the result that Reuss was forced to concede that Döderlein's 'psychiatric' explanation had been correct. As he wrote from Fasano on the shores of Lake Garda, where Feo was convalescing,

> It was such a remarkable business, this breakdown of the entire nervous system, & I still can't explain how it is possible that now everything has been so completely overcome. But Döderlein, the much-maligned, was right when he repeated time after time that there was no organic disorder, and that all that was needed was rest. If we had placed Babes in someone else's hands, or if she had not had the opportunity of fleeing speedily into the beloved clinic,

then I believe a disaster would have occurred. Döderlein is not only her gynaecologist, but also and above all her psychiatrist.[89]

Heinrich Reuss was surely right to express astonishment at the sudden discovery, by a gynaecologist, that Feo's painful abdominal symptoms – to cure which he had twice operated on her reproductive organs – were being caused solely by emotional upset! Even now, after her 'complete recovery', curious physiological symptoms continued to strike her down, as when, over Christmas, she felt sure she was dying of 'verdigris poisoning'. On the first day she had to dash to the toilet nineteen times, on the second ten, and on the third eight, as she told her grandfather. 'Towards the end all that came out was a white foam, on one of the days I also had a fever & felt as sick as a dog. But now I am up again & feel relatively well, my legs are still a bit funny, but I'm quite jolly & go for walks. The doctor here [in Fasano] is very surprised at my resilience.'[90] But then, five months after her 'complete recovery', just before her thirty-fourth birthday, Queen Victoria's great-granddaughter suffered another 'complete breakdown'.

On 5 May 1913 she wrote to Baroness Heldburg from a clinic in Dresden:

> There seems no life in me any more, I am sick of it, & all, & everything. I have battled against these feelings with all my might & main, till I crashed down completely, & thought I was going mad. I saw & heard all sorts of stupid things, was giddy & sick, & dead tired, only longed for sleep & rest. In the end my old man sent for a doctor, who is supposed to be good & he stuck me into this beastly Klinik, where I am treated with Arsenik & Torium Injections, *Kohlensaure* & *Electrische Bäder* [carbonic and electrical baths] & *Electrisieren* [electrotherapy]. This cure is to last for 6 weeks ... In all my pains & illness of the last years I wasn't a *single* minute *so* wretched as I am now.[91]

The feeling of mental debility was far worse than her lameness and all the physical pain she was suffering, she declared; on 19 May, however, she would be moving to a little villa in the grounds of the sanatorium at Hohenwiese in the Riesengebirge mountains where she hoped to find complete rest.[92] It was there that three decades later she would put an end to her life.

Both Döderlein and Reuss considered the treatment Feo had received in Dresden – the carbonic baths and electrotherapy were intended to 'strengthen the nerves', whereas the injections of arsenic and thorium were prescribed for dermatological problems[93] – to have been a success. Reuss stressed that, although the head of the Dresden clinic had again been a gynaecologist, he had not touched the internal organs, since 'these are in as good an order as can be expected after such a serious operation'.[94] But when Charlotte learnt of her daughter's treatment, she was again appalled. 'I fail totally to understand, besides being *more* than hurt, *never* having heard a word of this dangerous treatment Feo has undergone,' she wrote. 'And to what purpose', she asked, since Feo's 'inside [was] totally ruined?' 'I know these cures as being dangerously poisonous & of no avail, making people *after weeks* ill!'[95]

At Hohenwiese Feo's recovery was painfully slow. From time to time she accompanied her husband to the dilapidated Schloss Neuhoff just a mile away, but often she felt 'bad' and had to stay in bed. Not until the end of 1913, when they had moved into the renovated *Schloss*, did a slight improvement in her mood begin to make life seem tolerable again. 'This being among the living dead . . . was terrible, many many thousand times worse than the whole long period of pain of the earlier years,' she told her grandfather. 'Then one could still enjoy life, in spite of everything, & still had one's old energy. But this has taught me to understand others, & not to condemn out of hand other people with "nerves", & to regard them as lacking in energy & self discipline.'[96]

On 24 January 1914 Feo began to shiver with a high temperature; the local doctor gave her a powder which made her sweat profusely. After three days she 'felt better than I ever had, all last year'. She was sleeping 'like a top', she wrote, '& am happy all day long. Work, work, I *can* work again. Oh, it's such *incredible* joy . . . after the last *beastly* year.' Her husband was astounded by her happy disposition and joked that he would need time to get accustomed to having a fit wife again. He wrote to Döderlein to inform him of Feo's startling recovery, and the doctor was 'radiant', though warning that his patient would still need to avoid all excitement. 'He has been proved right, as always,' she wrote in triumph. On a visit to Berlin she took great pleasure in demonstrating to her royal aunts and uncles, including the Kaiser and Kaiserin, that Döderlein was not a 'spa charlatan', as they had all come to believe.[97] As late as March 1914, Feo was writing to Heldburg from Schloss Neuhoff: 'You can't think . . . *how* I enjoy *every trifle*, now that I am well again. If it *only* remains so, I *never* felt so strong & well in all my life before. Döderlein was right, after all!'[98]

That summer, as the lights went out all over Europe, Feo's private life darkened, too. With the death of her grandfather on 25 June 1914, her parents became the reigning Duke and Duchess of Saxe-Meiningen, but the rift between her and them only grew wider still.[99] Her husband served in the trenches on the Western Front, leaving her alone at Neuhoff, where she opened a small hospital for wounded soldiers. Her husband referred to this as a 'farce' which had not even served to distract her in her loneliness: she dressed up in an attractive matron's uniform but, as soon as problems arose, put herself to bed.[100] Gradually, she slipped into depression and further bouts of illness. 'I have been very ill,' she informed the widowed baroness in one of her rare wartime letters. 'First I had a severe bronchitis with fever, up again for a few days, then that terrible abdominal inflammation with a high temperature that came & went, & *incredible* pains . . . On one of the evenings I thought I wouldn't be able to bear it any longer. Morphine then helped somewhat . . . I was up again for a few days when I had another relapse.'[101]

These repeated attacks in the winter of 1914 finally broke Feo's optimistic spirit. As she wrote to Heldburg on 1 April 1915, in German now that war with England had broken out: 'The three feverish illnesses I had some months ago have brought me to the point of collapse. My stupid nerves don't want to go on any more, I can't do what I want or should. My energy is gone, & there's no point in fighting it . . . The old man doesn't know *how* ill I have been, even before this, & must not find out, otherwise he will worry.'[102] In actual fact, Heinrich Reuss *was* receiving disturbing reports of her depressed condition. She looked despondent, seemed overwhelmed by apathy, was spending far too much time in bed and not eating enough nor even washing herself properly. She had broken off almost all her correspondence and hardly ever saw anyone. A worried niece suggested that she needed to be seen by a psychiatrist.[103] As the war dragged on, Feo went from bad to worse. In May 1915, shortly after her thirty-fifth birthday, she once again became physically ill with a fever that forced her to take to her bed for several weeks; she was shaking and shivering so much that she was barely able to write.[104] She was so melancholic that Reuss – who was now a general – had to tell her that he was in the reserve, whereas in fact he was dangerously exposed in the ferocious fighting on the front line between Lille and Arras.[105] On 16 August 1915, Feo told Heldburg that for several days she had been 'in the claws of a horrid lumbago attack' which had made her 'totally stiff' and was continuing to trouble her.[106]

On 21 October 1915 Feo entered Döderlein's clinic for the fifth time, though her stay on this occasion was brief.[107] Döderlein declared himself 'very satisfied' with her condition and pronounced everything to be 'in good order'. But on her return to Neuhoff she reverted to spending most of the day in bed.[108] Then, in December 1915, she was admitted with 'severe influenza, a high temperature and a tormenting cough' to the Municipal Hospital at Hirschberg, where she was to stay for many months in the care of Dr M. Haedke. Shortly after her admission she developed bad pain on the left side of her stomach.[109]

A week later her pains got even worse. She had, she explained, been given peat baths to cure an inflamed nerve in her abdomen, but this had made her 'horrifically ill' with a temperature of 39.3°C. The pains, she said, were so indescribably severe that Haedke had given her an injection of an opium derivative, Pantapon, which they had found was more effective in her case than morphine. It was at this point that Feo discovered a 'swollen nerve' that stretched like a fine thread along the left stomach wall. With evident relish she now dictated in exact detail the miracle cure that appeared to have mastered her illness at a stroke. When she told Haedke of her 'discovery', he greeted it with enormous interest. 'He found the nerve straight away,' Feo reported triumphantly.

He said he could kill the nerve off, the way the dentist does it, if I agreed. In my joy I cried 'Yes'. 'Very well, then I'll do it tomorrow morning, and without pain. First I'll anaesthetise the skin with Novocain, then I'll inject the Novocain more deeply and anaesthetise the canal right up to the nerve. Finally, with a strong needle some 15 centimetres long . . . I'll enter the canal and kill off the nerve with an injection of alcohol . . . This morning I awoke fresh and alert, temperature 36.23°C, pulse 56, but still in pain. At 11.30 I was carried up into the operating room and the little operation was carried out. I felt only one little pinprick which hurt less than if you prick yourself in the finger while sewing . . . Yet quite suddenly the pains had gone. You can imagine how happy, joyful and thankful I am. I now have simply to lie quietly for three or four days, then I'll be able to get up . . . Soon there will be a perfectly healthy Babes again![110]

As so often in the past, Feo's triumph was premature. On the very next day she was forced to admit that her abdominal pain was worse than ever – 'the nerve', she imagined, was 'rebelling against death'. Haedke gave her another strong Pantapon injection and waited with her, holding her hands, until the drug finally took effect.[111] Though the evidence is ambiguous, her condition appears to have deteriorated further in the following weeks. She was readmitted to the hospital at Hirschberg, from where she reported that, though she had a clear head during the daytime, her temperature rose to over 40°C in the evenings, at which point she began to hallucinate and see 'ghastly things'. Haedke, she said, had pronounced her 'nervous system to be disordered'. Soon she was suffering from 'terrible pains and diarrhoea' as well, followed by 'heart cramps'. She begged Haedke, who diagnosed her as suffering from an irritation of the appendix which he thought could be cured with drugs, to perform an appendectomy, but he not only pronounced that this would be pointless but insisted that her husband should give his consent.[112] Haedke informed Prince Reuss that there were no signs of an inflammation of the appendix, as Feo claimed, and that an operation was wholly unnecessary; her abdominal pains and the high temperature were of a 'purely nervous kind', due solely to her 'hypernervous predisposition'.[113] As the doctor explained to the baroness, begging her to telegraph Reuss at the front to establish his views: 'Whereas a purely objective, medical judgement of the course of the illness and of the patient's present condition not only permits but actually dictates a passive, purely conservative treatment, Her Serene Highness urgently desires the operation and sees in such a step the only way to achieve a permanent cure.'[114] The baroness turned in her dilemma to another *protégée* of hers, Feo's cousin Princess Adelaide of Saxe-Meiningen (Patient A), now married to Prince Adalbert of Prussia, who was herself being treated for strange abdominal pains and lameness at a sanatorium at Bad Neuenahr in the Rhineland, and who answered full of sympathy: 'This is dreadful, the poor, *poor* creature! . . . She is a heroine, your Babes, & what a heroine! . . . I know what it means [to have] an operation in this state! If only Haz could come back, but perhaps the doctor even wouldn't allow [an operation] just now she is so ill?'[115]

Back on the battlefield in France, Reuss was in no mood to consent to an operation he regarded as worse than useless, the product simply of his wife's 'operation mania'.[116] His talks with Haedke had convinced him that Feo was a good-for-nothing, lazy dissembler who preferred to be in hospital because she was better cared for there than at home! 'Her illness consists mainly in complete lack of energy and total apathy,' he claimed unsympathetically in a letter to Heldburg.

> Her high temperature exists purely in her imagination, as Döderlein established long ago and as Haedke now thinks, too. Whenever she takes her own temperature she sometimes records 39°C, but whenever she forgets and someone else takes it she has no fever. When I visited her in the mornings I found her as happy as a lark, smoking, eating and laughing with the nurses, and if I then asked her how her night had been, she would say that she hadn't slept a wink and had had a high temperature. It's the same story with her heart symptoms. Her heart is completely normal, and the symptoms only appear when she is supposed to do something that doesn't suit her. She grossly exaggerates her illnesses and causes me and others quite unnecessary anxiety . . . The deadening of the nerve in the left side of the body, too, was a completely harmless & painless operation which need not have necessitated her staying in bed.

He was sad and angry that she was now back in the hospital at Hirschberg, and convinced that she had readmitted herself solely for her amusement and because she was too lazy to look after herself. Many upper-class German women were proving themselves wholly incapable of coping with the loneliness that war had brought and were spending their days in bed. 'What if we men were to do the same?' he asked.[117] (What indeed? The insane slaughter that was about to commence at Verdun and on the Somme might have been avoided, perhaps.)

In spite of his reservations, Haz grudgingly consented to his wife's operation.[118] Feo's pains had become quite unbearable, '*far* worse than that time with Döderlein, & that was bad *enough*', she contended. On 14 February 1916 she suffered from 'atrocious pains, 39.8°C in the daytime, terrible vomiting'. One night her pain was so severe that 'from 11 o'clock I thought I was going mad'. Haedke, who had been reluctant to the last to give in to her demands, at last agreed that the time had come for 'the knife to speak'. Again, Feo sang his praises. 'He is *so dreadfully* good to me, still warmer than Döderlein, he is the better man. I feel *so* safe in his hands, *no* fear *one bit.*'[119]

The result of the operation seemed to bear out the sceptics who had argued all along that it was unnecessary. The appendix was discovered to be so insignificantly affected that 'the pains of which she complained were in no way commensurate with the medical findings', her husband learnt from Haedke. Under normal circumstances, Feo should have been ready to leave the hospital in early March, 'but I have stopped measuring anything by the yardstick of normality and will let things take their own course, for I have no influence over her any more', Reuss sighed.[120] His demand that for the remainder of the war she should enter a sanatorium where an energetic doctor and good company would provide some mental stimulation was ignored.[121]

One month after the appendectomy Feo was again in great pain, this time from an 'inflammation of the nerves in the back and in the ribs on the right side'. The pains, she said, were so bad that she was unable to move and sometimes cried out loud. She had had, in addition, 'the most dreadful heart cramps, sometimes two or three a day', which had led to a traumatic visit from her parents. Her mother had behaved '*absolutely unbelievably*', refusing to visit the wounded or to distribute her signed photographs in the hospital and thereby causing great resentment among the soldiers and the staff. Feo had suffered 'terrible cramps' as soon as her parents were gone.[122]

By May 1916, however, the princess was back at Neuhoff and claimed to be her 'old self again'.[123] Reuss could hardly believe the dramatic and unprecedented mood swings that were now affecting his wife – she was ecstatic one moment and 'depressed unto death' the next.[124] In June 1916, when he was able to join her at Neuhoff, he reported to the baroness that 'your Babes is really in excellent health . . . She clambered about in the mountains with me for hours, has a wonderful appetite and sleeps well; not the slightest sign of heart or nerves.'[125] In July, while staying with Heldburg at her chalet in the Bavarian Alps, her behaviour was so reckless that both her hostess and her husband came close to despair.[126] Shortly after her return to Neuhoff she was once more laid low for two weeks by 'an internal chill which caused me unspeakable pain with a high fever'.[127] Thereafter she seems to have recovered her good health, at least until the end of the year.[128]

At this point, the correspondence with Baroness Heldburg breaks off abruptly, and we are left completely in the dark until that bleak day in August 1945 when the princess took her own life. At around Christmas 1916, Feo must have said or done something that offended even the infinitely patient old baroness, her mother-substitute for more than twenty years, and as she was too stubborn to apologize, their correspondence simply ceased.[129] But for those twenty years, her letters and those of her husband have enabled us to reconstruct her medical biography in a manner that would have been quite unthinkable had we been dependent on the handful of angry notes she exchanged with her real parents.

Over the decades during which we have been able to follow Feodora's history, a staggering catalogue of explanations for her periodic attacks of debilitating pain were advanced. Migraine, influenza, malaria, venereal disease, anaemia, appendicitis, heart disease, lumbago, cystic degeneration of the ovaries, congenital narrowing of the uterus, uterine colic, copper poisoning, a hyper-nervous predisposition, nervous breakdown and hypochondria were just some of the diagnoses advanced by the medical profession and others close to her. Some of them may indeed have been accurate in the short term, but their very number graphically demonstrates that none of them could stand the test of time, just as none of the attempted remedies – abdominal operations, arsenic-and-thorium pills and injections, carbonic baths, electrotherapy, complete rest in the mountains and so on and so forth – ever brought lasting relief. The pattern of Feo's illness, though slightly different from that suffered by her mother Charlotte and her grandmother Vicky – not least because, unlike them, she insisted that her pains must have an organic cause which could be eliminated through an operation – nevertheless emerges very clearly from our reconstruction. A more precise diagnosis, however, can only be made from an analysis of the patient's DNA.

CHAPTER 9

Ancient DNA

Genetic information that had seemed lost
forever turns out to linger in the remains
of long-dead plants and animals.
Svante Pääbo, Scientific American *November 1993*

A complementary approach to the compelling historical diagnosis
of porphyria within the royal houses of Europe would be to obtain
retrospective genetic evidence of the disease in historical figures
likely to be porphyric. Is this possible in a person long deceased?
Surprisingly, the answer today is yes, as long as some tissue or bone
material from the deceased person still exists. The method that is
used owes much to the pioneering work of a young Swedish
scientist, Svante Pääbo, working in Uppsala in the early 1980s.
Pääbo became intrigued with the possibility of reading the genetic
message, the so-called blueprint for life, in the DNA of extinct
species and in human remains. DNA does survive long after death,
particularly if the body is preserved in some way. Pääbo's initial
attempts with mummies, some from around 2000 years BC, met
with some measure of success – he managed to extract and analyse
the DNA from the mummified remains of a one-year-old Egyptian
boy.[1] He very soon realized, however, that he had a major problem
– only very small amounts of DNA could be recovered, and this was
degraded into very short fragments. Fortunately, a new technique
was just around the corner that would revolutionize molecular
biology and make the study of ancient DNA a reality.

The Polymerase Chain Reaction

The technique is the polymerase chain reaction (PCR), invented by Kary Mullis, a scientist working for the Cetus Corporation in Emeryville, California.[2] What this technique does is to generate billions of copies of a DNA fragment from as little as a single molecule. This is known as 'amplification'. Imagine a colony of bacteria that can grow and divide at will. Two cells will give rise to four, then four to eight, eight to sixteen and so on. After only thirty such cycles of growth and division, the original two cells will have grown to a staggering 2000 million. PCR works in much the same way, except that the cell division step in each cycle is replaced by the division of the normally double-stranded DNA molecule into two single strands (see Appendix for details of the structure of DNA), and the growth phase is the synthesis of a new strand of DNA, using each of the two separated strands as template. The information contained in DNA is encoded by combinations ('sequences') of four 'bases' known as A, C, G and T. It is these sequences of bases that molecular biologists study when comparing DNA from different sources.

Jurassic Park – The Study of Extinct Species

This technique could be used to solve the problem of DNA degradation in ancient tissues, and the study of ancient DNA has now emerged as a powerful approach for understanding the evolutionary relationships between living and extinct species. One example is the moa, a flightless bird that inhabited the islands of New Zealand. These giant birds could attain a height of 3.5 metres and weigh in at over two hundred kilograms. About one thousand years ago, the Polynesians first arrived on the islands and soon hunted them to extinction. Mummified soft tissues and bones of the moa have been found in caves and swamps and these have been used as a source of DNA for amplification. By comparing the sequences of amplified DNA from preserved moa tissue to those of the other flightless bird of New Zealand, the kiwi, it was discovered that, surprisingly, these two species are not closely related.[3] The moa and kiwi must therefore have evolved quite independently and have each separately lost the ability to fly.

The same technique was applied to a 47-thousand-year-old

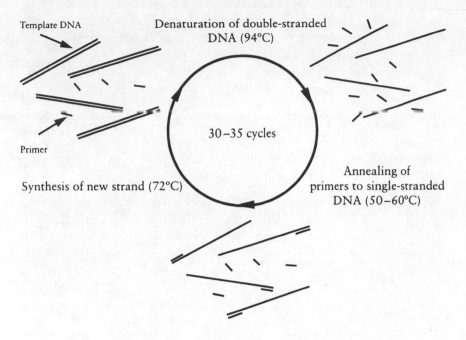

Template DNA

Primer

Denaturation of double-stranded
DNA (94°C)

30–35 cycles

Synthesis of new strand (72°C)

Annealing of
primers to single-stranded
DNA (50–60°C)

Principles of the Polymerase Chain Reaction

woolly mammoth, *Mammuthus primigenius*, found in the perma-frost of the Siberian tundra.[4] From this, DNA was amplified and the sequences compared to those of the Asian and African elephants of today in an attempt to establish which species was most closely related to the mammoth. Unfortunately, the short sequence obtained and the close similarity of all three species gave only an equivocal answer.

Another potential source of DNA from extinct species comes from insects preserved in amber (fossilized tree resin). In this case, however, although the hard exoskeleton of the insects is often remarkably well preserved, at over 20 million years old they are much older than the moa or the woolly mammoth, and the process of DNA degradation will be much more advanced. Nevertheless, some DNA has been amplified from the soft tissue from the preserved bodies of at least five different extinct species of insect.[5]

The isolation and amplification of DNA from insects preserved in amber forms the basis of the book *Jurassic Park* by Michael Crichton, subsequently made into a hit film by Steven Spielberg. The story deals with the regeneration of dinosaurs using DNA isolated from a blood-sucking insect that had supposedly fed, shortly before becoming submerged in tree resin, on dinosaur blood.

In reality, since all dinosaurs died out over 65 million years ago, any surviving DNA would be degraded into extremely short fragments. Notwithstanding this, a report appeared in the American scientific journal *Science* in November 1994 of the amplification of dinosaur DNA extracted from an 80-million-year-old bone fragment.[6] Unfortunately, when compared with other species, it showed closer similarity to the DNA of mammals than birds, the living descendants of the dinosaurs, and was probably of human origin.[7] This highlights a major problem of work with ancient DNA: given that only tiny quantities of DNA can be isolated, the possibility of contamination by DNA from other sources is very high.

A number of successful attempts at isolating and amplifying DNA from human remains have now been reported. One of the most remarkable is the amplification of part of the gene that encodes β-globin, one of the polypeptides that make up haemoglobin, from bone specimens that are up to twelve thousand years old.[8] Other successes include the amplification of DNA from corpses that range in age from seven thousand to over eight thousand years old recovered from a North American burial site at Windover in eastern central Florida,[9] and from the skeletal remains of Fremont Amerindians from the Great Salt Lake wetlands that range from four hundred to over 1300 years old.[10]

The Romanovs – A Case Study

Perhaps the best-known application of ancient DNA analysis to human remains is the identification of the bodies of the Romanovs, the Russian Imperial Family.[11] The final fate of the last Tsar, his wife and children, is largely undocumented but it was believed that Nicholas II, his wife Alexandra, their four daughters Olga, Tatyana, Maria and Anastasia, and their only son, Alexei, were executed, together with three servants and their physician, Dr Evgeny Botkin, by a Bolshevik firing squad in the cellar of Ipatiev House at Ekaterinburg, central Russia, on the morning of 16 July 1918. How their bodies were disposed of is a little uncertain but contemporary reports indicate that they were first transported to an area of old mineworkings in the nearby Koptiaki Woods. The corpses were then tipped down a disused mineshaft and grenades used in an unsuccessful attempt to collapse the shaft. This was, however, far from being a secure burial site, and on the morning of 18 July the Bolsheviks returned with the intention of moving the bodies to a much deeper mine. After the corpses were recovered the truck carrying them to their new burial site became stuck in the muddy roads of the forest. A decision was then taken to burn the bodies and the smallest, that of Alexei, was the first to be placed in the blaze. This was followed by a body identified at the time as that of Alexandra, although by this stage the bodies had been so badly damaged that considerable doubt was later raised. As it became clear that cremation would not destroy the bodies completely, the Bolsheviks finally decided to bury the remains in a shallow pit, no more than four feet in depth, that they dug in the middle of the road. Before dumping the remaining bodies in the grave, however, the corpses were further disfigured by having their faces stove in with rifle butts, and, in a final attempt to disguise the family's identity, sulphuric acid was poured over them.

Few people had witnessed the assassinations and fewer still knew the final resting place of the bodies. It is not surprising, therefore, that considerable doubt over the fate of the family remained. The burial site in Koptiaki Woods was first discovered in 1979 by Alexander Avdonin, a geologist, and Gelli Ryabov, a popular writer of crime stories. For fear of arrest and persecution, Avdonin and Ryabov kept their find a secret until the era of perestroika under President Mikhail Gorbachev. In July 1991, an international team uncovered nine skeletons in the shallow grave. But were these really the remains of the Russian Imperial Family? Using the natural sequence variation of DNA, the presence of a family group plus the remains of unrelated individuals (the servants and a doctor) was established, but proving individual identities was more complicated.[12] The sex of each skeleton was established by amplifying the DNA of a gene (amelogenin) that is present on both the X and Y sex chromosomes but differs in size. However, DNA is not limited to the nucleus of a cell but is also found in another cell organelle, the mitochondria, the so-called powerhouse of the cell. The unique feature of mitochondrial DNA is that it is inherited only from the mother; like nuclear DNA, it shows sequence variation that can be used to establish the pattern of inheritance, although in this case only through the maternal line.

The mitochondrial DNA of three living relatives of the Romanovs was used to determine whether the bodies in the Ekaterinburg grave possessed particular sequence variants that would establish a family relationship. One of the volunteers was HRH Prince Philip, the Duke of Edinburgh, who is a great-nephew of the Tsarina Alexandra via an unbroken maternal descent. The other two were descendants, again by unbroken maternal lines, from the Tsar's maternal grandmother, Louise of Hesse-Kassel. In all three cases, there was sufficient sequence identity with the mitochondrial DNA of the family group in the Ekaterinburg grave to confirm the probable identity of the bodies as those of the Tsar and his family.

The story does not end there, however. As long ago as the early 1920s, a woman called Anna Anderson had claimed to be the Grand Duchess Anastasia, and so began an investigation of passion and intrigue that continued well beyond her death in February 1984. Two bodies were missing from the grave at Ekaterinburg. Alexei's corpse was destroyed on the pyre, but it was not certain whether the second body disposed of in this way was Alexandra, Anastasia, or even the maid Anna Demidova. Could DNA analysis also authenticate Anderson's claim to be Anastasia, or eliminate her as a claimant by showing a lack of identity at the molecular level?

Anna Anderson's story began inauspiciously in Berlin in 1920, where she was admitted into a mental hospital after jumping off the Bendler Bridge into the Landwehr Canal. She refused to answer any questions about her identity and, after six weeks, she was removed to the Dalldorf lunatic asylum where she spent the next two years. The first claim that Anna Anderson was the Grand Duchess Anastasia, the sole survivor of the massacre of the Romanov family, came not from her but from another inmate of the asylum, Clara Peuthert, on her release in January 1922. The case was to occupy the world press, the historical profession and the legal system for the next six decades, not least because a claim to quite fabulous wealth was involved.

After Anna Anderson's death in 1984, any attempt at identification would have to rely on DNA evidence. She had been admitted into the Martha Jefferson Hospital in Charlottesville, Virginia, in 1979 to have a bowel operation, and small tissue samples were removed for histological analysis. These were fixed with formaldehyde, the conventional method for preserving tissue structure, and embedded in paraffin wax for the preparation of thin sections that could be viewed under a microscope. DNA is also preserved under these conditions. After extensive legal wrangles by representatives of the Russian Nobility Association and the supporters of Anna Anderson over the ownership of the specimens, two teams of scientists, one from the Forensic Science Service in the UK and the other from the Armed Forces DNA Identification Laboratory in the USA, undertook a series of tests on the bowel DNA and on DNA from six head hairs of Anna Anderson. The tests were designed to determine once and for all whether she was related to the Russian Imperial Family.

Mitochondrial DNA was used to look for a maternal link to the Tsarina by comparing the DNA sequence of Anna Anderson with that of the Duke of Edinburgh.[13] As shown in the following table, Anna Anderson's bowel and hair samples both gave the same result: her mitochondrial DNA sequence differed at six places from that of Prince Philip. It is highly improbable that Tsarina Alexandra was the mother of Anna Anderson.

Mitochondrial DNA Sequence Polymorphisms							
Origin of sample	DNA source	Position within mitochondrial DNA					
		16111	16126	16266	16294	16304	16357
Duke of Edinburgh	Blood sample	T	T	C	C	T	C
Anna Anderson	Bowel sample	C	C	T	T	C	T
Anna Anderson	Hair sample	C	C	T	T	C	T
Great-nephew of Franziska Schanzkowska	Blood sample	C	C	T	T	C	T

A second test used the presence of variable sequences in nuclear DNA to determine whether Anna Anderson could be the child of the Tsar and Tsarina. These sequences, called short tandem repeats

(STRs), are passed from parents to offspring in a normal Mendelian fashion, that is, one copy from the mother and one from the father. By comparing five STRs in Anna Anderson's DNA with those in the DNA of the Tsar and Tsarina, it became clear that Anna Anderson could not have been the Grand Duchess Anastasia. The romantic notion that Anastasia had somehow avoided the executioner in 1918 was therefore dispelled.

Size Variation in STRs					
	Tsar Nicholas		Tsarina Alexandra		Anna Anderson	
VWA	15	16	15	16	<u>14</u>	16
TH01	7	9.3	8	8	<u>7</u>	<u>9.3</u>
F13A1	7	7	3.2	5	3.2	7
FES/FPS	12	12	12	13	<u>11</u>	12
ACTBP2	11	32	32	36	15	<u>18</u>

The STRs that show that Anna Anderson could not be the daughter of the Tsar and Tsarina are underlined

Who then *was* Anna Anderson? Once again, DNA evidence can provide us with a clue. Soon after Anna first claimed to be Anastasia, a private detective hired by the Grand Duke of Hesse-Darmstadt, the brother of Tsarina Alexandra, had suggested that she was probably Franziska Schanzkowska, a Polish factory worker born around 1896 who had lived in Pomerania in north-eastern Germany. She had worked in a munitions factory in Berlin where she had been injured in an explosion. After admission to two mental hospitals, she disappeared in 1920, around the same time as the first appearance of Anna Anderson. A great-nephew of Franziska Schanzkowska, a man named Carl Maucher, was traced and a DNA test carried out on him. His mitochondrial DNA matches that of Anna's at all six positions where Anna's differs from that of the Duke of Edinburgh. This result therefore supports but does not prove the notion that Anna Anderson was Franziska Schanzkowska. A further twist to the tale is that Felix Schanzkowski failed to identify Anna Anderson as his sister in 1927 and again in 1938, this time along with his brother and sisters. Whether Anna Anderson was the lost Franziska Schanzkowska remains uncertain to this day. The entire episode does, however, provide an example of an important principle: DNA analysis can rule out relatedness if none exists, but it cannot prove that a relationship exists.

Mutation Detection in Ancient DNA

In this account of the analysis of ancient DNA, we have so far only looked at normal variation in the sequence of DNA. Porphyria, however, is a genetic disorder and, since the underlying defect in all inherited disease is a change in the DNA blueprint, the methodologies of ancient DNA analysis can be used to look for a change in the DNA that is responsible for an inherited disease. So far, however, this has been achieved only once. We refer to the work of David Hunt, one of the authors of this book, in collaboration with Dr John Mollon, a psychologist at the University of Cambridge.

The subject of their study was the celebrated British physicist and chemist John Dalton. Dalton's most important contribution to science was his theory that matter is composed of atoms of differing weights that combine in simple ratios. This atomic theory, which Dalton first advanced in 1803, is the cornerstone of modern physical science. A few years before this, in 1794, he had presented a paper to the Manchester Literary and Philosophical Society on what we now know as red-green colour blindness, a condition from which Dalton himself suffered.[14] His paper was the first detailed description of this form of colour blindness and, as a direct result, the condition is now known as daltonism in languages as diverse as Spanish and Russian.

Some form of red-green colour blindness afflicts about 7 per cent of all men but only about 0.5 per cent of women. The reason for this difference is that the genes that underlie this disorder, the genes that specify the visual pigments, are on the X chromosome. For a woman to have the disorder, she must inherit two X chromosomes with defective genes, one from her mother and the other from her father, whereas a man needs to have only a single defective X chromosome inherited from his mother.

John Dalton's explanation for his own colour vision defect, namely that his eyes must contain a blue filter, was to prove controversial. In the hope of settling the controversy at some later stage, John Dalton instructed his medical attendant, Joseph Ransome, to remove his eyes on his death so that the 'blue filter' might be observed. He died on 27 July 1824, and his eyes were duly removed and dissected, but no filter was found. However, the remains of one eye was placed between two watch-glasses. It subsequently passed into the possession of the Manchester Literary and Philosophical Society and survives to this day in the care of the Manchester Museum of Science and Industry.

The opportunity therefore existed to carry out the first retrospective diagnosis of a genetic disease using ancient DNA techniques on a historical character with a well-characterized disorder. Humans have three colour vision genes which have been assigned to the perception of red, green and blue light. The type of colour blindness that afflicted Dalton arises from the absence of either the red or the green visual pigment gene on the X chromosome. He was therefore a 'dichromat', but was it the red or the green photoreceptor that was absent from his retina? Permission was granted by the Manchester Literary and Philosophical Society for small samples to be taken from the dried eye tissue,* although these were to be kept to a minimum so as not to damage the eye (a curious stipulation for a specimen that had already suffered the ravages of time and now resembled a hard dried prune). These small fragments proved sufficient for the task and the DNA of John Dalton's visual pigment genes was successfully amplified. The resulting gene fragments were fully analysed in order to determine whether one or other of the red or green genes was missing.[15]

The results of five different tests were all consistent in showing that Dalton completely lacked the gene for the green visual pigment. Could these molecular findings be reconciled with the historical accounts of his defect? Two contemporaries of Dalton, the physicists Sir John Herschel and Sir David Brewster, had each questioned him and both reported that he did not see the spectrum as foreshortened at long wavelengths, as expected in a dichromat who lacks the long-wave red receptor,[16] and the scientific publisher Richard Taylor records in a footnote of 1846 that 'Dr Dalton has never stated that the spectrum he saw was *shorter* than the spectrum seen by others'. In other words, although the green visual

---

* It is perhaps worth pointing out that *any* surviving tissue, and not just that from the eyes, could have been used since all cells of the body contain the same DNA.

pigment was absent from John Dalton's retina, the presence of the red visual pigment meant that he was sensitive to the same part of the spectrum as people with normal colour vision. Within this spectral range however, his perception of colours was inferior, particularly in the red/green region.

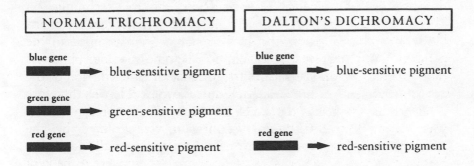

Molecular Basis of Normal Trichromatic and Dichromatic Colour Vision

The work on John Dalton's DNA demonstrates the power of ancient DNA analysis not only to identify the presence of a genetic defect but also precisely to classify a disorder.

CHAPTER 10

Blood and Bones:
The Search for the Royal Mutation

To prove the diagnosis, the physician today
would examine urine and stool for the
characteristic abnormal constituents. This is, of
course, not possible for George III . . .
Ida Macalpine and Richard Hunter, 1969

DNA analysis would clearly give us the information that we needed about porphyria in the Royal Family, but where could we obtain suitable samples? George III lies buried in St George's Chapel in Windsor and, although we fleetingly considered asking for permission to exhume him, the possibility seemed very remote that it would be granted. Since we are dealing with an inherited disorder, however, the defective gene, if there is one, will obviously also be present in at least some of George III's relatives. Our course of action was therefore very clear: if we wanted to prove beyond reasonable doubt that porphyria was and perhaps still is present in the royal houses of Europe, then we needed to find a relic from either an ancestor or a descendant of George III's who had a medical history suggestive of porphyria, and to subject that remnant to DNA analysis. But where could such relics be obtained? Three possibilities presented themselves.

King Charles I and His Ancestors

In the course of their research on George III, as we have seen, Macalpine and Hunter discovered strong evidence of porphyria in James I and VI, the son of Mary Queen of Scots by her second husband, Henry Stewart, Lord Darnley. Mary herself is described as 'one of the great invalids of history'. She almost certainly suffered from gastric ulcers, rheumatism and hysteria, and from her late teens she had frequent bouts of abdominal pain, lameness, fits and mental disturbance, a combination of symptoms which is itself suggestive of porphyria. She suffered two serious attacks, one in 1566 when she was twenty-four years old and the second in 1570. In both cases, she developed an excruciating pain in her side, vomited continuously, became delirious with fits, and even lost her sight and power of speech. She eventually lost consciousness and was thought for a time to be dead.[1] One interpretation that has been put on her symptoms is that she suffered from a gastric ulcer. However, in her authoritative biography of Mary, Antonia Fraser states that 'It certainly seems far easier to relate these symptoms [of porphyria] rather than those of gastric ulcer,'[2] to the case of Mary. There is no recorded suggestion that Mary's urine had the tell-tale discoloration of porphyria, but this was certainly the case with her son, James I and VI, who, according to the detailed notes made by his doctor Sir Theodore Turquet de Mayerne (1573–1655) in 1613, often 'likened the colour of his urine to the dark red colour of Alicante wine'.

James I was a sorrowful ruler who 'exhibited to the world stammering, slobbering, shedding unmanly tears, trembling at a drawn sword, and talking in the style alternately of a buffoon and a pedagogue'.[3] Although the New Zealand medical historian A. W. Beasley prefers the diagnosis of cerebral palsy for James's condition, even he is forced to suggest that the Stuart monarch must have been suffering from porphyria as well, as only this illness would account for the reports of flatus, vomiting, severe abdominal colic and black-red urine.[4] It is significant that many of these symptoms were also present in his mother.

James I died in 1625 and was succeeded by his second son, Charles I (1600–49). There is no evidence that Charles himself suffered from porphyria, but the symptoms of his father and grandmother returned to plague his youngest daughter, Henrietta Anne, Duchess of Orleans (1644–70). She suffered a number of mild attacks of colic, vomiting, indigestion, headache and mood changes and died unexpectedly at the age of twenty-six after a short illness, the main features of which were severe abdominal pain, vomiting, respiratory weakness, incontinence and coma.[5]

The evidence for porphyria in the lineage from Mary Queen of Scots to Henrietta Anne is therefore quite compelling, with only Charles I showing no signs of the disease. However, if the diagnosis of porphyria in his daughter is correct, then Charles must be one of the many cases where the defective gene was present but asymptomatic.

Charles I was certainly a controversial character. He was embroiled for much of his reign in disputes with Parliament that culminated in 1642 in the Civil War between the parliamentary forces, the Roundheads, and the forces loyal to the King, the Cavaliers. Charles gave himself up to the Scottish Army in 1646 but was delivered to the English Parliament in June of the following year. He was eventually tried as a tyrant, murderer and enemy of the nation in 1649, convicted and sentenced to death. He was executed by beheading at Whitehall on 30 January 1649. It is inevitable that the clothing worn by Charles at his execution would have been heavily bloodstained, and such soiled garments would have been removed from his personage at burial. If any such garments could be found, we reasoned, perhaps in a collection of the King's relics, then we would have a potential source of Charles I's DNA.

One of the many advantages of working in the collegial atmosphere of the British university system is that colleagues are frequently a mine of amazing information. A chance conversation between John Röhl and Dr John Gurney, a fellow historian at the University of Sussex, on the possibility of finding a useful royal relic brought the immediate response that the shroud in which Charles I was wrapped after his execution was kept only a few miles from the university at Ashburnham Place, a stately house in a hamlet just a few miles west of Battle, Sussex.

John Ashburnham and his brother William were loyal servants of Charles I, and it was John who acquired the relics of Charles, which included the linen shirt worn by the king on the scaffold. It was John Ashburnham's wish that these items be bequeathed 'to those persons to whom the Manor of Ashburnham shall descend'.

We presented ourselves at the house on the afternoon of 22 January 1996 and were given the privilege of seeing the relics. They are contained in a glass display case, neatly folded to show each item. On closer examination, they appeared much as they had been described in 1888 by the Reverend Rose Fuller Whistler, the then Vicar of Ashburnham, as consisting of a watch with ribbon; a shirt marked with the initials C. R. in small red characters and an embroidered crown; a pair of silk undergarments; and a sheet which had purportedly been thrown over the King's body after he was beheaded. The Revd Whistler had reported in 1888 that bloodstains were still apparent on the sheet.[6] More than a hundred years later, we could see that a number of very faint stains of uneven outline were still present. In places, they appeared to be splash marks. We soaked a number of the stained patches in a DNA extraction solution, taking care not to handle the cloth directly. Samples were also taken from unstained regions of the cloth to provide a means of assessing the level of background contamination.

We were now left with a number of imponderables. Were these really the garments Charles I had worn at his execution in 1649? How many others had handled (and possibly contaminated) the items over the intervening centuries? We knew that getting DNA from these samples would not be an easy task, although preliminary tests did give a positive result. But, such difficulties apart, we now had our first ancient royal sample.

The Bones of Princess Feodora

A major breakthrough in our quest for samples came in late 1995, when we discovered that Princess Feodora of Reuss was buried near the small town of Kowary in present-day Poland. In order to obtain the samples that we needed for our tests, two obstacles needed to be overcome: we had to establish the exact location of Feodora's grave, and obtain permission to exhume her remains. To expedite the former, we contacted the Burgomaster of Kowary, Marek Jiruska, suggesting that he place an article in the local newspaper explaining our interest in the descendants of Queen Victoria (but carefully avoiding any mention of porphyria). In this way, we hoped to jog local memories and find someone who recalled the circumstances of the princess's death. We also wrote to Professor Julian Kornobis, an expert in forensic medicine at the University of Wroclaw, asking for his help, as a colleague, in securing permission for the exhumation. In this letter, we explained the nature of our interest and invited him to join us as a collaborator in our research. We received no reply – and were soon to realize that approaching Professor Kornobis had been a grave mistake.

In late July 1996, the Burgomaster contacted us to say that placing an article in the local press would not, in his view, be the best way to proceed, as it would only revive earlier rumours that the princess's grave contained buried treasure. He had, however, made discreet enquiries and now had information on both the location of Feodora's grave and the circumstances surrounding her death. Most important of all, he was willing for us to proceed with the exhumation. We made arrangements to travel to Poland as soon as possible. Just before we left, however, we received the disturbing news that a professor from the Institute of Forensic Science at Wroclaw University, together with several of his assistants, had arrived in Kowary with a warrant demanding to be shown the location of Princess Feodora's grave. We could only surmise that the professor, whose name was Tadeusz Dobosz, had learnt of our intentions from the letter we had written earlier to Professor Kornobis. There was worse news to come: the team from Wroclaw had opened the grave and removed skeletal remains that included a jawbone containing a gold tooth, a piece of pelvis with some tissue still attached, and a number of smaller bones. This had happened while the Burgomaster was away from Kowary, so no detailed record of exactly what had been recovered from the grave was kept. There were yet more complications to come, however, for it now emerged that Feodora's grave had been opened and vandalized by would-be grave robbers on a number of occasions since 1945. It also seemed possible that, in the catastrophic circumstances of 1945, she had not received a proper burial. There was, we were warned, no coffin and no skeleton as such. To protect the grave from further inquisitive visitors, a stone slab had now been placed over it.

Fortunately for us, Burgomaster Jiruska was staunchly on our side and had succeeded in having everything returned from Wroclaw to Kowary. When we arrived, he told us that he had persuaded Professor Dobosz and his team to return the remains by intimating that 'the family in England was dismayed by the news that Feodora's remains had been removed to Wroclaw'. The reference to the British Royal Family and the implied threat of an international incident, however improbable, had had the desired effect.

Our first opportunity to visit the grave site came in the late afternoon of 19 August 1996. We had expected to find a normal, earth-dug grave with a temporary stone covering, but instead the grave turned out to be a very solid double vault, built with bricks into the top of a large mound. Both Feodora and her husband Prince Heinrich, who died in 1939, had been buried there, hence the two vaults. The burial site was certainly no temporary resting place but a purpose-built family grave. These were worrying discrepancies between the information that had been passed to us before we left England and the sight that now met our eyes.

The grave consisted of two interconnecting vaults, one presumably for Feodora and the other for her husband, with a large stone slab covering each entrance, both of them unmarked. The slab that covered the left-hand grave was undamaged but the other slab had been chipped and broken at one corner, sure signs that the grave had been opened many times before. An intensive search unearthed a few oddments only – some fragments of bone later identified as a rib and part of a femur, together with some metal artefacts that looked like handles and rests from a coffin. Since Feodora had been buried without a proper coffin, we surmised that these were probably from her husband's casket. For all these reasons, then, the results of the exhumation which had taken so much trouble to arrange were meagre and extremely disappointing. But what of the bones that had been returned from Wroclaw? Burgomaster Jiruska had brought one box with him containing a number of bones, neatly labelled and bagged. The jawbone with the gold tooth was certainly there, together with the fragment of pelvis with soft tissue attached. We were told of a second box, but this was said to contain just metal objects, probably from the coffin. However, when we eventually got the opportunity to inspect this box ourselves, we found that, in addition to the metal artefacts, it contained several long bones, which seemed much more promising. Both boxes were put into the boot of one of the cars for later sampling.

The final task was to take samples from the bones. With a disposable hacksaw blade we cut segments from each bone and, where possible, material was also scraped from the internal marrow cavity. As expected, some bones were represented twice, evidence that we were dealing with at least two skeletons, although many bones were clearly missing, presumably as a result of grave-robbing over the years.

Our main concern, as we returned to England with our unusual cargo, was whether the bones from which we had taken samples really were Feodora's. In view of all the confusion at the time of the burial and later, and not least in the foregoing few weeks, the provenance of our evidence was unfortunately less than assured. We were now more determined than ever to explore other avenues for the collection of samples.

The Grave of Princess Charlotte

As documented in Chapter 7, it was the letters of Feodora's mother Princess Charlotte of Saxe-Meiningen to her physician Professor Schweninger that first alerted us to the possible presence of porphyria in the German Imperial Family. Charlotte, granddaughter to Queen Victoria and sister to the last Kaiser, died on 1 October 1919 in Baden-Baden in south-western Germany, but there was no record of her being buried there. The trail leading to her grave was far from easy to follow. Indeed, at one stage we nearly abandoned all hope of ever finding it, as we were informed that the family crypt which was the burial place of the Dukes and Duchesses of Saxe-Meiningen for centuries had been opened in 1977. The Communist authorities, we were told, had incinerated all the ducal remains and then buried the ashes in an unmarked mass grave in the municipal cemetery.

The records of the cemetery revealed that eleven bodies had been taken from the crypt for reburial in 1977, but the names of Princess Charlotte and her husband Duke Bernhard III of Saxe-Meiningen were not among them. Further enquiries established that neither Charlotte nor Bernhard had ever been buried in the Meiningen crypt. Instead, they had chosen the grounds of their favourite castle, Schloss Altenstein, some thirty kilometres to the north of Meiningen, just outside the tiny resort of Bad Liebenstein, as their final resting place. The grave was located on a hill overlooking the beautiful little *Schloss*. Charlotte and her husband were buried in separate vaults, each covered with a massive stone slab. Both graves were inscribed and wonderfully intact, but the chance of obtaining permission to move the stone slabs and examine the remains seemed very remote.

Undaunted by this seemingly insurmountable difficulty, we approached the Thuringian authorities. Their answer was enlightened and co-operative: they accepted the scientific legitimacy and public interest of our enquiry, they replied, but they were bound by law to secure the written permission of living descendants before an exhumation could take place. We in turn explained that, since Charlotte had only had one child, Feodora, who in turn had died by her own hand without issue in 1945 (we were able to submit a copy of her death certificate), there were no living descendants for us to approach. On 12 May 1997, we finally received permission for the exhumation to proceed when the authorities decided that the ducal grave at Schloss Altenstein was in any case due for a thorough routine inspection.[7]

The date for the exhumation was set for the morning of Friday, 4 July 1997. By the time we arrived at the graveside in Altenstein, about a dozen officials and workmen were busily inspecting and repairing the grave. Heavy lifting gear had been used to move the stone slab – weighing over three tons – covering Charlotte's grave. The vault was around five feet in depth, with the metal lining of the coffin – intact except for some water damage at one point near the top – raised slightly from the bottom on supports. The wooden outer casket had rotted away completely, but a regimental banner from the 1870–1 Franco–Prussian War with its emblem of the cross of the Teutonic Knights had survived the passage of time, and remained dramatically draped over the coffin.

The water-damaged area was used as our point of entry and a six-inch-square hole was cut by an expert craftsman, sufficient to examine the body with the aid of a flashlight. The skeleton was completely intact; no soft tissue remained but Charlotte's funeral dress was still present and the stems of a flower posy that had been placed in her hands could still be seen. The left femur was carefully extricated from the skeleton and removed from the coffin. Samples were collected from a wedge-shaped cut made in the top of the bone, from the marrow cavity, and from a drill hole made in the knee joint. Finger digits were scattered in the midriff region where they had fallen, and two of these were also taken for analysis.

DNA *Sequence Analysis*

Of the three 'royal' samples we were able to collect, we can be confident of the authenticity of only one, the bone samples from Princess Charlotte's grave. The sheet at Ashburnham, although purportedly the shroud in which the body of King Charles I had been wrapped, was not otherwise authenticated, and we remain uncertain about the true identity of the bones from Princess Feodora's grave since it had clearly been disturbed many times over the years and the bones that we sampled had been collected not by us but by the team from the University of Wroclaw.

The method we adopted for extracting DNA from our collection of bone samples involved an initial and very careful cleaning of the outer surface to remove all traces of soil and any contaminating DNA from contact by others, although, in the case of Princess Charlotte, such contamination is not possible since her remains have been undisturbed until her grave was opened for repair and maintenance in our presence in July 1997. The task of extracting DNA is made more difficult by the age of the material which, although not old by ancient DNA standards, is nevertheless, in the case of Princess Charlotte, nearly eighty years old. DNA is a robust molecule but it does degrade into ever shorter pieces. The rate of this process seems to be unpredictable but may be accelerated by humid conditions. Feodora's grave was very damp and, as could be seen from damage to the slab that covered the grave, it had clearly been opened many times in the past. In contrast, Charlotte's grave was in relatively good condition and had remained sealed since her burial in 1919.

Bone samples were reduced to a fine powder by the rasping action of either a small hacksaw blade or a grinding bit in an electric drill. The powder was then extracted using standard methods. As is often the case with ancient samples, no DNA could actually be seen during this extraction process. PCR is, however, an extremely sensitive technique that will amplify a product from the tiniest amount of starting DNA template. As explained in Chapter 9, if operating at maximum efficiency PCR will generate millions of copies from each starting strand of DNA. This also means that the smallest contamination from the handling of material both before and after extraction may give erroneous results. In all our procedures, we took all possible precautions to avoid contamination. All PCRs were set up in an uncontaminated area of the laboratory and all reagents and equipment used in preparing and measuring the solutions were continuously monitored for contamination.

The Romanov study identified twelve positions in the 'D-loop region' of the mitochondrial DNA that are identical in all maternal line descendants from Queen Victoria.[8] We limited our study to three of these, at positions 16111, 16126 and 16169, since a difference at any site would be sufficient for us to conclude that the particular bone sample did not originally come from one or other of the royal princesses. As we have seen, mitochondrial DNA can be used to establish family relationships so long as there is a continuous maternal line of descent. Tsarina Alexandra and Princess Charlotte were first cousins and, more importantly, they were both daughters of Queen Victoria's daughters: Alexandra was the daughter of Princess Alice (1843–78) and Charlotte was the daughter of Princess Victoria (1840–1901). Alexandra, Charlotte and Charlotte's daughter, Feodora, would all have inherited the same mitochondrial DNA from Queen Victoria. Prince Philip is a great-nephew of the Tsarina via an unbroken maternal descent: hence the value of the information in the Romanov study.

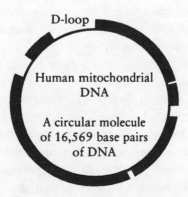

D-loop

Human mitochondrial DNA

A circular molecule of 16,569 base pairs of DNA

As anticipated from the condition of the two graves, amplification of mitochondrial DNA from the bones collected from Charlotte's grave proved to be more straightforward than with those from Feodora's. Nevertheless, an amplified product was eventually obtained from both and this was sequenced using standard methods. The bases at the three key sites, compared to the corresponding sequence of the Duke of Edinburgh's DNA, are as follows.

Origin of sample	Sites in mitochondrial DNA		
	16111	16126	16169
Princess Charlotte's grave	T	T	C
Princess Feodora's grave	C	T	C
HRH Duke of Edinburgh	T	T	C

The important site is 16111. As expected, Princess Charlotte and the Duke of Edinburgh are identical, whereas the DNA extracted from the bones recovered from Princess Feodora's grave gave a different result. We can only conclude therefore that the latter samples are not from Princess Feodora. Whether they are from her husband, who was buried in the same grave, or from some other source, must remain unresolved.

The mitochondrial DNA result from Princess Charlotte's bones meant that we could proceed in our search for a porphyria mutation in her DNA secure in the knowledge that the bones belonged to Princess Charlotte.

Genetic Basis for Porphyria

As detailed in the Preface, the porphyrias are a group of diseases that primarily affect the production of haem, a critical component of the oxygen-carrying blood protein, haemoglobin. Prior to the major advances in recent years in molecular genetics that have revolutionized the study of inherited diseases, the only way of demonstrating the presence of porphyria in an individual was to measure either the activity in blood samples of the enzymes involved in the production of haem, or the excessive accumulation in stool samples of metabolic intermediates from the haem biosynthetic pathway. Diagnosis was limited therefore to the living, and a retrospective diagnosis from the remains of a deceased person was impossible. Modern techniques of molecular biology have changed all that.

In their original paper published in 1966, Macalpine and Hunter suggested the diagnosis of acute intermittent porphyria (AIP) to account for the disorder that afflicted George III but, largely as a result of Rimington's influence, they changed the diagnosis in their later 1968 report to variegate porphyria (VP). The genetic basis for these two diseases is now understood and, in view of the doubt over the diagnosis, we chose to test for the presence of both diseases in Princess Charlotte's DNA.

A reduction in the level of the enzyme protoporphyrinogen oxidase (PPOX) has been known for some time to be the cause of VP. This is the penultimate enzyme in the haem biosynthetic pathway and accounts for the excessive accumulation and excretion of protoporphyrin in affected individuals. The report of the identification of the PPOX gene appeared as recently as 1995.[9] The gene consists of 5751 base pairs of DNA and, like many genes, the sequence is subdivided into alternate protein-determining regions (exons) and non-coding regions (introns) which do not contribute to the making of the protein. In the case of PPOX, the gene is interrupted by thirteen introns to give a total of fourteen exons.[10] Since this initial discovery, seven mutations have been discovered in different families suffering from VP, one in exon 2, two in exon 3, and one each in exons 6, 7, 10, and 13.[11]

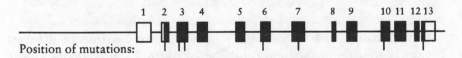

Position of mutations:

The open boxed regions indicate transcribed exons or part of exons that do not contribute to the protein

Structure of the PPOX gene showing numbered exons, separated by introns, and position of known mutations

Mutations in porphobilinogen deaminase (PBGD), the third enzyme in the haem biosynthetic pathway, are responsible for AIP. It is around ten thousand base pairs in length and composed of 13 exons, flanked, as in PPOX, by introns. By late 1996, over sixty different mutations had been identified.[12]

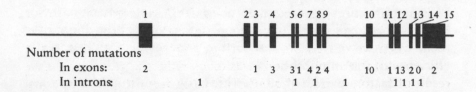

Structure of the PBGD gene showing numbered exons, separated by introns, and position of known mutations

Sequencing of the PPOX and PBGD Genes

If either VP or AIP is present in the royal families of Europe, it most likely arose from a single mutation that has been passed on from generation to generation, frequently through asymptomatic carriers. We would therefore expect to find the same mutation in all affected individuals. As detailed in the previous chapter, the identification of a genetic mutation in ancient DNA that is responsible for an inherited disease has so far been achieved only once, namely the absence of the green visual pigment gene as the cause of John Dalton's colour blindness. In the present case, we are looking not for the *absence* of a gene but for a base change in the sequence of a gene. This is therefore a much more difficult endeavour since, in essence, we are looking for a small typographical error rather than a complete deletion, and the task is made more complicated in the present case by the multiple coding and non-coding regions, the exons and introns, of the PPOX and PBGD genes. Since ancient DNA is usually at least partly degraded, we can expect to amplify only small sections of DNA at a time, requiring a large number of different PCR amplifications and, unless the reagents and conditions used in each PCR amplification are exactly suited to the ancient DNA template, little or no amplification will take place.

The laborious process of amplifying the PPOX and PBGD genes, exon by exon, from extracts of Charlotte's bones was carried out by Dr Anna Evans in the laboratory at University College London. So that the complete sequence of each exon could be obtained, the amplified region included part of the two flanking introns. Each PCR amplification was optimized using DNA isolated from a fresh blood sample collected from a non-diseased normal person. Even then, when we moved on to Charlotte's DNA, we found that the efficiency of the amplifications was much reduced, presumably as a result of factors extracted along with DNA from the decomposing bone tissue. This meant that on most occasions no amplified DNA could be seen at the end of the initial PCR, and the process had to be repeated using a small quantity of the first PCR solution before any product could be visualized. If present, the amplified DNA was then sequenced using standard methods, details of which are beyond the scope of this book.

Since the symptoms described by all of our royal patients fit better with VP than with AIP, we concentrated our efforts on amplifying PPOX, the gene for VP. In fact, due to limited time, the analysis of PBGD, the gene responsible for AIP, was restricted to only a few exons and no mutations were found. We started our investigation of the PPOX gene by looking at those exons where mutations had previously been reported, since it is not uncommon to find that the same disease-causing mutations are widely spread in the population. At the time of this work, these were exons 2, 3, 6, 7, 10 and 13. After overcoming the considerable difficulties of obtaining an amplified product, each of these exons from Charlotte's DNA was sequenced. Unfortunately, no mutations were found.

The analysis was then enlarged to include the remaining exons, with the exception of exon 1 which does not contribute to the PPOX protein and is less likely therefore to contain a disease-causing mutation. This left six exons for us to work through systematically. Exons 5 and 11 proved impossible to amplify from Charlotte's DNA. For reasons that are not entirely clear, these two exons are difficult to amplify even from DNA isolated from fresh blood. The four remaining exon fragments were successfully amplified and sequenced. To our great excitement, sequencing revealed a mutation in one of these, the exon 8 fragment. The change, a T to C substitution, is, however, not in the exon itself but eighteen bases into the adjoining intron. Nevertheless, any change within the first twenty bases of an exon/intron boundary must be considered a serious candidate for a disease-causing mutation.

Boundary of exon 8 with intron 8
The T to C substitution in Charlotte's gene is underlined

	Exon 8	Intron 8
Normal sequence	-AGCTTCAG ‖	GTAATGGAATAGCCACCTTCC-
Charlotte's sequence	-AGCTTCAG ‖	GTAATGGAATAGCCACCCTCC-

When the DNA products from PCR are analysed by separation in an electric field they usually give a single band representing a single product. However, PCR amplificaton from DNA that contains one normal and one mutant gene (as found in the DNA from a person with a dominant disease) sometimes gives two bands when separated in this way. Satisfactorily for us, analysis of exon 8 of the PPOX gene amplified from Charlotte's DNA resulted in the appearance of two bands.

As detailed in Chapter 9, DNA sequences are inherently variable; it is this variability that provided the basis for example of the identification of the Romanovs in the grave in Ekaterinburg and for dismissing Anna Anderson's claim to be the Princess Anastasia. Even for genes like PPOX that specify proteins, on average about one base in every thousand differs between unrelated individuals. These differences or 'polymorphisms' mostly do not cause any change in the resulting protein (they are called silent substitutions), they are generally without deleterious effects, and each occurs at a frequency of more than 1 per cent. It is possible therefore that the change identified in Charlotte's DNA is such a natural variation. To answer this, we screened the DNA from over a hundred unrelated normal individuals (equivalent to over 200 genes) for the mutation but none were found to possess this change. The mutation in Charlotte's DNA is not therefore a commonly found variation.

Is it sufficient, however, to cause VP? As explained earlier, intron regions of genes do not contribute to the amino acid sequence of the protein but are removed by a process that simultaneously deletes the introns and joins (splices) the exons together. This must be done very precisely since the failure to remove all or part of an intron or the inadvertent removal of all or part of an exon, will be catastrophic for the protein. The signals that determine the position of each splice are contained in the DNA sequence at the exon-intron boundary. The first six bases within the intron are critical for correct splicing, but there is evidence from mutations in a number of genes that changes in the sequence beyond this can result in inherited disease. In AIP, for example, a mutation more than twenty bases into an intron of the PBGD gene is known to cause the disease.[13] However, in other cases such sequence changes in introns are not disease-causing. It is therefore impossible to predict with any certainty whether a particular change will disrupt splicing and thereby result in the production of a severely altered protein. Since we are unable to assess directly the effect of the mutation in Charlotte's PPOX gene on the activity of the protein, we cannot be completely certain that we have identified a disease-causing mutation.

Some level of corroboration would have come from the presence of the same mutation in Feodora's DNA but, given the doubtful provenance of the bones that we sampled in Poland, such corroboration has so far proved impossible. This left the samples that we had obtained from Charles I's blood-spattered shroud. Exon 8 was successfully amplified but found not to contain this mutation. If the provenance of the shroud can be trusted and this is the disease-causing change, this result would imply that the mutation was not passed on through Charles I to his sons, Charles II and James II.

Overall, the DNA analysis had been successful in identifying a novel mutation in the PPOX gene of one of our royal patients. However, because of the nature of the mutation, we remain unsure as to whether it would cause VP. This was not the unequivocal answer that we were seeking but, bearing in mind the catalogue of symptoms of porphyria from which Charlotte suffered throughout her life, the discovery of a mutation in the VP gene must be considered significant. Confirmation of VP in the royal houses of Europe was, however, to come from another source.

CHAPTER 11

The Ghosts of Windsor

I think there can be little doubt that George III suffered
from periodic attacks of a metabolic illness.
HRH Charles, Prince of Wales, April 1972

King George III spent the last ten years of his increasingly lonely
and removed existence in Windsor Castle. The guards on the North
Terrace could see the white-bearded monarch shuffling past his
window although, by then, the 'retired' King could neither see nor
hear his soldiers. After his death in January 1820, the guards still
reported seeing a bearded figure in white at the window of the old
King's room, and so the legend of George III's ghost was born.[1]
However, as we were to find out, it was not his ghost which was
haunting the present incumbents of the castle, but his porphyric
gene.

In the course of our research, we naturally had to consider
whether any member of the present-day British Royal Family had
inherited the Royal Malady. We knew that the porphyria theory
advanced by Macalpine and Hunter had prompted considerable
discussion in royal circles and that the family had had themselves
tested for the condition (see Chapter 2). Moreover, Prince Charles
had also taken a personal interest in Farmer George, his curiosity
leading him to spend much of his spare time researching the history
of his great-great-great-great-great-grandfather in the Royal
Archives at Windsor Castle. So interested was he, indeed, that he
wrote the foreword to John Brooke's biography of George III, in
which he argued that previous historians had treated the King quite
unfairly. Prince Charles also accepted the porphyria theory because
it corresponded so closely to historical reality. In fact, Charles

appeared to accept the diagnosis with an unusual air of authority, writing: 'I think there can be little doubt that George III suffered from periodic attacks of a metabolic illness.'[2] Was he merely convinced by the arguments put forward by Macalpine and Hunter, or was his confident acceptance of their theory perhaps based on his knowledge of a family secret? We suspect the latter.

As with Macalpine and Hunter thirty years before, it would have aided our cause considerably if we had had access to a living and co-operative family member with porphyria. With the assistance of such a patient it would have taken only a matter of months to determine the exact type of porphyria involved and discover the causative mutation. So far, only one definite diagnosis of porphyria within the European royal family has been made, that of Princess Adelaide, which we described in Chapter 2. The identification of another European royal family member with the illness, preferably from a different branch of the family, would therefore have significant implications. If the individual concerned were to belong to the British Royal Family, it would also help establish our theory that the mutant porphyria-causing gene had been passed through Queen Victoria. If, as we suppose, Queen Victoria passed the mutant porphyria gene on to her daughter Vicky, then there would be a 50 per cent chance that each of her other children would also have inherited the disorder. For the gene to be still present within the British Royal Family, King Edward VII would also have to have inherited it, and to have passed it on to George V.

The Case of Alice and George de Mellet de Bonas

As one might expect, during our investigation into the porphyria theory we came across a number of rumours regarding people who were thought to be porphyric descendants of King George III. Some of these were supposedly illegitimate descendants, products of the common Hanoverian practice of consorting with a concubine. If such people existed, it would make our task of proving the porphyria theory so much simpler, but the idea seemed almost too good to be true.

Almost by accident, however, we came across a mother and son who claimed descent from Edward, Duke of Kent, the father of Queen Victoria. Originally from Ireland, Mrs de Mellet de Bonas could trace her family tree back only two generations, since the records were destroyed in the 1916 Easter uprising. However, it is unlikely that they were descended from the Duke of Kent because it is well established that Edward only had two children, the future Queen Victoria (born 24 May 1819), and another infant girl born some thirty years earlier called Adelaide Victoire Auguste.[3]

The future Queen Victoria was a result of Edward's marriage to Victoire, the widowed Princess of Leiningen. Prior to his marriage, he had lived with a mistress, Mme de St Laurent, for twenty-seven years, and it appears that they had no children.[4] It has been suggested that his mistress was, in fact, sterile.[5] However, before his relationship with Mme de St Laurent, Edward had a brief relationship with a young Frenchwoman, Adelaide Dubus. The young lady became pregnant but tragically died in childbirth on 15 December 1789. The baby girl was cared for by her mother's sister and was christened Adelaide Victoire Auguste, but unfortunately she too died a few months later.[6] Thus, Edward only had one child who lived to maturity, and any connection that Mrs de Mellet de Bonas might have with the Royal Family must be through some other liaison.

The only reason we report the case is that Alice de Mellet de Bonas bears a striking physical resemblance to Queen Victoria, and her son George is remarkably similar in appearance to the young Edward VII. They even act as professional doubles for the royal pair, and Mrs de Mellet de Bonas has appeared as Queen Victoria in the comedy TV programme *Red Dwarf*, brandishing a machine gun! Although the link to the Royal Family is dubious, there is no doubt that both Alice de Mellet de Bonas and her son are porphyric. She has suffered a number of attacks which have caused severe abdominal pain and mental confusion. George, on the other hand, is a latent porphyric. They both have the clinically important 50 per cent reduction in the level of the enzyme PBGD and are therefore prone to attacks of acute intermittent porphyria. However, despite their uncanny resemblance to Queen Victoria and her son, in the absence of any firm family link to the Hanoverian line we must leave their case for now.

Rumours on the Grapevine

In a short article written in 1985, Professor Ian Christie, a retired historian from University College London, revealed that Macalpine and Hunter had contacted him in 1966 for advice on the historical aspects of their research. They shared their confidential information with him and he was highly impressed by the quality of their research.

In the course of an interview with us in 1996, Ian Christie provided the tantalizing information that, subsequent to the publication of their book in 1969, Macalpine and Hunter had heard through the medical grapevine of three further cases of porphyria in another branch of the family. Moreover, Christie stated, 'in two of these three families a pattern emerged of actual illness in two successive generations'. So impressed was he by these further cases that he emphatically propounded the porphyria theory in his writings 'as an established fact'.[7]

Professor Christie made another important disclosure when we spoke to him. He told us that around 1969 Ida Macalpine had had a visit from the eminent Oxford historian J. Stephen Watson, who was also writing a book on George III. On a trip to Malta, Watson had met with Prince Charles and their conversation had turned to the subject of the Hanoverian monarch. The prince told Watson that the porphyria theory put forward by Macalpine and Hunter was a wonderful achievement and then volunteered the comment: 'You know, it's still in the family!' Although the prince could have been referring to the German princesses (Patients A and B), Macalpine interpreted the statement as meaning that porphyria was still present in the House of Windsor.

If porphyria still afflicted the British Royal Family, then who had developed the disorder and how had it been diagnosed? We now know to whom the prince was probably referring, but before we discuss that case and the evidence for the diagnosis, we should first address another persistent rumour concerning another British Royal who has been dogged by ill-health.

Princess Margaret

In his book *Margaret: The Tragic Princess*, James Brough recounted an extraordinary story that had been told to him by two Fleet Street reporters. One of the reporters had heard a rumour around the time of the break-up of Princess Margaret's marriage in the mid-1970s that she had been treated for porphyria by a leading specialist.[8] Could Princess Margaret have had, or still have, porphyria? Brough attempted to explain her character and activities in the light of the rumoured diagnosis of porphyria. He noted that she always wore special make-up for protection against the sun, suggesting that, like certain porphyrics, she was hypersensitive to sunlight. It is known that she avoided taking sleeping pills even though she often had trouble sleeping, perhaps because she knew that the barbiturate-based tablets would provoke an acute attack. The princess had a spell in hospital in 1967 which was attributed, in part, to excessive weight loss through dieting. Maintenance of a constant carbohydrate intake is recognized as an important aspect of controlling porphyric attacks and reducing diets are known to be precipitating factors in porphyria. If this were the case, then she would have been advised to embark on a high-carbohydrate diet in order to prevent future attacks of porphyria, and this could explain the princess's subsequent weight gain. Needless to say, this was all conjecture on the part of the biographer.

James Brough also wonders whether Prince Charles's interest in and admiration for George III might be related to his sympathy for his aunt's condition. This is unlikely, especially if Princess Margaret were not diagnosed until the mid-1970s, several years after the prince wrote his foreword to John Brooke's biography. It is far more probable that the Prince of Wales's public acceptance of the porphyria theory stemmed from the revelation that another close relative of his was clinically diagnosed with variegate porphyria in 1968.

A Second Clinically Diagnosed Case of Porphyria

In Ida Macalpine's correspondence we came across a reference to Professor Ian Magnus, an expert on erythropoietic porphyria, whom Claude Rimington suspected of having inside information on a member of the royal family of Hesse who had served in the same regiment as him. We contacted Professor Magnus, who now lives in retirement in Suffolk, and he informed us that Rimington must have been mistaken. However, he did say that he had heard a story of an RAF physician who was thought to have seen several members of the Royal Family about porphyria and even knew his name, which he subsequently passed on to us. He warned us, however, that the doctor concerned was considerably older than himself, and that there was therefore every possibility that he would no longer be alive.

Nevertheless, we duly wrote to the officer in question, Dr Henry Bellringer. He responded promptly and in his letter stated that he had indeed examined several members of the Royal Family, in 1968, and found symptoms in one of them which were equivalent with porphyria. The patient was Prince William of Gloucester, at that time seventh in line to the throne.

Porphyria and Prince William of Gloucester

Henry Bellringer became involved in the case when he was asked by HRH the Duchess of Gloucester (now Princess Alice) if he would see her son, Prince William, in August 1968. The Duchess of Gloucester had become worried about a rash that William had had on and off for the past three years, which had started while he was a diplomat in Nigeria. It was urgent that Bellringer see William as soon as possible because, as a keen flyer, he was about to pilot his own plane to Japan, where he was to join the embassy staff in Tokyo. The consultation between the prince and Dr Bellringer took place at Barnwell Manor, the Gloucesters' family home, on 17 August 1968. William was then approaching his twenty-seventh birthday.

The prince explained to Dr Bellringer that three years earlier, in December 1965, shortly after his arrival in Lagos, he had suddenly felt weak and dizzy and rapidly developed a sharp fever. Prior to his departure for Nigeria he had been given chloroquine to prevent malaria. The prince felt sick and bilious, and the symptoms of jaundice appeared. He continued in this condition until mid-January, and although he then felt better, he still became very tired as soon as he attempted anything strenuous. Malaria was suspected. It was about this time that he noticed the rash, which he described as blisters appearing on his face, especially on his forehead. The rash at times appeared on the back of his hands and chest and occasionally, though rarely, on his back. The blisters were 'quite large', and when they dried they left a dark patch before they cleared. Individual spots took a long time to clear and some left scars. 'Ever since, the rash has fluctuated in severity.'[9] There had been more blisters than usual in the previous three months, which he had spent in this country, May to June 1968, although the weather for this period had been quite dull with most areas of the country experiencing less than average sunshine.

Initially, the prince had attributed his blistery rash to knocks and bumps he received during his outdoor activities, which included polo, water-skiing and tinkering about in the new aircraft he had bought some months after his arrival in Lagos. He abstained from alcohol for twelve months, partly presumably because of the jaundice, but also because it took the best part of a year before he was his old self again. He also reported that at irregular intervals his urine was quite dark for a few days.

As Prince William was about to set off for Japan, there was no time to carry out extensive tests before his departure. Dr Bellringer therefore tentatively diagnosed variegate porphyria, and advised the prince about potentially harmful drugs which could precipitate a porphyric attack, even giving him a card to carry on his person warning physicians about his condition. The card also warned surgeons to regard acute abdominal pain with caution. He was given some cream to help alleviate irritation and prevent bleeding from the superficial ulcerations. Uvistat cream was also given to provide some degree of protection from sunlight and to hide the blemishes which had caused his mother such concern. Dr Bellringer then arranged to see the prince on his return from Japan and also informed his mother of his diagnosis.

Upon his return to Britain in August 1970, Prince William was again examined by Dr Bellringer. By now he had quite a number of small scars across his forehead, and on the back of his hands and forearms. They were also present on his chest where an open shirt had exposed the area to sunlight. Present, too, were quite large fluid-containing blisters (bullae) on the forehead and back of the hands. Some dry, star-shaped, pigmented scars remained. A skin test revealed that it showed fragility, and slid under pressure. The prince reported that the rash seemed to improve during the less sunny time of the year, but said he had not made any conscious effort to avoid exposure to the sun.

Tests carried out on specimens provided by the prince revealed that the specimens contained porphyrins 'greatly in excess of normal', and a similar test carried out by another physician produced a similar result. Another sample sent later to Abraham Goldberg's laboratory in Glasgow gave normal results, but by that stage the prince was in remission.

Prince William was examined for a second opinion by Dr Arthur Rook and his colleagues at Addenbrookes in 1970. They concluded that he was suffering from variegate porphyria in relative remission. Some time later, Prince William revealed to Henry Bellringer that he had also been examined by Professor Ishihara in Tokyo, who also concluded that the prince had porphyria.

A quick review of Prince William's symptoms reveals that they bore the by now all-too-familiar characteristic hallmarks of porphyria: bilious attacks, general malaise, muscle weakness, fragile skin, sun sensitivity, elevated excretion of porphyrins and production of dark urine. No wonder Dr Bellringer was left with little alternative but to write in his notes that 'there can be scarcely any doubt that this is a case of porphyria'. The mixture of acute and dermatological symptoms pinpoints the disease type as variegate porphyria. The fact that the diagnosis was confirmed independently by two other physicians makes the case convincing beyond a shadow of doubt.

Prince William of Gloucester – a Tragic Tale[10]

Prince William of Gloucester was born on 19 December 1941 at Hadley Common in Hertfordshire. William was born by caesarean section and thus both mother and baby remained in the nursing home for two weeks before they were allowed to return to Barnwell Manor. The estate and its surroundings contributed to William's happy childhood and it was here that he came to appreciate the outdoor life with which he was always to be associated. After preparatory school he went to Eton where, although he was described as academically very capable, he was easily distracted by outdoor pursuits and leisure activities. In his final year at Eton, William was accepted by Cambridge University, and in the gap between leaving school and going up to Magdalene College he took his first flying lessons, an activity for which he quickly developed a passion.

Despite twice failing the Civil Service entrance examination, Prince William eventually joined the Foreign and Commonwealth Office and in the summer of 1965 was posted to Lagos as Third Secretary to the British High Commission. He set sail for Nigeria on 19 November, determined to learn as much as possible about Africa and its heritage. Shortly after his arrival in Lagos he took delivery of a Piper Comanche twin-engined aircraft which provided him with a mode of transport to explore the country. As we now know, as William's twenty-fourth birthday and his first Christmas in Nigeria approached, he suffered his first overt attack of porphyria. In one of his first letters home he describes this unhappy time. 'I am afraid that I had an absolutely rotten birthday and Christmas,' he wrote.

> The day before my birthday, I felt rather weak and dizzy and went to bed in the afternoon. By the evening I was running quite a fever. I spent the next three days in bed and then got up as I felt better. Nobody, including the doctor, seemed to know what I had had, some thought malaria. By Christmas eve I was worse again and went to bed that afternoon. I got up on Christmas morning to go to church, where I felt frightful, and on my way out, a friend took one look at me and said: 'There is no doubt what you have got, its jaundice'. My eyes were bright yellow! In any case, I have felt like death for the last two days.[11]

The prince was at least not troubled by insomnia, for he reported, 'I have seldom slept better when feeling so rotten,' but he was clearly quite ill as he 'could not eat because I was unable to keep anything down'.[12] His illness persisted until mid-January 1966, but even afterwards he was easily tired if he tried anything strenuous. As we know from Bellringer, he did not feel right for about another year.

In June 1968, Henry Duke of Gloucester suffered a stroke, prompting William to think in earnest about his role in the management of the family estate and home. He resigned from his diplomatic post and returned to Barnwell Manor, where he set about restructuring the estate and taking an interest in methods of farming. It would be misleading, however, to suggest that he buried himself in the affairs of the family business, for he still carried out his royal duties and travelled whenever the opportunity arose. He also developed a keen interest in competitive light aircraft racing. The prince had sold his twin-engined Piper Comanche aircraft in Japan and now purchased a single-engined Piper Arrow. In 1970 he obtained a competition licence which allowed him to fly in air rallies. He became the first British Royal to race an aeroplane.

On 28 August 1972, he entered the Goodyear International Trophy, which started at the Halfpenny Green Airfield in Staffordshire, England. The co-pilot for this race was Commander Vyrell Mitchell and together they took off side by side with another aircraft in the competition. For reasons which are not fully understood, William's aircraft took off flying very low and entered upon a very steep turn at a comparatively low speed. The aircraft lost height and its left wing hit a tree. The plane continued flying but rolled over and crashed in a ball of flame. Both William and his co-pilot were killed instantly. The detailed crash investigation which followed found no fault with the plane and thus the accident was attributed to pilot error. However, those who knew William and his co-pilot found it difficult to accept that he would willingly have undertaken such a dangerous manoeuvre, even under the pressure of a competitive race.

William was remembered as an outstanding young man, adventurous, independent and courageous. He preferred to be judged by his own achievements rather than as a member of the Royal Family. He has also been described to us as 'wilful', as a person who wanted to be treated as royal on some occasions and in an extremely private manner on others. William was a loyal son who held his parents in great esteem and, needless to say, his mother was heartbroken at his sudden death. William's father, who had been ill for some time, died in 1974, and his younger brother Richard inherited the family title and estate.

Dr Bellringer's last meeting with William was a couple of days before the prince's death, since, at the insistence of his mother, he had continued to attend the prince at monthly intervals after his return from Japan. Bellringer greatly admired his patient and described him as a 'likeable friendly man, with a keen sense of humour, a genuine concern for his fellow men and a love of animals, especially his labrador dogs who worshipped him. He had an agile intelligence, with all his wits about him. It had been a great privilege to have been able to serve and know him and so intimately. What a tragic loss.'[13]

Henry Bellringer was aware of the work of Macalpine and Hunter, and when we asked him whether he had made Prince William's diagnosis of porphyria with their research in mind, he answered that he had tried not to let it influence him. As he pointed out, with all the symptoms, he was left with little option but to diagnose the prince's condition as porphyria. On the theme of the Royal Malady, he did highlight that both of William's parents were descended from Mary Queen of Scots, so genetically he could have inherited the disorder from either of them. However, it seems much more likely that he inherited it from his father, especially as rumours had been circulating that the Duke of Gloucester had also been diagnosed with porphyria. For example, in his book *The Madness of Kings*, Vivian Green states that Macalpine and Hunter suspected that an uncle of Queen Elizabeth II might have the disease.[14] Whether the old Duke of Gloucester really did have porphyria is a question which will be answered whenever the appropriate records are released.

The diagnosis of William of Gloucester's porphyria was confirmed to us by a number of other sources, including several people who had worked closely with the prince. They described the disorder as an inconvenience rather than a problem, the persistent skin rash being the most irksome symptom.

Immediately after his first consultation with Prince William, Henry Bellringer wrote to the head of the royal physicians, Sir Ronald Bodley Scott, and informed him of the provisional diagnosis he had just made. According to Bellringer, Sir Ronald was not best pleased at the news, presumably because it meant that he would now have to screen the rest of the Royal Family. There was little further correspondence between the two physicians and we do not know if Sir Ronald instigated the wider family screen, let alone whether any further porphyrics were identified.

Dr Bellringer died in 1997, shortly before the completion of this book, in his ninety-first year. A man of strong moral fibre, he had great compassion for his patient. He remained lucid despite his great age, and was clearly aware of the potential problem in telling us the story of Prince William's condition. Partly because of his respect for William, and partly because of the suffering he knew could be caused by porphyria, he overcame his 'anxious thoughts and reservations' to tell us what he knew.

We have presented the case of Prince William of Gloucester to several of the country's leading porphyria experts who agree that the diagnosis of porphyria in remission was absolutely correct. The final clinching evidence would of course have been a DNA analysis, but for obvious reasons that is not possible. We also described the evidence to Sir Abraham Goldberg, who said that the case would give a whole new momentum to the porphyria hypothesis. Finally, we met in Dublin with Dr Geoffrey Dean, described by Ida Macalpine as a member of the debunking South African 'axis' because of his continued objection to her theory. He, too, found the evidence of porphyria in Prince William most convincing, and added wryly that, while his was clearly not the South African form, Macalpine and Hunter might have been right all along in diagnosing variegate porphyria in George III!

Conclusion

With the clinical determination of variegate porphyria in a grandson of King George V, we have reached the end of our extraordinary multidisciplinary journey. Taking as our starting point the brilliantly intuitive and carefully researched, but unfortunately incomplete, work of Ida Macalpine, Richard Hunter and Claude Rimington in the 1960s on the 'madness' of George III and some of his relatives, we set out to try to verify – or if need be falsify – their stunning hypothesis that many of the kings and queens who have ruled over us in the past four hundred years were afflicted with a rare hereditary illness that is associated with attacks of physical debility and mental confusion. Reflecting in part our diverse scholarly backgrounds, the approach we adopted was essentially threefold: historical, genetic and detective.

There is a widespread misconception that historical evidence is somehow 'softer' or less reliable than 'hard' clinical data that can be subjected to repeated analysis in the laboratory. Since we have followed both paths in our quest for certainty, it is perhaps worth making the point that, deliberate forgery apart, there is nothing uncertain about the evidence of the archives, which can be inspected by doubters and critics. No one spends a lifetime writing letters to their mother, doctor or close confidant describing painful and embarrassing symptoms unless they actually suffer from those symptoms, just as no one who is married to such a person keeps a diary record of their spouse's distressing attacks unless those attacks actually occur. Our research in the archives brought to light literally hundreds of letters and diary entries generated by different people in various parts of Europe over very many decades. Each such source corroborates the other. Together they do not lie. From the Sergeant King of Prussia and George III of Great Britain and Ireland in the eighteenth century through to Princess Adelaide of Saxe-Meiningen and Prince William of Gloucester in the twentieth, the distressing story they tell is always the same: bouts of acute abdominal pain, peripheral neuropathy, skin fragility and blistering, dark red urine, agitation, insomnia, weakness and – sometimes – mental confusion. The one thing that is missing from the otherwise overwhelming historical evidence – the actual naming of the disease by a competent clinician – could not have been found for the simple reason that porphyria was not recognized as a specific metabolic disorder until the 1920s and 1930s.

It was to achieve complete certainty in our findings, and to convince even the most doubting sceptic, that parallel to our archival investigations we embarked upon the search for the DNA of deceased royals. From the beginning of our collaboration in November 1995 it was clear that this was going to be the most daunting of the problems facing us. Not only did it seem virtually out of the question that we would ever gain access to suitable relics, but even if we did, the task of actually identifying the porphyria mutation in ancient DNA was bound to prove unbelievably difficult. The strongest individual case we were able to put together on the basis of the archival record was that of 'Charlotte the Brat', as the Kaiser's sister liked to sign herself in her correspondence with her British cousins. Now, having located her grave, found her coffin and taken samples from one of her bones, we have painstakingly analysed her DNA. From this, we have identified a novel mutation within her PPOX gene. Similar mutations in other families are known to cause porphyria.

The certainty that our reading of the historical record was indeed correct was provided, at the last, not only by the white-hot technology of DNA sequencing, but also by the more traditional investigative methods favoured by Sherlock Holmes. By establishing the true identity of 'Patient A' as Adelaide Princess of Prussia, who was born a princess of Saxe-Meiningen and had been diagnosed as porphyric by the distinguished physician Professor Alfred Vannotti, we were able to reconstruct her painful early life with the help of the documents in the archives, and to speak to her close relatives, who confirmed our diagnosis of her illness. Our efforts to obtain samples for analysis from her children and grandchildren proved as futile as had the efforts of the original proponents of the theory thirty years earlier, however. All the more significant, consequently, was the discovery, after painstaking detective networking within the British medical profession, that Prince William of Gloucester, a cousin of Queen Elizabeth II, had been diagnosed with variegate porphyria at the very time that Macalpine, Hunter and Rimington were engaged in their pioneering work. Though in his case the illness mercifully manifested itself in a relatively moderate form, and was more of an irritation than a life-threatening condition, there is absolutely no doubt, in view of the information passed on to us by the late Dr Henry Bellringer, that William of Gloucester had inherited variegate porphyria. The diagnosis was made independently by three physicians in different parts of the world, all of them using the standard biochemical tests to establish porphyrin levels in the prince greatly in excess of normal.

It seems clear, from the historical evidence presented in this book, that apart from George III himself several of his siblings and some of his Continental relatives – the Sergeant King of Prussia and the Elector Wilhelm I of Hesse-Kassel in particular – were sufferers, as were many of George's children, both male and female. To judge from their medical biographies, which are so painful to read, it is also beyond dispute that Crown Princess Vicky of Prussia-Germany, the tragic Empress Frederick, and her daughter Charlotte and granddaughter Feodora had the disease, for what else could have caused their terrible attacks of lameness and abdominal pain and skin rashes – and in Charlotte's case dark red urine? And if they had inherited porphyria, the implication is quite compelling that the faulty gene must have passed to them via Queen Victoria, whose own symptoms, though by no means negligible, were somewhat less specific and acute. By similar reasoning, we are almost bound to conclude that, since Prince William of Gloucester is known to have had variegate porphyria, the mutation must have come down to him via Edward VII and George V.

As for the question of how porphyria in the royal families of Europe might have affected the course of history, we imagine that the eventual answer will *in most cases* be couched in terms of weakness and failure rather than of commission. In the light of our conclusions, historians may wish to consider afresh the extent to which George III's attempt to establish his personal rule was vitiated by his periodic attacks of physical debility and mental derangement, for example, and to ask how far Parliament's ascendancy over the Crown was promoted by his illness and that of his two sons who followed him on the throne. Would Victoria and Albert's ambitious eldest daughter Vicky have achieved more of her aim of turning first Prussia and then a united Germany into a modern parliamentary monarchy in close alliance with Britain if she had not been struck down every few weeks by episodes of excruciating pain? Would Princess Charlotte, the Kaiser's sister, have made more progress with her plan of December 1908 to save Germany and Europe from impending disaster by replacing her brother's authoritarian rule with a collective regency of all the German princes had she been in better health?[1]

If Vicky had porphyria and passed it on to her daughter Charlotte, did she not also pass it on to some of her other children, two of whom died in childhood? Most crucially, did she not perhaps pass it on to her eldest son, Kaiser Wilhelm II? Could some of the last German Kaiser's notorious speeches and irrational actions be attributed to the gene of George III? Admittedly, he showed none of the *physical* symptoms of porphyria and felt exceptionally well and pleased with himself throughout his life. However, many of his contemporaries, Bismarck included, considered him to be 'not quite sane' and to have inherited his mental disorder from his British or Russian forebears. Some expressly blamed his 'English' or 'Coburg' blood. In 1888, shortly before Wilhelm's accession, the eminent British specialist Sir John Erichsen informed Lord Salisbury that the new German monarch 'was not, and never would be, a normal man', that 'he would always be subject to sudden accesses of anger' and would, at such times, be 'quite incapable of forming a reasonable or temperate judgment', and that though he would probably not become clinically insane, 'some of his actions would probably be those of a man not wholly sane'.[2] Was this a coded reference to porphyria? Twenty years later, in November 1908, after the Kaiser had given plentiful grounds for thinking that Erichsen's dire prognosis might well be correct, Lord Esher, one of King Edward VII's closest friends, remarked of

Wilhelm II: 'I am sure that the taint of George III is in his blood.'[3] If nothing else, Esher's terse comment is testimony to the fact that, one hundred years after the onset of George III's final illness, the Royal Family's purple secret was still a matter of deep concern at the Court of St James.

Science, Tetrapyrroles and Porphyria

Man cannot give a true reason for the grass
under his feet, why it should be green rather
than red, or any other colour.

Sir Walter Ralegh, 1614

Why grass is green, or why our blood is red
are mysteries which none have reached unto.

John Donne, 'Of the Progress of the Soul', 1612

Background

Before giving a description of what porphyria is and how it occurs,
a brief introduction to some biological processes is required. In
particular, for any inheritance study, it is important to comprehend
the concept of biology's central dogma, that is, the relationship
between the genetic material of all organisms (DNA) and the
molecules that act to regulate and organize the cell (the proteins).[1]
This is fundamental to understanding how genetic material is
passed from generation to generation and how inborn errors arise
and, rather than being eliminated, are maintained and propagated.
This appendix also includes a concise review of the role of one of
Nature's most colourful discoveries, a family of biological molecules called the modified tetrapyrroles. More specifically, it will
outline how haem, the compound which gives blood its brilliant red
colour, is made in humans. Against this basic scientific backdrop
the molecular basis of the porphyria disease will be explained and
related to the symptoms and discomfort which sufferers experience
and endure.

In 1962, Jim Watson, Francis Crick and Maurice Wilkins were awarded the Nobel Prize in Physiology and Medicine in recognition of their work on the structure of deoxyribose nucleic acid (DNA), which was determined in 1953.[2] Their work represented an enormous landmark in twentieth-century biological science because it signalled the dawn of a new discipline, that of molecular biology. Prior to their discovery, a major problem existed in understanding how cells could pass on their genetic information from generation to generation. The likelihood that DNA was the genetic material became apparent in a series of classic experiments in the 1940s. In these experiments, researchers demonstrated that DNA from a strain of bacteria (*Pneumococcus*) which caused a deadly infection in mice could be used to induce a similar deadly trait in a related, though non-lethal, strain of bacteria.[3] The simple inference from these experiments was that the non-lethal bacteria had been given new instructions to make them lethal. These instructions could only have come from the added DNA. The answer to how DNA could bestow the transfer of information came from the elucidation of the structure of DNA. Using data collected by Maurice Wilkins and Rosalyn Franklin in King's College London, Watson and Crick proposed a model for the structure of DNA. The structure provided a wonderfully clear and simple explanation for how DNA could act as the genetic material.

DNA is essentially a chain ('polymer') of repeating units. These repeating units consist of a sugar (called deoxyribose) and a base. There are four possible bases, thymine (T), cytosine (C), guanosine (G) or adenine (A). The repeating units are linked together through a group of atoms called a phosphate such that they form very long polymers consisting of millions, or tens of millions, of these units. This polymer of repeating units is referred to as a strand of DNA.

Human DNA contains somewhere around four billion bases; the complete sequence could be written in the abbreviated form reflecting the order of As, Cs, Gs and Ts into a book of a million pages. This book is already under construction in the world-wide effort to determine the complete human DNA sequence, the human genome project. The DNA and all the genes of a particular organism are called a genome. In more complex organisms, the genome is so large that it is packaged in a number of discrete bundles, called chromosomes, and there are twenty-three such chromosomes in human cells. In this respect, our one-million-page book can be divided into twenty-three chapters. The chromosomes are held in a part of the cell called the nucleus. By necessity DNA is a very long molecule, as it contains a large amount of information, but because the molecule is comparatively thin, it can be packaged into a very small volume. If one were to unravel all the DNA from a single human cell and attach it end to end, it would measure two metres in length. Considering that there are something like 10 trillion cells in the human body, unravelling and attaching the DNA end to end from all these cells would create a length of DNA which could be wrapped around the earth half a million times, although this would produce a line only one centimetre wide.

DNA is rarely found as a single stranded chain of units. More commonly it is found in a double-stranded state, where two single strands are wound around each other to give a helical appearance,

P   O   Base: A

P   O   Base: C

O   Base

P   O   Base: G   A-C-G-T

P   O   Base: T

SINGLE BASE   DNA CHAIN   DNA SEQUENCE

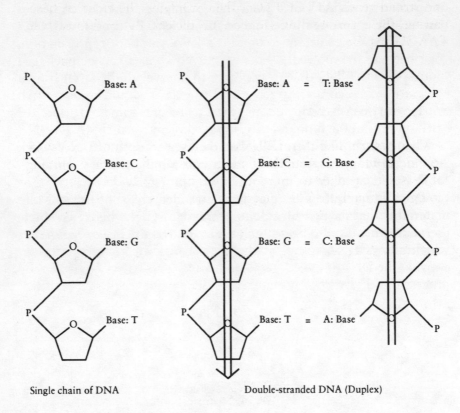

Single chain of DNA   Double-stranded DNA (Duplex)

rather like the twisted strands of a length of string. The two strands of DNA which make up the double helix (also referred to as a duplex) form a very stable structure because of the way they interact with each other. To form the helix, the two strands of DNA must line up in opposite directions, an orientation which allows the bases on one strand of the DNA to interact with bases on the other strand of DNA. This interaction is known as base-pairing and it is very specific as adenine (A) can only base-pair with thymine (T) and cytosine (C) can only base-pair with guanine (G).

The consequence of this is that, knowing the sequence of bases on one strand of the DNA molecule we can deduce the sequence on the opposite (complementary) strand. For instance, if the sequence on one strand reads ATTCCTTGG then, applying the rules of base-pairing, the corresponding sequence on the other strand must read TAAGGAACC.

-A-T-T-C-C-T-T-G-G-

⋮ ⋮ ⋮ ⋮ ⋮ ⋮ ⋮ ⋮ ⋮

-T-A-A-G-G-A-A-C-C-

When written like this, DNA has the appearance of a molecular zip, and in many respects the analogy of a zip is quite appropriate, for it is the capacity to unzip the molecule which is crucial to its biological function. The most essential feature of any genetic material is that it must be able to be copied and then passed on to the next generation. The ability to base-pair is the major property which allows DNA to act as the genetic material. The process of copying the DNA is called 'replication' and is co-ordinated with the process of cell division. When the cell divides the resulting two cells

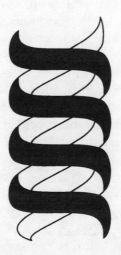

Helical structure of duplex DNA

each contain an exact copy of the DNA. If the DNA molecule is thought of as a molecular zip, then it is easy to visualize how the DNA is replicated. From one end, the duplex is unzipped or separated, thereby exposing two single strands of DNA. The exposed strands act as a template for the synthesis of a new strand. Thus while the 'parent' DNA is being unzipped, the two exposed strands are copied to give two new zips. The two new zips each therefore contain one parental DNA strand and one newly synthesized strand of DNA. Only when the process of replication is complete does the cell divide. DNA replication is carried out with great accuracy and the cell rarely makes mistakes during this process, but if mistakes are made, the cell has mechanisms to correct these.

However, occasionally such mistakes are not corrected and errors are introduced into the DNA sequence which can have grave consequences. Once inserted, the errors – 'mutations' – are propagated from one generation to the next. Why mutations occur and why they are not immediately eliminated is an involved subject area in itself and will not be dealt with here.

This brief description of DNA replication does not reflect the many complications that the cell has to overcome to undertake this task, nor does it document the enormous number of factors which are required for the process. The information for life is stored within the DNA and can be likened to the software programs which are required to run a computer. In DNA, these programs are arranged into discrete regions which are called genes. Generally, each gene contains information about a unique protein. It is proteins which control and regulate cellular function. In the simplest organisms such as bacteria the DNA contains enough information for between

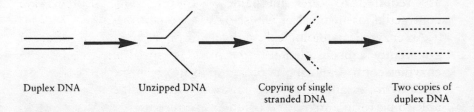

Duplex DNA   Unzipped DNA   Copying of single stranded DNA   Two copies of duplex DNA

three and four thousand genes, corresponding to three to four thousand different proteins. The information within the genes is stored in the form of a code, the genetic code. Thus the order of the bases (A, C, G and T) within a gene contains the information for the composition of a particular protein. The genetic code has now been 'cracked', meaning that it is possible to predict the composition of the protein for which the gene encodes. Furthermore, it is also possible to determine the composition of a protein when an error, or mutation, has been introduced into the gene.

A primary function of any genetic material is that it should be very stable. As with a computer, if the software becomes corrupted or breaks down then the computer malfunctions. If the DNA (the cell's genetic software) were seriously corrupted then the cell would either have no instructions to follow or would observe the wrong instructions. Comparatively speaking, DNA is extremely stable, so much so that it can remain intact long after the organism has died.

Within the cell, decoding the information held within the genes into specific proteins is performed by two processes which are referred to as transcription and translation. Proteins are synthesized from building blocks called amino acids. In the same way that DNA is a polymer of units each containing one of four different bases, so proteins are polymers made from twenty different types of amino acids. Proteins can consist of a few amino acids or they may consist of several thousand amino acids linked together. On average, however, proteins contain around three hundred amino acids. The size of the protein and its amino acid composition is determined by the sequence of bases within the gene. The composition of the protein allows it to fold into a very defined shape and structure which is crucial to its proper functioning.

There is a vast range of different proteins in a cell, responsible for performing many different tasks. Some proteins are structural and are required to offer mechanical support; some proteins are contractile, as in muscle; whilst others are enzymes.

An enzyme is a biological catalyst, a protein that has the effect of apparently causing chemical reactions to speed up. In the cell, enzymes control all aspects of metabolism, from the breakdown of carbohydrates and fats to the synthesis of antibiotics. Enzymes are able to perform a myriad of complex chemistry at very fast rates. In a simple bacterium there are many hundreds of different enzymes where each enzyme is specific for only one reaction. Thus, for instance, one of the basic processes by which living systems generate energy, the breakdown of glucose into carbon dioxide and water, requires twenty different enzymes which reflect the twenty different steps in the process. These enzymes are used only for this process and are not used for any other metabolic process.

The Modified Tetrapyrroles – the Pigments of Life

As quoted at the beginning of this chapter, both Walter Ralegh and John Donne pondered why grass was green and blood red. The compounds which make grass green, chlorophyll, and give blood its red appearance, haem, are part of a family of compounds which have been dubbed 'the pigments of life'.[4] This family of compounds are all modified tetrapyrroles. As the word implies, tetrapyrroles are composed of four pyrroles. A pyrrole can be envisaged as a chemical pentagon with a central nitrogen atom. When four of these small five-membered ring structures are joined together they make a larger, macrocyclic, ring structure. These macrocyclic ring structures have a number of properties which have endeared them to Nature such that they have been commandeered to fulfil a wide range of diverse and extremely important biological functions. In fact, tetrapyrroles have greatly influenced life from its earliest primordial beginning, through the catastrophic environmental pollution associated with the onset of photosynthesis, up to the more subtle variations in recent times which, as the evidence presented in this book demonstrates, have plagued the royal houses of Europe.

Nature has utilized four major tetrapyrrole derivatives, namely chlorophyll, haem, coenzyme F_{430} and vitamin B_{12}. The first and most striking observation about these molecules is that they are highly coloured. Chlorophyll is the green pigment found in algae and higher plants that is required for the process of photosynthesis. Coenzyme F_{430} is a yellow pigment found in a class of bacteria responsible for the generation of methane gas. Vitamin B_{12}, an essential human dietary supplement, is involved in several aspects of metabolism and is red in colour. Haem, the compound which gives blood its colour, is required for respiration and oxygen transport.

What are the properties of these molecules that allow them to be

Chlorophyll-a

Mg

Uro'gen III

Co

Vitamin B$_{12}$

Ni

Fe

Coenzyme F$_{430}$

Haem

used for so many different roles? Firstly, the tetrapyrrole macro-molecular structure is able to accommodate a metal ion at its centre, allowing it to participate in further chemistry. For instance, in blood, oxygen is carried by the 'haem group' (of atoms) by attaching the oxygen to the central iron atom. Second, the tetrapyrrole itself has a number of chemical properties which allow it to partake in reactions. In the case of photosynthesis, for example, chlorophyll is able to absorb light and convert it into chemical energy.

Life on earth has existed for between 3 and 3.5 billion years but, up until the point that the process of photosynthesis evolved, about 2 billion years ago, life on earth had existed largely in an oxygen-free environment. As there was no oxygen, living systems did not breathe, they merely fermented. Oxygen was a highly toxic substance and cells probably took precautions to remove it from their immediate environment. Now organisms had to evolve new ways of dealing with the ever-increasing concentrations of oxygen in the atmosphere. This resulted in the development of the process of 'respiration' where oxygen is used in the process of combustion (in which energy is obtained from sugars). Nature has found two roles for haem in the process of respiration. First of all, the complete combustion of sugars and carbohydrates requires that the smallest components of these materials, the protons and electrons, are transferred on to oxygen atoms. This 'electron transport' system is used to generate the majority of the energy which is released during the breakdown of sugars. Major components of this electron transport system are called cytochromes, which are proteins enclosing a haem group (which is then known as a 'bound haem group'). Because of the central metal ion, haem is able to participate in electron transport. The second role for haem in respiration is that of oxygen transport. Larger systems require that oxygen be transported to respiring tissue, for instance in muscles during exercise. This is one of the roles of haemoglobin, the major proteinaceous component of blood. Haemoglobin is made of a protein called globin with a bound haem group. Oxygen binds to the haem group and is transported around the body to where it is required. Furthermore, haemoglobin also transports carbon dioxide away from actively respiring tissue. Haemoglobin has proved to be a wonderful model for the study not only of the action of haem but also of proteins in general.

Natural history evolved over a 4-billion-year period but the porphyria hypothesis relates to how one member of this tetrapyrrole class, haem, has influenced history over a very much shorter period of time, a mere four hundred years of European and world history. To appreciate this we now have to turn our attention to how humans make haem, because our understanding of the process of haem synthesis is essential not only in understanding the molecular basis of porphyria but also in understanding some of the symptoms of the disease.

The construction, or 'biosynthesis', of all natural products is organized into pathways. These pathways can be envisaged as small factories within the cell. The factory is based on a production line with a starting raw material. As the raw material is passed along the production line it is modified and transformed by a number of processes that occur in a specific order until the final product is made. As with factories, Nature's production line responds to consumer demand. Thus, for instance, to increase production the factory would require more starting material, increase the work-force and thereby expand output. Conversely, if too much product is being made, less starting material would be required and the number of workers reduced. There is really no difference between this and the process of biosynthesis in cells.

Haem Biosynthesis[5]

The starting point for haem synthesis is a small molecule called aminolaevulinic acid (ALA). ALA contains five carbon atoms and one nitrogen atom. Overall the pathway takes eight molecules of ALA and converts them into one molecule of haem, which contains thirty-four carbon atoms and four nitrogen atoms. Thus during the transformation six carbon atoms are removed, as carbon dioxide, and four nitrogen atoms are lost as ammonia.

The first stage in the pathway is the welding of two molecules of ALA into a pyrrole building block, called porphobilinogen (PBG). The pyrrole is a pentagonal-shaped molecule. The enzyme that carries out this reaction is called ALA dehydratase (because it removes a molecule of water during the reaction). To help in the catalytic process the enzyme requires the use of zinc. The metal is easily displaced from the protein by another metal, lead, which consequently inactivates the protein.[6] The effects of lead and its relationship to porphyria will be discussed later.

The second step in the haem biosynthetic pathway is the linking of four of the pyrrole building blocks to form a linear tetrapyrrole. This is a very complicated reaction as it requires a number of different chemical processes. One of the consequences of this step is that four of the nitrogen atoms located on the side arm of the molecule are lost as ammonia. The enzyme that performs this reaction is called PBG deaminase (because it removes ammonia from PBG). The structure of the enzyme allows an insight into why certain known mutations prevent the enzyme functioning normally.[7]

The third step in the pathway is the closing of the linear tetrapyrrole into a cyclic tetrapyrrole. This sounds a very simple process but is made more complex by the inversion of the terminal ring of the tetrapyrrole with respect to the other three rings. The product of this reaction is an intermediate called uroporphyrinogen III and the enzyme which catalyses the reaction is called uroporphyrinogen III synthase.

The subsequent two steps in haem biosynthesis relate to the removal of some of the carbon groups which are located on the periphery of the molecule. Initially four carbon groups are removed by the enzyme uroporphyrinogen decarboxylase and subsequently two more are removed by the enzyme, coproporphyrinogen oxidase. These transformations convert uroporphyrinogen III into protoporphyrinogen via coproporphyrinogen.

Up until this stage all the intermediates in the pathway have been colourless. The next enzyme performs a reaction whereby protopor-phyrinogen is reacted with oxygen (oxidation) to yield protopor-phyrin, with the generation of a deep red colour. This process introduces three new double bonds into the infrastructure of the pyrrole and it is this that leads to the development of colour. Thus, protoporphyrin is the first porphyrin. The gene which encodes for this step is called protoporphyrinogen oxidase and it was the last gene of haem biosynthesis to be identified, with the publication of the sequence in 1995.[8]

The final step in haem biosynthesis is the conversion of protoporphyrin into haem. This process requires the insertion of iron into the centre of the molecule, a process which is carried out by the enzyme ferrochelatase. Once this task has been accomplished the haem molecule becomes available for incorporation into globin and the cytochromes.

The whole pathway is tightly regulated. The cell employs a number of techniques to ensure that haem is maintained at the appropriate levels. In humans, haem is synthesized at different rates in different tissues. Higher levels of haem are required by liver and bone-marrow cells, the latter being subsequently converted into the red blood cells. Conversely, in cells which do not require much haem, the levels of haem-synthesizing enzymes are kept low. It is important to remember that the regulation of the pathway can be affected by mutations which regulate the level of a particular enzyme as well as by mutations which affect the structure and activity of the enzyme itself.

In total there are seven enzymes and six intermediates between ALA and haem. An understanding of this pathway, the enzymes, the genes and the intermediates allows a detailed comprehension of the disorders associated with the pathway, the porphyrias.

The Porphyrias[9]

The porphyrias encompass the class of disorders that affect haem biosynthesis. They can be inherited or acquired; in other words, either the disorder is found within the family, passed from generation to generation, or the disorder is caused by an external source such as a chemical or drug. Either way, interfering with the

Name	Enzyme dysfunction	Type	Inheritance pattern	Major symptoms	Excretion pattern
Aminolaevulinic acid dehydratase porphyria	Aminolaevulinic acid dehydratase	Hepatic	Recessive	Acute	Increased ALA
Plumbism (lead poisoning)	Aminolaevulinic acid dehydratase	Hepatic	Acquired	Acute	Increased ALA
Acute intermittent porphyria	Porphobilinogen deaminase	Hepatic	Dominant	Acute	Increased ALA and PBG
Congenital erythropoietic porphyria	Uroporphyrinogen III synthase	Erythropoietic	Recessive	Dermatological	Increased ALA, PBG and uroporphyrin
Porphyria cutaneatarda	Uroporphyrinogen decarboxylase	Hepatic	Acquired or Dominant	Dermatological	Uroporphyrin
Hereditary erythropoietic porphyria	Uroporphyrinogen decarboxylase	Hepatic	Dominant	Dermatological	Uroporphyrin
Hereditary coproporphyria	Coproporphyrinogen oxidase	Hepatic	Dominant	Mixed	ALA, PBG and coproporphyrin
Variegate porphyria	Protoporphyrinogen oxidase	Hepatic	Dominant	Mixed	ALA, PBG, coproporphyrin & protoporphyrin
Erythropoietic porphyria	Ferrochelatase	Erythropoietic	Dominant	Dermatological	Protoporphyrin

haem biosynthetic pathway at any one of the seven enzymes we have just discussed leads to a particular type of porphyria. The major types of porphyria are reviewed here, with particular attention paid to the types of porphyria which are thought to have caused the Royal Malady.

The common link between all the porphyric disorders is that they affect the haem pathway and cause accumulation of intermediates within the pathway. It is the accumulation of intermediates, rather than the lack of haem, which gives rise to the two major clinical symptoms associated with all porphyrias, neurophysiological and dermatological features. Generally, the early intermediates ALA and

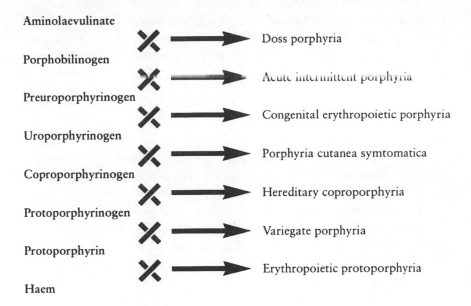

Aminolaevulinate

Porphobilinogen

Preuroporphyrinogen

Uroporphyrinogen

Coproporphyrinogen

Protoporphyrinogen

Protoporphyrin

Haem

Doss porphyria

Acute intermittent porphyria

Congenital erythropoietic porphyria

Porphyria cutanea symtomatica

Hereditary coproporphyria

Variegate porphyria

Erythropoietic protoporphyria

PBG give rise to the neurophysiological conditions whereas the later intermediates (porphyrins) cause the dermatological problems.

The inherited porphyrias give rise to five hepatic porphyrias and two erythropoietic porphyrias. The hepatic porphyrias are largely associated with what are known as acute porphyrias, in which the disorder sets in rapidly, with severe symptoms but of comparatively short duration. These attacks are manifested in the form of abdominal pain with vomiting and constipation, sometimes with a neuropsychiatric (mental) involvement such as anxiety, depression, disorientation, confusion and delirium. Further dysfunction of the nervous system may also occur such as weakness and numbness (peripheral neuropathy), respiratory difficulty and *grand mal* seizures. Most of the hepatic porphyrias are also associated with elevated porphyrin levels which may result in a skin disorder. This is described in more detail below.

The erythropoietic forms of the disorder are associated more with dermatological features, which include skin rashes and blistering, rather than acute attacks. This is due to the accumulation of porphyrins within the blood, bone marrow and other organs. The porphyrins exert a severe photodynamic effect leading to chronic inflammation, blistering and lesions on exposed skin areas such as the hands and face. The lesions tend to become infected and are slow to heal, leaving a marked scarring pattern on the individual.

Inheritance Pattern

Inherited diseases are genetic forms of a disease that are passed from one generation to the next. Genetic defects are normally associated with mutations within genes. These mutations lead either to loss of production of the protein encoded by a gene, or to malfunctioning of the protein. Humans have two copies of nearly every gene, reflecting the fact that we have two copies of every chromosome, one copy inherited from our mother and one from our father. The exceptions relate to genes carried on the sex chromosomes, as males have an X and a Y chromosome whereas females have two X chromosomes.

As there are two copies of every gene, apart from those located on the sex (X and Y) chromosomes, the double gene dosage ensures that enough of the encoded protein is made. If one of the genes is mutated, so that it produces an inactive protein, then only half the amount of normal protein will be made. In many cases this 50 per cent level is sufficient for normal cellular activity. However, in some cases a 50 per cent reduction can lead to a bottleneck in cellular metabolism or development. In this case, the defect in the gene causes what is known as a 'dominant' disorder. An inherited disorder is referred to as a dominant disorder if the presence of only one copy of the faulty gene is enough to endow the individual with the disease symptoms, or phenotype. In fact, most of the porphyrias are inherited as dominant disorders. A recessive disorder occurs when a disease requires the inheritance of two faulty copies of the gene. This explains why recessive diseases are more uncommon in families than dominant disorders.

As genetic disorders of porphyrias are generally dominant, the affected individuals carry one normal copy of the gene and one defective copy. This implies that in normal healthy individuals both copies of the gene contribute towards the biosynthesis of haem and that a drop in the level of a particular enzyme leads to a constriction in the flow of intermediates through the pathway. In fact, many people are able to carry a defective gene in haem biosynthesis and are not affected by porphyria. Why is this? It appears that humans can tolerate lower levels of haem biosynthetic enzymes so long as the pathway is not stimulated. The constriction in the pathway is not noticed until the pathway is required to work maximally. In the same way that a river with weakened banks will flow normally until a period of heavy rain, at which point the weakened banks burst and cause a flood, so, with porphyria, the pathway can be considered as merely weakened, until it bursts under pressure of increased metabolic activity. In the case of porphyria, the overflow from the pathway allows large quantities of the toxic intermediates to circulate. It is the intermediates in the pathway which cause the symptoms of porphyria.

The factors which affect the metabolic activity of the haem biosynthetic pathway are multiple and complex; in part, they are determined by the genetic background of the individual, but precipitating agents such as diet, alcohol, hormones and, particularly, certain drugs also contribute. This means that individuals can carry the disease but be asymptomatic and that the disease can appear to skip generations. It also means that individuals who have been asymptomatic can suddenly have an attack triggered if they are administered certain drugs. These drugs include barbiturates and sulphonamides. It is a sad fact that, due to the severity of certain forms of porphyria, the first attack can be fatal, especially if the cause is not diagnosed early on.

Acquired Porphyrias

As was mentioned earlier, some porphyrias are not inherited but are acquired through exposure to certain chemicals. If one of the enzymes of the haem biosynthetic pathway becomes modified in some way, for example by a chemical agent, then this may affect the ability of the enzyme to function properly. One type of such interference comes from lead poisoning. In this case lead, which is a common heavy metal contaminant, interferes with the first enzyme in the haem biosynthetic pathway, called ALA dehydratase. In fact, Sir George Baker in 1760 deduced that an outbreak of colic in the West Country, referred to as the Devonshire Colic, was due to lead contamination of the local cider from cider presses.[10] The symptoms of lead poisoning include anaemia, from reduced haem synthesis; abdominal pain; constipation; and peripheral neuropathy.[11] The latter symptoms are probably due to the increase in concentrations of circulating ALA. It is quite a coincidence that Sir George Baker was involved in the Devonshire Colic episode, as the symptoms of the victims would have been very similar to those suffered by his most famous patient, King George III.

More recently, it has been suggested that the ill-fated Franklin Arctic expedition was a victim of lead poisoning.[12] The Franklin expedition left London after meticulous preparation on 19 May 1845, to map the Northwest Passage. It consisted of two ships, 129 enlisted men and five officers under the command of Sir John Franklin. Although the two ships reached Beechey Island, none of the men were seen alive again. Records suggest that the Franklin expedition became disorderly and confused. It has now been suggested that lead poisoning and its consequential neurological problems were to blame for the demise of the trip, as elevated levels of lead were found in the frozen remains of some of the crew. Lead was to be found in plenty aboard the ship, from tableware to food wrappings. The high levels of lead found in the remains of the crew and the erratic behaviour of the members of the expedition before their death is very suggestive that plumbism (lead poisoning) was the cause. Lead poisoning has also been used as a contributory explanation for the fall of the Roman Empire.[13] Apart from using lead to line their water systems, the Romans used lead in wine-making and, in the form of lead salts, as artificial sweeteners. It has been estimated that the Roman upper class, the patricians, consumed five times the normal intake of lead, resulting in a high level of insanity among the Roman aristocracy.

Another well-known example of an acquired porphyria comes from the use of the fungicide hexachlorobenzene which was used with disastrous consequences in south-east Turkey in 1956.[14] The chemical was sprayed on to fields of wheat but ended up in the food chain, ultimately in bread. The chemical interferes with the enzyme uroporphyrinogen decarboxylase and prevents its normal functioning. This episode gave rise to an outbreak of cutaneous hepatic porphyria which was manifested in liver disease and photosensitivity and caused the deaths of a number of patients.

The Myth of Werewolves and Vampires[15]

Some of the symptoms of the porphyria sufferer, including mental derangement, anaemia, photophobia, skin scarring and discoloration as well as hypertrichosis (increased body hair), which can be associated with certain porphyrias, have led to reports that such sufferers were the basis of legends of vampires and werewolves. Certainly, pictures of individuals who are unfortunate enough to suffer with these disorders bear a close resemblance to the modern concept of a werewolf. There is no real evidence that porphyrics were the werewolves of legend, however, and the propagation of such stories has a detrimental and demeaning aspect and does little to inform the public as to the true suffering and discomfort which the disorder inflicts. As with all such stories, however, if they are repeated often enough some people will come to accept them as true.

The Royal Porphyrias

The porphyria from which King George III is likely to have suffered is thought to have been either acute intermittent porphyria (AIP) or variegate porphyria (VP). In their first research article on the Royal Malady, Ida Macalpine and Richard Hunter diagnosed AIP as the cause of his illness, as they initially found no evidence of photosensitivity.[16] However, in their second research article on the occurrence of porphyria in the European royal families, they changed their diagnosis because they had found several royal patients with skin fragility and sensitivity.[17] In essence, in the absence of a thorough biochemical analysis of the patient, the only difference between the symptoms of AIP and VP is the skin sensitivity. However, as we have seen, the evidence available to Macalpine and Hunter for skin sensitivity in the royal patients was rather weak, and we have been careful to consider both major types of porphyria in our investigation into the porphyria hypothesis.

Acute Intermittent Porphyria (AIP)

Acute intermittent porphyria (AIP) is the most common of the inherited porphyrias and is caused by a deficiency in the enzyme porphobilinogen deaminase (PBGD). A deficiency in this enzyme leads to the accumulation of the early pathway intermediates porphobilinogen (PBG) and ALA, which are excreted in the urine of patients during an attack. The excretion of PBG can give rise to the presence of coloured urine, usually red or brown. More often, the colour of urine develops with time after it is left to stand. AIP is normally triggered by factors such as diet, hormones and drugs. The disorder is generally expressed after puberty and with a higher incidence in women than in men, perhaps reflecting the greater fluctuation in hormonal levels.

There have been a number of clinical studies on the incidence of the symptoms of AIP. In all cases, around 90 per cent of patients suffer from abdominal pain, with a majority also suffering from vomiting and constipation. Patients were also found to suffer from limb, head, neck or chest pains, muscle weakness, hypertension and tachycardia and to display mental symptoms. In addition, some patients reported convulsions, sensory loss, breathing difficulties and fever. The abdominal pains are often severe enough to warrant surgical exploration. If this is accompanied by a barbiturate-based anaesthetic, it often makes the attack of AIP more acute and can lead to death. In severe cases, the urine of the patient has a port-wine colour due to the high concentration of excreted PBG and its chemical derivatives.

Patients can become hypersensitive, anxious, restless, insomniac, paranoiac or depressed and, in some cases, have been labelled as hysterical. The high incidence of AIP patients in psychiatric institutions shows how easy it is to misdiagnose the disorder. All of the major symptoms of AIP are thought to be caused by the effect of the early pathway intermediates on the nervous system, causing it to function incorrectly. However, the exact cause and site of the dysfunctions are still unknown.

AIP is thought to occur in about one in ten thousand of the population, although the actual frequency may be even higher than this. One of the problems in assessing the level of occurrence of AIP is that about 90 per cent of people who carry the defective gene for AIP never display any symptoms. The reasons why so many carriers remain asymptomatic is unclear. One point which is certain is that AIP can be induced in carriers by a number of factors, including certain drugs, alcohol and hormones. The main effect of these factors is to increase the level of activity of the enzyme which makes ALA, the starting point of haem biosynthesis. The increased concentration of ALA leads to an increase of flow of intermediates through the haem pathway, an increase which most healthy individuals can cope with. However, AIP patients have a reduced level of PBGD and thus the pathway in these individuals cannot cope with the increase in rate and a bottleneck forms at this point. An increase in ALA and PBG occurs and these elevated levels consequently lead to the neurophysiological problems associated with an AIP attack.

Progesterone and oestrogen, endocrine hormones associated with women's menstrual cycles, are also known to influence AIP attacks. On the whole, AIP is rarely manifested before puberty and there is a drop in the level of AIP attacks in post-menopausal women. Overall, AIP is more common in women than men (a ratio of three women to two men suffer with AIP) and women are more susceptible to AIP attacks at the start of their period. A number of women AIP sufferers have reported a periodicity of attacks which reflects their menstrual cycle. Certain contraceptive pills also cause attacks in women carriers of the disorder.

Poor diet is also a major influence on AIP attacks. In general it is thought that a low calorific diet can increase the likelihood of an attack and, consequently, AIP sufferers are more likely to precipitate an attack if they go on a crash diet.

Variegate Porphyria

Variegate porphyria arises from a dysfunction in the enzyme protoporphyrinogen oxidase (PPOX), the penultimate enzyme of the haem biosynthetic pathway. As the name implies, variegate porphyria is a mixed porphyria in which sufferers display symptoms of acute (neurovisceral) porphyria and/or photosensitivity. The photosensitivity is due to the accumulation of protoporphyrin.

Variegate porphyria occurs with a much higher incidence in South Africa than the rest of the world. As explained in Chapter 1, this was a result of the marriage between two Dutch settlers at the Cape of Good Hope in 1688.[18] The relative isolation of the community where they settled allowed for a rapid propagation of the mutant gene for variegate porphyria. Biochemical studies have shown that carriers of the mutant variegate porphyria gene have a 50 per cent reduction in PPOX. More recently, with the isolation of the gene, it has been possible to determine the actual mutation which caused the South African porphyric malady.[19] PPOX contains 477 amino acids and the mutation within the gene changes just one of these amino acids (the amino acid at position 59 is changed from an arginine to a tryptophan). Through this seemingly innocuous change of just one amino acid, the enzyme is rendered completely inactive. However, as predicted nearly thirty years ago, variegate porphyria patients in Europe do not have the same mutation, thus explaining why sufferers in Europe do not exhibit exactly the same symptoms as those in South Africa. Overall, variegate porphyria should be considered a world-wide problem occurring with only a slightly lower incidence than AIP.

In terms of its symptoms, variegate porphyria is very similar to AIP except that photosensitivity is much more common. Thus patients describe a very similar range of neurovisceral symptoms to those observed in acute porphyria, including acute abdominal pain, peripheral muscular weakness and psychiatric symptoms. The photosensitivity results in the appearance of vesicles and bullae, increased skin pigmentation, hair growth and skin fragility. The skin fragility means that if the skin is pushed under pressure it appears to slide. As one might expect, photosensitivity is more marked in countries where there is a good deal of sunshine.

The major biochemical finding associated with variegate porphyria is the excretion of large amounts of protoporphyrin in the faeces. Faeces of variegate porphyria sufferers appear fluorescent when viewed under ultraviolet light, and this was a basic diagnostic test for variegate porphyria in the early days.

The same factors which influence AIP attacks also influence variegate porphyria. Thus barbiturates, contraceptive steroids and dietary changes all have an effect on either starting or exacerbating variegate porphyria attacks.

Treatment for AIP and VP

The major treatment, as for most porphyrias, is the avoidance of precipitating factors. Patients should have an adequate nutritional intake, especially increasing the carbohydrate component of their diet. A strong analgesic medication would probably be prescribed to combat the severe pain. Beta blockers are sometimes prescribed in response to hypertension and tachycardia. A compound called haematin is often administered intravenously in order to reduce the levels of the intermediates from the pathway. The idea behind the administration of the drug is to reduce the metabolic activity of the haem pathway by mimicking haem. Protection against photo-sensitivity can be achieved by the use of protective clothing. Administration of light-quenching reagents such as beta carotene may be of some benefit.

The History of Porphyria[20]

The history of the porphyrias goes hand in hand with the history and development of medicine and science. Although porphyria was not recognized as a disease until the start of the twentieth century, it is possible to identify porphyric patients from old case notes, such as those of Hippocrates, the Greek 'father of medicine' (460–370 BC). He identified a patient who suffered from an attack with severe pain, had convulsions, mental disturbance, was talkative and passed dark urine.[21] However, an understanding of what porphyria is and why it occurs requires an understanding of the science of porphyrins, and these studies did not start until 1840.

In the mid-nineteenth century, haem, as a component of blood, was first studied by German chemists who were able to isolate the red pigment from blood treated with sulphuric acid. They were able to remove the iron and found that the coloured material also fluoresced when viewed under ultraviolet light. The iron-free material was called haematoporphyrin (literally 'purple blood'). Shortly after this, in the later nineteenth century, the first clinical porphyrin studies were undertaken, when porphyrin from a patient's urine was found to be similar to haematoporphyrin. In a view that was sixty years ahead of its time, the chemist Dr F. Baumstark hypothesized that the excretion was due to an error in haemoglobin synthesis.

However, the introduction of sulphonal drugs (1886) and barbiturates (1903) had the greatest effect on clinical porphyrin studies, as the drugs produced a large influx of porphyric patients whose urine provided a chemical soup of porphyrins for chemists to study. Thus by the end of the nineteenth century the porphyric trinity of symptoms were recognized – dark urine, severe abdominal pain and muscular weakness. The photodynamic effect of porphyrins was shown by Dr F. Meyer-Betz, a physician working in Munich who started an unhealthy tradition amongst researchers of using themselves as guinea pigs for their own research. Previously, it had been shown that iron-free haem (haematoporphyrin) was toxic to micro-organisms but only in the presence of light. Meyer-Betz took the experiment a stage further when he injected himself with a similar porphyrin solution. In the dark he was fine, but when he exposed himself to sunlight he developed skin blisters and rashes; erythema (flushing of the skin due to capillary dilation), oedema (swelling due to accumulation of fluid) and pain followed quickly.

Work on the disease in the early twentieth century was also dominated by German researchers. Hans Günther (1884–1956) coined the phrase *Haematoporphyrie* for porphyrin metabolism, and from a comparatively large collection of porphyric patients made the first attempts at classifying the disorder. He recognized that some patients had the disease from birth (congenital), some developed the disease after taking certain drugs (acute toxic) and some developed acute attacks spontaneously (acute genuine). Günther is thus credited with realizing that porphyria belongs to a group of disorders which could be described as inborn errors of metabolism.

One of Günther's patients, Hans Petry, who suffered with a very rare form called congenital erythropoietic porphyria, went on to work for another remarkable German chemist, Hans Fischer. The urine which Petry excreted provided a rich supply of porphyrins for

Fischer to experiment with. Fischer took a methodical, step-by-step approach to the study of porphyrins and was instrumental in determining their chemical structures. For his outstanding research, he was awarded the Nobel Prize in 1930, and his laboratory spawned many eminent scientists who also went on to make a notable contribution to the study of porphyrins and porphyria. Among these was Jan Waldenström, a physician who studied acute porphyria in Sweden and showed that the disease was inherited in a dominant manner even though it was frequently latent.

By the mid-twentieth century, attention was focused on elucidating the haem biosynthetic pathway. In this area of research an American chemist, Dr David Shemin, led the way, although he too used himself as a guinea pig for his investigations. He ingested isotopically labelled chemicals to show that haem was made from chemicals readily available in the body. Moreover, he showed that 5-aminolevulinic acid (ALA) was the first intermediate in the pathway. Eventually the whole pathway was completely elucidated, with Rimington playing a key role in the identification of porphobilinogen (PBG), the second intermediate in the pathway. Once the pathway was fully worked out, it became apparent that all the forms of hereditary porphyria were associated with lesions in specific enzymes of the pathway. The larger group studies of porphyric families led to a greater understanding of inheritance patterns and a slightly better understanding of the precipitating factors.

One by one during the 1980s and 1990s, the genes for all the human haem biosynthetic enzymes were isolated and sequenced. There is still a great deal to be learnt about how these genes are controlled and regulated, factors that are very important for a full understanding of porphyria. However, the identification of the genes has led to the determination of some of the mutations which cause the various forms of porphyria. Several structures (shapes) of the enzymes for haem biosynthesis have been elucidated, allowing an insight into how these enzymes work. Moreover, the structures also provide a molecular explanation as to why the mutant enzymes are defective.

Very recently, techniques in molecular science have allowed the construction of specific animal models for porphyria (mainly mice – referred to as 'transgenic' or 'knockout' mice). The animal models appear to have similar symptoms to humans and thus represent an important tool not only for further understanding the factors which cause porphyric attacks but also for finding a cure.[22] The latter will depend upon the development of drugs which have the effect of calming the haem pathway and prevent the accumulation of the toxic intermediates.

Advances in science have allowed the basis of the porphyrias to be understood at the molecular level. Now it is the aim to convert this knowledge into a practical therapy for this debilitating disorder.

Notes

PREFACE

1. Princess Elizabeth to Lady Harcourt, 20 April 1813, printed in P. C. Yorke, ed., *Letters of Princess Elizabeth of England, Daughter of King George III, and Landgravine of Hesse-Homburg* (London, 1898), pp. 60f. Full details of the exhumation and the condition of King Charles's remains are given in William Munk, *The Life of Sir Henry Halford* (London and New York, 1895), pp. 53–62.
2. Munk, op. cit., pp. 61f.

CHAPTER 1: *The Porphyria Controversy*

1. I. Ray, 'Insanity of King George III', *American Journal of Insanity*, vol. 12 (1855), p. 1.
2. J. H. Plumb, *The First Four Georges* (London, 1956), p. 95.
3. M. Guttmacher, *America's Last King: An Interpretation of the Madness of George III* (New York, 1941).
4. Plumb, op. cit., p. 104.
5. Ibid., p. 92.
6. John Brooke, *King George III* (London, 1972), p. 23.
7. Ida Macalpine and Richard Hunter, 'The Insanity of King George III: A Classic Case of Porphyria', *British Medical Journal* (1966), pp. 65–71.
8. Ida Macalpine, Richard Hunter and Claude Rimington, 'Porphyria in the Royal Houses of Stuart, Hanover and Prussia: A Follow-up Study of George III's Illness', *BMJ* (1968), pp. 7–18.

9. Ida Macalpine and Richard Hunter, 'Porphyria and King George III', *Scientific American*, July 1969, pp. 38–46.
10. Ida Macalpine and Richard Hunter, *George III and the Mad Business* (London, 1969).
11. *Porphyria – a Royal Malady* (St Albans, 1968).
12. Ida Macalpine and Richard Hunter, 'A Clinical Reassessment of the Insanity of George III and Some of its Historical Implications', *Bulletin of the Institute for Historical Research*, vol. 40 (1967) p. 166.
13. Macalpine and Hunter, 'The Insanity of King George III'.
14. Ibid.
15. Macalpine, Hunter and Rimington, op. cit.; see also, for the most recent discussion of James's numerous curious symptoms, A. W. Beasley, 'The Disability of James VI & I', in *Seventeenth Century*, vol. X, no. 2 (Autumn 1995), pp. 151–62. Beasley accepts the suggested diagnosis of porphyria in James as 'impressive', but argues that the King suffered in addition from cerebral palsy.
16. The medical history of Augustus and his brothers and sisters is examined further in Chapter 4.
17. Macalpine, Hunter and Rimington, op. cit.
18. Hugh Trevor-Roper, *BMJ*, 13 April 1968, p. 1105.
19. C. E. Dent to Ida Macalpine, 10 January 1966, Macalpine-Hunter Papers (MHP)/Cambridge University Library (CUL).
20. Lennox Eales and Eugene B. Dowdle, *BMJ*, 30 March 1968, pp. 841–2.
21. Ibid.
22. G. Dean, *The Porphyrias: A Story of Inheritance and Environment* (London, 1971).
23. G. Dean, *BMJ*, 17 February 1968, p. 443.
24. G. Dean, *BMJ*, 27 April 1968, p. 224.
25. Abraham Goldberg, *BMJ*, 24 February 1968, pp. 509–10.
26. G. Dean, *Porphyria Variegata*. Acta Dermatovener, suppl. 180, pp. 81–5.
27. C. E. Dent to Ida Macalpine, 18 January 1966, MHP, CUL; C. E. Dent, *BMJ*, 3 February 1968, pp. 311–12; W. N. Arnold, *The Lancet* (1966), 347, pp. 1811–13.
28. Ibid.
29. C. E. Dent, *BMJ*, 13 April 1968, p. 118.
30. Ida Macalpine, *Scientific American*, August 1969, pp. 8–9.
31. Ibid.
32. C. E. Dent, *BMJ*, 3 February 1968, pp. 311–12.
33. G. Dean, *BMJ*, 17 February 1968, p. 443.
34. L. Eales and E. B. Dowdle, *BMJ*, 30 March 1968, pp. 841–2.
35. C. E. Dent, *BMJ*, 3 February 1968, pp. 311–12.
36. L. Eales and E. B. Dowdle, *BMJ*, 30 March 1968, pp. 41–2.
37. C. E. Dent, *BMJ*, 3 February 1968, p. 311–12.
38. G. Dean, *Scientific American*, July 1969, p. 8.

39. L. Eales and E. B. Dowdle, *BMJ*, 30 March 1968, pp. 41–2.
40. C. E. Dent to Macalpine, 18 January 1966, MHP, CUL; also see C. E. Dent, *BMJ*, 3 February 1968, pp. 311–12.
41. Ida Macalpine to C. E. Dent, 24 January 1966, MHP, CUL.
42. C. E. Dent, *BMJ*, 13 April 1968, p. 118.
43. A. L. Cochrane, *BMJ*, 17 February 1968, p. 444.
44. A. Goldberg, *BMJ*, 4 May 1968, pp. 509–10.
45. C. E. Dent to Ida Macalpine, 18 January 1966, MHP, CUL.
46. Ida Macalpine to C. E. Dent, 24 January 1966, MHP, CUL.
47. Ida Macalpine to Dr A. Gajdos, 22 April 1968, MHP, CUL.
48. Ibid.
49. A. Gajdos, *BMJ*, 18 May 1968, pp. 430–1.
50. Ibid.
51. See for example Jean Bernard, *Le Sang et l'Histoire* (Paris, 1983); Donald P. Tschudy, 'Porphyrin Metabolism and the Porphyrias', in G. G. Duncan, ed. *Duncan, Diseases of Metabolism*, (Philadelphia, 1974).
52. Dr M. M. Salzmann to the authors, 6 June 1997.
53. Compare Antonia Fraser's *Mary Queen of Scots* (London, 1993) and Jenny Wormald's *Court, Kirk and Community in Scotland* (Edinburgh, 1991).
54. 'King of America', *Guardian*, 25 February 1995. See also the report by Bruno Cabanes on the film and its implications, 'Le Roi Fou de Windsor', in *L'Histoire*, no. 192 (October 1995), pp. 9–11.
55. Tony Scull, *Guardian*, 26 February 1995.
56. Ibid.
57. John Röhl, *Guardian*, 26 February 1995.
58. See Chapter 7.

CHAPTER 2: *On the Trail of Living Descendants*

1. C. Rimington, 'A biochemical fantasy' in M. R. Moore, K. E. L. McColl, C. Rimington and A. Goldberg, *Disorders of Porphyrin Metabolism* (New York, 1987).
2. Macalpine, Hunter and Rimington, 'Porphyria in the Royal Houses'.
3. Cecil Woodham Smith, *Queen Victoria: Her Life and Times* (London, 1972), vol. 1, p. 41.
4. Ibid., p. 43.
5. Macalpine, Hunter and Rimington, *BMJ*, 1968, 1, pp. 7–18.
6. Report of the Examination of the Body of His Late Royal Highness the Duke of Kent, 25 January 1820, Royal Archives (RA), 46638–9.
7. See Chapter 4 for the Duke of Kent's medical history.
8. T. K. With to Claude Rimington, 10 April 1967, MHP, CUL.
9. Ida Macalpine to Abraham Goldberg, 6 May 1967, MHP, CUL.
10. Ida Macalpine to Claude Rimington, August 1967, MHP, CUL.
11. Claude Rimington to Ida Macalpine, 10 August 1968, MHP, CUL.

12. G. Dean, *BMJ*, 17 February 1968, p. 443.
13. Stadtarchiv of the City of Nürnberg to the authors, 2 April 1997.
14. Letter to the authors, 20 August 1996.
15. *Lives of the Fellows of the Royal College of Physicians* (Oxford, 1982), pp. 304–5.
16. Gordon Wolstenholme (ed.), *Lives of the Fellows of the Royal College of Physicians* (Oxford, 1984), pp. 292–3.
17. Claude Rimington, *International Journal of Biochemistry*, vol. 25 (1993), pp. 1347–50.
18. Richard Hunter to Abraham Goldberg, 8 July 1966, MHP, CUL.
19. Ida Macalpine to Claude Rimington, 29 December 1966, MHP, CUL.
20. Claude Rimington to Ida Macalpine, 30 December 1966, MHP, CUL.
21. Claude Rimington to Ida Macalpine, 18 August 1967, MHP, CUL.
22. Claude Rimington to Ida Macalpine, 14 February 1967, MHP, CUL.
23. A. Vannotti, *Porphyrins: Their Biological and Chemical Importance* (London, 1954).
24. A. Vannotti to Claude Rimington, 11 May 1967, MHP, CUL.
25. Claude Rimington to A. Vannotti, 8 May 1967, MHP, CUL.
26. Ida Macalpine to Dr de Saussure, 26 May 1967, MHP, CUL.
27. Ibid.
28. The Swiss physician Dr Paul Niehans (d. 1982) had attained some notoriety by pioneering live-cell therapy which, though widely used in Europe, is forbidden in the United States. Pope Pius XII and Princess Adelaide's sister Feodora were among his many patients.
29. Ida Macalpine to Dr de Saussure, 18 June 1967, MHP, CUL.
30. A. Vannotti to Claude Rimington, 6 July 1967, MHP, CUL.
31. P. Niehans to A. Vannotti, 13 June 1967, MHP, CUL.
32. In response to our enquiry, the Policlinique Médicale Universitaire at Lausanne kindly informed us in a letter of 24 September 1997 that it was their practice to preserve current records for ten years, and important dossiers for twenty years. Princess Adelaide's wartime file would thus have been shredded by 1965 at the latest.
33. Ellen Franz, the later Baroness Heldburg, was born in Naumburg in central Germany on 30 May 1839. Her father was Dr Hermann Franz, the director of a commercial college in Berlin; her mother was born Sarah Grant, of Essex, England. Ellen Heldburg conducted almost all of her correspondence with the three women whose medical history we shall explore – Adi, Charlotte and Feodora I – in English.
34. Ada Princess of Saxe-Meiningen to Ellen Heldburg (EH), 25 November 1904, Thüringisches Staatsarchiv Meiningen (ThStaMgn), Hausarchiv (HA) 376 III.
35. Friedrich Prince of Saxe-Meiningen to EH, 3 May 1906, ThStaMgn, HA 375 IV.
36. Friedrich to his father, 11 May 1906, ThStaMgn, HA 375 IV.
37. Friedrich to his father, 1 July 1906, ThStaMgn, HA 375 IV.
38. Ada to EH, 28 June 1906 and summer 1907, ThStaMgn, HA 376 IV.

39. Ada to EH, 30 December 1906, ThStaMgn, HA 376 IV.
40. Ada to EH, 21 March 1907, ThStaMgn, HA 376 IV. 'The deafness disappeared as mysteriously as it had arrived in September 1907.'
41. Friedrich to EH, 29 April 1907, ThStaMgn, HA 375 IV.
42. Friedrich to his father, 5 June 1908, ThStaMgn, HA 375 IV; Ada to Georg II, Duke of Saxe-Meiningen, 6 June 1908, ThStaMgn, HA 376 IV.
43. Ada to EH, 28 May 1911, ThStaMgn, HA 376 IV.
44. Adalbert Prince of Prussia to EH, 26 and 29 July 1914; Adalbert to Adi Princess of Saxe-Meiningen, 30 July, 1 and 8 August 1914, ThStaMgn, HA 409 I; Ada to EH, 22 August 1914, ThStaMgn, HA 376 IV.
45. Adi Princess of Prussia to EH, 20 and 28 January 1916; ThStaMgn, HA 410 III.
46. Adalbert to EH, 20 February 1916, ThStaMgn, HA 410 III.
47. Kaiserin Auguste Viktoria to EH, 19 and 28 February 1916; Adalbert to EH, 19 February 1916, ThStaMgn, HA 410 III.
48. Adalbert to EH, n.d. (February 1916), ThStaMgn, HA 410 III.
49. Adi to EH, 27 April 1916, ThStaMgn, HA 410 III.
50. Adi to EH, 7 May 1916, ThStaMgn, HA 410 III.
51. Adalbert to EH, 18 May 1916, ThStaMgn, HA 410 III.
52. *Feuille d'avis de Vevey et des cercles de La Tour-de-Peilz et de Corsier*, 27 April 1971.
53. M. Ware to Ida Macalpine, 18 June 1967, MHP, CUL.
54. The name Lingen was used as an incognito by many in the Hohenzollern family, including Queen Victoria's daughter Vicky and Victoria-Marina's mother, Princess Adi.
55. Donald Tschudy was to become one of the leading proponents of the porphyria theory in the United States. See his article entitled 'Porphyrin Metabolism and the Porphyrias', in *Duncan, Diseases of Metabolism* (Philadelphia, 1974).
56. D. Tschudy to Claude Rimington, 7 September 1967, MHP, CUL.
57. Ibid.
58. Cripps to Ida Macalpine, 16 August 1967, MHP, CUL.
59. Ida Macalpine to Cripps, 21 August 1967, MHP, CUL.
60. Abraham Goldberg to Ida Macalpine, 18 September 1967, MHP, CUL.
61. Ida Macalpine to Claude Rimington, 1 July 1968, MHP, CUL.

CHAPTER 3: *'Madness' and King George III*

1. For a medical reference to mental disorders, see for instance Peter J. McKenna, *Schizophrenia and Related Syndromes* (London, 1997).
2. M. Guttmacher, *America's Last King*.
3. Sir L. Namier, 'King George III: A Study of Personality', in *Crossroads*

of Power, (London, 1962), p. 139; see also Brooke, *King George III*, p. 334.

4. Plumb, *The First Four Georges*.
5. H. C. Erik Midelfort, *Mad Princes of Renaissance Germany* (Charlottesville and London, 1994).
6. Ibid., p. 26.
7. V. H. H. Green, *The Madness of Kings: Personal Trauma and the Fate of Nations* (Stroud, 1993). See also J. M. Post and R. S. Robins, *When Illness Strikes the Leader: The Dilemma of the Captive King from George III to Ronald Reagan* (New Haven, 1993).
8. Based on the account given in Green, op. cit., and references therein.
9. Ibid.
10. Based on the account given in Ida Macalpine and Richard Hunter, *George III and the Mad Business* (London, 1969, 1991, 1995).
11. I. Macalpine and R. Hunter, *Bulletin of the Institute for Historical Research*, vol. 40 (1967), pp. 166–85.
12. Macalpine and Hunter, op. cit., p. 3.
13. Brooke, *King George III*, p. 323.
14. Macalpine and Hunter, *George III*, p. 4.
15. Ibid., p. 11.
16. Ibid., p. 15.
17. Ibid., p. 17.
18. Ibid., p. 17.
19. Ibid., p. 19.
20. Ibid., p. 25.
21. Ibid., p. 27.
22. Ibid., p. 29.
23. Such legends are probably inventions to spice up eighteenth-century pamphlets. See Brooke, *King George III*, p. 392.
24. Macalpine and Hunter, op. cit., p. 52.
25. Ibid., p. 53.
26. Ibid., p. 56.
27. The reports of the King's physicians, 1810–19, RA, 22 July 1811.
28. Macalpine and Hunter, op. cit., p. 53.
29. Brooke, *King George III*, op. cit., p. 335.
30. Macalpine and Hunter, *George III*, pp. 73–4.
31. Ibid., p. 86.
32. Ibid., p. 112.
33. Ibid., p. 116.
34. Ibid., p. 151.
35. Brooke, *King George III*, op. cit.
36. Ibid., p. 341.
37. Stanley Ayling, *George the Third* (London, 1972), p. 124.
38. Nesta Pain, *George III at Home*, (London, 1975), p. 99.
39. John W. Todd, *BMJ*, 17 February 1968, p. 444.
40. Brooke, *King George III*, xviii.

41. Christopher Hibbert, *George IV Prince of Wales 1762–1811* (London, 1972), p. 81.
42. Antonia Fraser, *Mary Queen of Scots*, pp. 445–6.
43. *Porphyria – A Royal Malady*, p. 49.
44. Hans Roeseler, 'Friedrich Wilhelm I: 1688–1740', in Willy Andreas and Wilhelm von Scholz, eds., *Die Grossen Deutschen, Neue Deutsche Biographie* (Berlin, 1935), vol. 2, p. 117.
45. Gerhard Oestreich, *Friedrich Wilhelm I. Preussischer Absolutismus, Merkantilismus, Militarismus* (Göttingen, 1977), p. 73.
46. Hans-Joachim Neumann, *Erbkrankheiten in europäischen Fürstenhäusern* (Berlin, 1993), pp. 148–57.
47. Kurt R. Spillmann and Kati Spillmann, 'Friedrich Wilhelm I. und die Preussische Armee: Versuch einer Deutung auf psychoanalytischer Basis', paper delivered at the 16th International Historical Congress, Stuttgart, 26 August 1985.
48. Claus A. Pierach and Erich Jennewein, 'War der Preussische König Friedrich Wilhelm I. (1688–1740) an Porphyrie erkrankt?' in *Internationale Zeitschrift für Geschichte und Ethik der Naturwissenschaften, Technik und Medizin*, forthcoming. We are grateful to the authors for permission to draw on their work.
49. Ibid., p. 10.
50. Ibid.
51. Rainer von Hessen, ed., *Wir Wilhelm von Gottes Gnaden: Die Lebenserinnerungen Kurfürst Wilhelms I. von Hessen 1743–1821* (Frankfurt/Main and New York, 1996).
52. Nils Minkmar, 'Der Fürst als Volontär. Überleben bei Hofe: Das Empfindsame Journal des Kurfürsten Wilhelm I. von Hessen', *Die Zeit*, no. 46, (November 1996), p. 8.
53. Hessen, op. cit., pp. 98f.
54. Ibid., pp. 134ff.
55. Ibid., p. 147.
56. Ibid., pp. 153f.
57. Ibid., pp. 225f.
58. Ibid., p. 222. See also pp. 365, 330.
59. Ibid., p. 238.
60. Ibid., p. 296.
61. Ibid., pp. 302f.
62. Ibid., p. 318.
63. Ibid., pp. 329, 335f., 336f., 340, 352, 354, 365, 381, 385, 398, 416, 422, 426f.; see also the extracts from his calendar almanach, p. 555.
64. P. Fitzgerald, *Royal Dukes and Princesses of the Family of George III: A View of Court Life and Manners for Seventy Years* (London, 1882), vol. 2, pp. 200ff.
65. Ibid., pp. 202ff.
66. Ibid., p. 205.

67. Dorothy Margaret Stuart, *The Daughters of George III* (London, 1939), p. 251.

CHAPTER 4: *The 'Family Complaint': The Fifteen Children of King George III*

1. Quoted in Stuart, *The Daughters of George III*, p. 251.
2. Hibbert, *George IV Prince of Wales*, vol. 1, pp. 248ff.
3. Hibbert, op. cit., vol. 2, p. 15.
4. Woodham Smith, *Queen Victoria*, vol. 1, p. 77.
5. V. Delves Broughton, *Court and Private Life in the Time of Queen Charlotte: Being the Journals of Mrs. Papendiek* (London, 1887), vol. 1, p. 50.
6. Macalpine and Hunter, *George III and the Mad Business*, pp. 232f.
7. See Hibbert, op. cit., vol. 1, p. 250, vol. 2, p. 15.
8. Hibbert, op. cit., vol. 1, p. 24.
9. Henry B. Wheatley, ed., *The Historical and Posthumous Memoirs of Sir Nathanial William Wraxall* (London, 1884), vol. 5, p. 363.
10. A. Aspinall, ed., *The Correspondence of George, Prince of Wales, 1770–1812* (London, 1963–71), vol. 4, p. 44.
11. Hibbert, op. cit., vol. 1, p. 38; see also Munk, *The Life of Sir Henry Halford*, pp. 172–4.
12. Hibbert, op. cit., vol. 1, p. 233.
13. Ibid., p. 62.
14. Aspinall, *The Correspondence of George, Prince of Wales*, vol. 2, p. 160.
15. Hibbert, op. cit., p. 249.
16. Aspinall, *The Correspondence of George, Prince of Wales*, vol. 2, p. 352, vol. 4, p. 41.
17. Macalpine, Hunter and Rimington, op. cit., p. 41.
18. Ibid.
19. Ibid.
20. Earl of Ilchester, ed., *The Journal of Elizabeth, Lady Holland, 1791–1811* (London, 1908), vol. 2, p. 49.
21. Hibbert, op. cit., vol. 1, p. 160.
22. Ibid., p. 171.
23. P. Fitzgerald, op. cit., vol. 1, pp. 375ff.
24. Hibbert, op. cit., vol. 1, p. 250.
25. Ibid., p. 251; Roger Fulford, *George the Fourth* (London, 1935), p. 93.
26. James Grieg, ed., *The Farington Diary* (London 1922–8), vol. 4, p. 54.
27. Hibbert, op. cit., vol. 1, p. 252; Grieg, op. cit., vol. 4, pp. 130f., vol. 5, p. 237.
28. Hibbert, op. cit., vol. 1, p. 254.
29. Castalia Countess Granville, ed., *Lord Granville Leveson Gower (First Earl Granville): Private Correspondence, 1781–1821* (London, 1916), vol. 2, pp. 297f.

30. A. Aspinall, ed., *Letters of the Princess Charlotte* (London, 1949), p. 16; Macalpine and Hunter, op. cit., p. 230; Macalpine, Hunter and Rimington, op. cit., p. 40; Hibbert, op. cit., vol. 2, pp. 13ff.; Fulford, op. cit., p. 118.

31. Aspinall, op. cit., p. 16; Macalpine and Hunter, op. cit., p. 230; Roger Fulford, *Royal Dukes: The Father and Uncles of Queen Victoria* (London, 1933), p. 210; Hibbert, op. cit., vol. 2, pp. 13f.; Joanna Richardson, *George IV: A Portrait* (London, 1966), p. 113.

32. A. Aspinall, ed., *Mrs. Jordan and Her Family, Being the Unpublished Correspondence of Mrs. Jordan and the Duke of Clarence, Later William IV* (London, 1951), pp. 222f.

33. John Gore, ed., *Creevey* (London, 1948), p. 91.

34. Hibbert, op. cit., vol. 2, pp. 13ff.

35. Quoted in Macalpine, Hunter and Rimington, op. cit., p. 41.

36. Aspinall, *Letters of the Princess Charlotte*, p. 112.

37. Hibbert, op. cit., vol. 2, pp. 20f.

38. Gore, op. cit., pp. 116f.

39. Fulford, op. cit., p. 216; Fulford, *George the Fourth*, p. 287; Hibbert, op. cit., vol. 2, pp. 78ff., 309. See also Philip Whitwell Wilson, ed., *The Greville Diary* (London, 1927), vol. 1, pp. 193f.

40. Gore, op. cit., pp. 160f.

41. A. Aspinall, ed., *The Letters of King George IV* (Cambridge, 1938), vol. 2, p. 223.

42. Munk, op. cit., pp. 174ff; Fulford, *Royal Dukes*, pp. 69, 78; Richardson, op. cit., p. 196; Wilson, op. cit., vol. 1, p. 110; Hibbert, op. cit., vol. 2, p. 145; Fulford, *George the Fourth*, pp. 191f.

43. Hibbert, op. cit., vol. 2, pp. 192, 216f.

44. Wilson, op. cit., p. 116; Hibbert, op. cit., vol. 2, p. 340; Richardson, op. cit., p. 282.

45. Peter Quennell, ed., *The Private Letters of Princess Lieven to Prince Metternich 1820–26* (London, 1948), p. 121; Richardson, op. cit., p. 245.

46. Gore, op. cit., p. 230.

47. Hibbert, op. cit., p. 255.

48. Quennell, op. cit., pp. 205, 215; Hibbert, op. cit., vol. 2, p. 256.

49. Fulford, op. cit., p. 251.

50. Hibbert, op. cit., p. 255.

51. Ibid.

52. Lytton Strachey and Roger Fulford, eds., *The Greville Memoirs* (London, 1938), p. 25.

53. Richardson, op. cit., p. 266.

54. Hibbert, op. cit., vol. 2, pp. 279ff.; Fulford, *Royal Dukes*, p. 80; Richardson, op. cit., pp. 299f.

55. Hibbert, op. cit., vol. 2, pp. 223, 281f.; see also Fulford, op. cit., pp. 221, 226.

56. Quoted in Hibbert, op. cit., vol. 2, p. 326.

57. Fulford, *George the Fourth*, pp. 251ff.; Richardson, op. cit., p. 309; see also Hibbert, op. cit., vol. 2, pp. 93, 280; Aspinall, *Letters of the Princess Charlotte*, p. 224.
58. Macalpine, Hunter and Rimington, op. cit., p. 42.
59. Hibbert, op. cit., vol. 2, p. 301; Fulford, op. cit., p. 282.
60. Gore, op. cit., p. 285.
61. Fulford, op. cit., pp. 289f.
62. Wilson, op. cit., vol. 1, p. 121.
63. Hibbert, op. cit., vol. 2, pp. 224, 230f., 238, 304f., 323; Macalpine, Hunter and Rimington, op. cit., p. 42.
64. Hibbert, op. cit., vol. 2, p. 323; Richardson, op. cit., p. 331.
65. See Hibbert, op. cit., vol. 2, p. 308.
66. Wilson, op. cit., vol. 1, p. 116.
67. Edward Law, ed., *Lord Ellenborough, A Political Diary, 1828–1850* (London, 1881), vol. 1, p. 370; vol. 2, pp. 231f.
68. Wilson, op. cit., vol. 1, p. 134; see also p. 184.
69. Hibbert, op. cit., vol. 2, pp. 326ff.; Woodham Smith, *Queen Victoria*, vol. 1, p. 78.
70. Hibbert, op. cit., vol. 2, p. 330.
71. Bulletin, 15 April 1830; Sir Henry Halford to the Duke of Wellington, 27 April 1830, Royal Archives (RA), Add. 3/18.
72. Halford to the Duke of Wellington, 1 and 4 May 1839; Halford to the Duke of Clarence, 2 May 1830, RA, Add. 3/18.
73. Richardson, op. cit., pp. 328, 337f., 340.
74. Halford to Duke of Wellington, 3 May 1830, RA, Add. 3/18. See also Munk, *The Life of Sir Henry Halford*, pp. 176–8.
75. At the autopsy the doctors reported that 'the Anasarca had disappeared excepting some slight remains of it in the thighs' – Halford, Tierney, Cooper and Brodie, 'An Account of the Appearances which were observed in the Inspection of the Mortal Remains of His Majesty George the 4th', RA, Add. 21/27.
76. Law, *Lord Ellenborough*, vol. 2, pp. 328f.
77. Halford to Duke of Wellington, 29 April 1830, RA, Add. 3/18.
78. Halford to Duke of Wellington, 30 April 1830, RA, Add. 3/18.
79. Halford to Duke of Wellington, 6 and 7 May 1830, RA, Add. 3/18.
80. Halford to Duke of Wellington, 9, 10 and 11 May 1830, RA, Add. 3/18.
81. Halford to Duke of Clarence, 12 May 1830, Halford to Duke of Wellington, 11, 14–17 May 1830, RA, Add. 3/18.
82. Halford to Duke of Wellington, 17 May 1830, RA, Add. 3/18.
83. Halford, Tierney, Cooper and Brodie, op. cit.
84. Strachey and Fulford, op. cit., p. 49; *Porphyria – A Royal Malady*, p. 42.
85. Niedersächsisches Hauptstaatsarchiv to the authors, 30 December 1996, 13 January 1997. Dr Zimmermann's records bear the reference Dep. 84 KG and Dep. 103.

86. *Porphyria – A Royal Malady*, p. 50.
87. Ibid.
88. Dr J. G. Zimmermann to Gen. Richard Grenville, 27 August 1787, 1 February 1788, RA, Add. 15/110, 15/117.
89. Macalpine, Hunter and Rimington, op. cit., p. 50.
90. Ibid.
91. Roger Fulford writes of the Duke of York's death: 'It was heart trouble, aggravated by dropsy' – Fulford, *Royal Dukes*, p. 77. Christopher Hibbert also believes that the cause of the duke's final illness was 'dropsy' – Hibbert, op. cit., vol. 2, p. 283.
92. Fitzgerald, op. cit., vol. 2, pp. 156f.
93. Wilson, op. cit., vol. 1, pp. 61f.; Fitzgerald, op. cit., vol. 2, pp. 156–79; Munk, op. cit., pp.158–68.
94. Philip Ziegler, *King William IV* (London, 1971), pp. 58f.
95. Ibid., p. 63.
96. Ibid., p. 131.
97. Aspinall, ed., *Mrs. Jordan and her Family*, p. 146.
98. Ibid., p. 150.
99. Ibid., pp. 192f.
100. Ibid., pp. 235f.
101. W. Gore Allen, *King William IV* (London, 1960), p. 125. See also pp. 192f.
102. See for example Aspinall, op. cit., pp. 248, 252f., 282.
103. Wilson, op. cit., vol. 1, pp. 272f.; Strachey and Fulford, op. cit., pp. 30–41; Allen, op. cit., pp. 78, 191.
104. Strachey and Fulford, op. cit., p. 121.
105. Allen, op. cit., p. 83.
106. Wilson, op. cit., vol. 1, p. 391.
107. Ibid., p. 465.
108. Law, op. cit., p. 193.
109. Woodham Smith, op. cit., p. 131.
110. Ziegler, op. cit., p. 271.
111. Fulford, op. cit., p. 125.
112. Wilson, op. cit., vol. 1, p. 557.
113. Ibid., p. 20.
114. Ibid., p. 273.
115. Fulford, op. cit., pp. 124–8.
116. Allen, op. cit., p. 226. On the King's last illness see also Munk, op. cit., pp. 186–93.
117. Ziegler, op. cit., pp. 270f., 289.
118. Stuart, op. cit., pp. 63f.
119. Ibid., p. 63.
120. Fitzgerald, op. cit., p. 272.
121. Ibid.
122. Stuart, op. cit., p. 65.
123. Ibid.

124. Ibid., pp. 65f.
125. Ibid., p. 67.
126. Dr Du Vernoy to King Friedrich I of Württemberg, 9 April 1811, Hauptstaatsarchiv Stuttgart, Hausarchiv, Bestand G 245 Bü 11. We are most grateful to the archivist Dr Franz J. Moegle-Hofacker for drawing our attention to this correspondence.
127. Dr Du Vernoy to King Friedrich, 12 October, 2 and 5 November 1814, Hauptstaatsarchiv Stuttgart, Hausarchiv, Bestand G 245 Bü 11.
128. Fulford, op. cit., p. 166.
129. Zimmermann to Grenville, 3 July 1787, RA, 11607.
130. Aspinall, *Later Correspondence of George III*, vol. 1, p. 382.
131. Ibid., p. 507.
132. *Porphyria – A Royal Malady*, p. 52.
133. Aspinall, *The Correspondence of George, Prince of Wales*, p. 124.
134. Gen. F. A. Wetherall to Sir B. Bloomfield, 18–22 January 1820, RA, 46618–30.
135. Victoire Duchess of Kent to her mother, 29 February 1820, RA, M3/25. Cf. Woodham Smith, op. cit., pp. 40ff.; Fitzgerald, op. cit., pp. 237ff.
136. Samuel Lascombe, 'Report of the Examination of the Body of His late Royal Highness The Duke of Kent, Wednesday, January 26 1820', RA, 46638–9.
137. Stuart, op. cit., pp. 88f.
138. Ibid., p. 106.
139. Yorke, *Letters*, pp. 267f.
140. Sir Henry Halford to Lord Melbourne, 27 August, 2, 6 and 12 September 1840, RA, MP 122/95–101.
141. Sir Henry Halford to Lord Melbourne, 16, 20 and 22 September 1840, RA, MP 122/104–7.
142. Mrs Delany's Diary, 1 December 1785 to 3 January 1786; Queen Charlotte to Mrs Delany, 4 January 1786, in Yorke, op. cit., pp. 10–12.
143. Quoted in Stuart, op. cit., p. 141.
144. Countess of Bute to Mrs Delany, 7 January 1786; Countess of Stamford to Mrs Delany, 10 January 1786, in Yorke, op. cit., p. 13.
145. Fitzgerald, op. cit., vol. 1, pp. 68f.
146. Yorke, op. cit., pp. 14f.
147. Mrs Delany to Mrs Hamilton, 25 December 1786; Yorke, op. cit., pp. 15f.
148. Yorke, op. cit., pp. 16f.
149. Stuart, op. cit., p. 141.
150. Fitzgerald, op. cit., vol. 1, p. 85.
151. Stuart, op. cit., p. 104; see also p. 149.
152. Ibid., p. 175.
153. Hibbert, op. cit., vol. 1, p. 262.
154. Yorke, op. cit., pp. 130f.; Axel Albrecht Freiherr von Maltzahn,

Elisabeth Landgräfin von Hessen-Homburg, Königl. Prinzessin von Großbritannien und Irland (Homburg, 1908), p. 38.

155. Yorke, op. cit., pp. 148–50.
156. Ibid., pp. 159ff.
157. Ibid., pp. 162f.
158. Ibid., pp. 174ff.
159. Ibid., pp. 179ff.
160. Ibid., pp. 212, 218, 223, 234, 250.
161. Ibid., pp. 332ff.
162. Ibid., pp. 336f.
163. Ibid., pp. 267f.
164. Ibid., pp. 201ff.
165. Ibid., pp. 242ff.
166. Ibid., pp. 249ff.
167. Ibid., pp. 314ff.
168. Ibid., pp. 318ff.
169. Ibid., pp. 322f.
170. Ibid., pp. 343ff.
171. Ibid., pp. 346f.
172. Johann Georg Hamel, 'Chronik, Jahrgang 1840', Stadtarchiv Bad Homburg, Bestand E 1 (Nachlass Hamel), Bd. 5, pp. 1–22.
173. Stuart, op. cit., p. 199.
174. Ibid.
175. Maltzahn, op. cit., p. 448.
176. Gerta Walsh, 'Von der Königlichen Prinzessin zur Landgräfin in Homburg', in: *Ich Schreibe, Lese und Male ohne Unterlass ... Elizabeth, Englische Prinzessin und Landgräfin von Hessen-Homburg (1770–1840) als Künstlerin und Sammlerin* (Bad Homburg/Greiz, 1995), pp. 10f., 21f.
177. Grieg, *The Farington Diary*, op. cit., vol. 5, p. 70.
178. Fitzgerald, *Royal Dukes and Princesses*, vol. 2, p. 46. See also Yorke, op. cit., p. 14.
179. Drs von Zimmermann, Stromeyer, Richter and Fischer in the Hanover archives, quoted in *Porphyria – A Royal Malady*, p. 51.
180. Zimmermann to King George III, August 1786, quoted in *Porphyria – A Royal Malady*, p. 51.
181. Fulford, op. cit., pp. 253, 258f.
182. Ibid., p. 267.
183. Aspinall, *Mrs Jordan and Her Family*, p. 200.
184. Fulford, op. cit., p. 277.
185. Hibbert, op. cit., vol. 1, p. 180.
186. Fitzgerald, op. cit., vol. 2, p. 95; Fulford, op. cit., p. 283.
187. Fulford, op. cit., p. 277.
188. Ibid., p. 283.
189. William Frederic Chambers and others, 'Report on the Dissection of the late Duke of Sussex', 23 April 1843, RA, M51/117.

190. See p. 8.
191. Fulford, op. cit., p. 301.
192. Yorke, op. cit., p. 212.
193. See Fulford, op. cit., p. 301.
194. Stuart, op. cit., p. 213.
195. Ibid., pp. 208, 269.
196. Sir Henry Halford to the Prince of Wales, 15–19 December 1810, RA Reports, King's Physicians, November 1788–February 1811.
197. Stuart, op. cit., p. 253.
198. Ibid., p. 255.
199. Ibid., p. 261.
200. Ibid., pp. 267f.
201. Ibid., pp. 106, 220f.
202. Ibid., pp. 276, 288.
203. Fitzgerald, op. cit., vol. 1, p. 265. See also Stuart, op. cit., pp. 285, 288f.
204. Stuart, op. cit., pp. 265, 288.
205. Ibid., pp. 312ff.
206. Ibid., p. 318.
207. Ibid., pp. 135, 262.
208. Ibid., pp. 90f., 269; see also p. 317.
209. Ibid., pp. 280f.
210. Ibid., p. 245; see also p. 288.
211. Ibid., p. 302.
212. Ibid., pp. 327f.
213. Ibid., p. 329.
214. Ibid., p. 331.
215. Ibid., p. 351.
216. Ibid., pp. 329, 332.
217. Ibid., p. 332.
218. Ibid., p. 339.
219. Ibid., p. 334.
220. Hibbert, op. cit., vol. 1, p. 265.
221. Stuart, op. cit., pp. 351, 355.
222. Princess Amelia to George Prince of Wales, 28 July 1810, RA, Add. 14/202.
223. Stuart, op. cit., pp. 351f.
224. Ibid., p. 361.
225. Ibid., pp. 355f.
226. Princess Amelia to King George III, 9 May 1810, RA, Add. 14/173. The doctors' reports to the King are also preserved in the Royal Archives.
227. Stuart, op. cit., pp. 367ff., 375.
228. Ibid., p. 365.
229. Sir Henry Halford to King George III, 24 May 1810, RA, Add. 14/185.

230. Dr David Dundas to King George III, 19 May 1810, RA, Add. 14/179; Sir Henry Halford to Queen Charlotte and King George III, 20, 22, 27 and 30 May 1810, RA, Add. 14/181, 183, 188, 191; Dr Matthew Baillie to King George III, 19, 21, 26 and 29 May 1810, RA, Add. 14/180, 182, 186, 190.
231. Princess Amelia to King George III, 3 June 1810, and the King's reply, RA, Add. 14/196–7.
232. Princess Amelia to King George III, 9 May 1810, and the King's reply, RA, Add. 14/173–4.
233. Sir Henry Halford to King George III, 10 May 1810, RA, Add. 14/175.
234. Sir Henry Halford to King George III, 16 and 18 May 1810, RA, Add. 14/177–8.
235. Dr Matthew Baillie to King George III, 23 May 1810, RA, Add. 14/184.
236. Sir Henry Halford to King George III, 26 May 1810, RA, Add. 14/187.
237. Sir Henry Halford to King George III, 28 May 1810, RA, Add. 14/189.
238. Dr Pope to Lt-Col Tayler, 31 May and 3 June 1810, RA, Add. 14/192, 195. The sentence 'the pain in the side remains as usual' recurs in Pope's letter to Tayler of 27 June 1810, RA, Add. 14/200.
239. Sir Henry Halford to King George III, 5–8 October 1810, RA, Add. 14/206–9.
240. Sir Henry Halford to King George III, 9–14 October 1810, RA, Add. 14/210–15.
241. Sir Henry Halford to King George III, 15–26 October 1810, RA, Add. 14/216–27.
242. Sir Henry Halford to George Prince of Wales, 28 October–2 November 1810, RA, Add. 14/228–30.
243. Fitzgerald, op. cit., vol. 1, p. 221.
244. Ibid., p. 222.
245. Stuart, op. cit., pp. 367ff., 375.
246. Ibid., p. 376.
247. Ibid., p. 366.
248. Ibid., p. 342. See also Fulford, op. cit., p. 63.

CHAPTER 5: *The 'Hereditary Malady': The 'Peculiarities' of Queen Victoria*

1. Woodham Smith, *Queen Victoria*, vol. 1, pp. 77f.
2. Elizabeth Longford, *Victoria* (London, 1964), p. 311.
3. Roger Fulford, ed., *Dearest Child: Private Correspondence of Queen Victoria and the Princess Royal, 1858–1861* (London, 1964), pp. 113ff., 174, 194, 206; Hector Bolitho, ed., *Further Letters of Queen*

Victoria (London, 1938), p. 101.

4. Roger Fulford, ed., *Dearest Mama: Private Correspondence of Queen Victoria and the Crown Princess of Prussia, 1861–1864* (London, 1968), pp. 239, 257.

5. Roger Fulford, ed., *Darling Child: Private Correspondence of Queen Victoria and the German Crown Princess* (London, 1976), p. 219.

6. Longford, op. cit., p. 503.

7. Ibid., p. 83.

8. Woodham Smith, op. cit., vol. 1, pp. 162f., 177; Longford, op. cit., p. 89.

9. Woodham Smith, op. cit., vol. 1, p. 92.

10. Ibid., pp. 93f., 96, 100f.

11. Ibid., p. 102f.

12. Longford, op. cit., p. 384. See also Roger Fulford, ed., *Your Dear Letter: Private Correspondence of Queen Victoria and the German Crown Princess, 1865–1871* (London, 1971), pp. 187f.

13. Woodham Smith, op. cit., vol. 1, pp. 104–8, 446n; Longford, op. cit., pp. 48f., 384.

14. Woodham Smith, op. cit., p. 151.

15. Ibid., p. 161. Cf. Longford, op. cit., p. 89.

16. Woodham Smith, op. cit., vol. 1, pp. 162f., 177; Longford, op. cit., p. 89.

17. Longford, op. cit., p. 200; see also p. 203; Strachey and Fulford, op. cit.; Wilson, op. cit., vol. 2, pp. 368f.

18. Wilson, op. cit., vol. 2, p. 130.

19. Woodham Smith, op. cit., vol. 1, pp. 205, 229; Longford, op. cit., p. 160; Fulford, *Dearest Child*, p. 142.

20. Wilson, op. cit., pp. 201f.

21. Ibid., p. 283.

22. Woodham Smith, op. cit., vol. 1, pp. 228, 232; Fulford, *Dearest Mama*, p. 303.

23. Fulford, *Dearest Child*, p. 77.

24. Woodham Smith, op. cit., vol. 1, p. 329; Longford, op. cit., p. 78.

25. Bolitho, op. cit., p. 49.

26. Woodham Smith, op. cit., vol. 1, p. 329.

27. Strachey and Fulford, *The Greville Memoirs*, vol. 7, p. 388; cf. Wilson, op. cit., vol. 2, p. 584. See also Longford, op. cit., p. 272, and Fulford, op. cit., pp. 136–8.

28. Woodham Smith, op. cit., vol. 1, pp. 397, 329–31.

29. Longford, op. cit., pp. 261, 266.

30. Ibid., p. 273.

31. Philip M. Magnus, *King Edward the Seventh* (London, 1964), p. 15.

32. Longford, op. cit., pp. 278, 292f.; Woodham Smith, op. cit., p. 400.

33. Fulford, op. cit., pp. 48, 54.

34. Ibid., p. 56; see also p. 122.

35. Longford, op. cit., pp. 290f.

36. Bolitho, op. cit., p. 117.
37. Fulford, op. cit., pp. 319f.
38. Ibid., pp. 324f., 327.
39. Ibid., pp. 330–3.
40. Ibid., p. 342.
41. Ibid., pp. 362f.
42. Vicky to Prince Albert, 7 June 1861, RA, Z 4/21; Hector Bolitho, *The Prince Consort and His Brother* (London, 1933), p. 212. See Longford, op. cit., p. 292, and Hannah Pakula, *An Uncommon Woman: The Empress Frederick: Daughter of Queen Victoria, Wife of the Crown Prince of Prussia, Mother of Kaiser Wilhelm* (New York, London, Toronto, Sydney, Tokyo, Singapore, 1995), p. 152.
43. Longford, op. cit., p. 292n.
44. Fulford, op. cit., pp. 364ff.
45. John Van der Kiste and Bee Jordaan, *Dearest Affie ... Alfred, Duke of Edinburgh, Queen Victoria's Second Son 1844–1900* (London, 1984), p. 40.
46. Bolitho, *Further Letters*, pp. 133f.
47. Ibid., pp. 134f.
48. Longford, op. cit., pp. 311–13, 321.
49. Fulford, *Dearest Mama*, pp. 200f; see also p. 259.
50. Ibid., p. 257.
51. Bolitho, op. cit., pp. 135f.
52. Fulford, op. cit., pp. 74f.
53. Ibid., pp. 164f., 168f.
54. Ibid., pp. 216f.
55. Ibid., pp. 280, 287.
56. Ibid., p. 301.
57. Ibid., p. 305.
58. Ibid., pp. 319, 322, 326f.
59. Fulford, *Your Dear Letter*, p. 236.
60. Ibid., p. 31.
61. Ibid., p. 146.
62. Ibid., pp. 150, 162f.
63. Ibid., p. 177.
64. Ibid., pp. 181f; see also pp. 227, 236.
65. Ibid., pp. 187f.
66. Ibid., p. 200.
67. Ibid., p. 195.
68. George Villiers, *A Vanished Victorian: The Life of Lord Clarendon by His Grandson* (London, 1938), p. 315.
69. Arthur Ponsonby, *Henry Ponsonby, Queen Victoria's Private Secretary, His life from his Letters* (London, 1942), pp. 73–6; Longford, op. cit., p. 380.
70. Ponsonby, op. cit., pp. 75f.
71. Longford, op. cit., p. 385.

72. Ibid., pp. 383f.
73. Fulford, *Darling Child*, p. 25.
74. Longford, op. cit., p. 385.
75. Fulford, op. cit., p. 25.
76. Longford, op. cit., p. 386.
77. Ibid., p. 387.
78. Ibid., pp. 416, 444; see also Fulford, op. cit., pp. 33, 47.
79. Longford, op. cit., pp. 79, 81; see also p. 114.
80. Queen Victoria to Vicky, 28 February and 1 April 1874, ibid., pp. 130, 134f; see also p. 210.
81. Roger Fulford, ed., *Beloved Mama: Private Correspondence of Queen Victoria and the German Crown Princess, 1878–1885* (London, 1981), p. 83.
82. Ponsonby, op. cit., p. 129.
83. Fulford, op. cit., pp. 141f.
84. Longford, op. cit., pp. 451–3, 461.
85. Fulford, op. cit., p. 157.
86. Ibid., p. 177.
87. Ponsonby, op. cit., pp. 234f.
88. Longford, op. cit., p. 474; see also Agatha Ramm, ed., *Beloved and Darling Child: Last Letters between Queen Victoria and Her Eldest Daughter 1886–1901* (Stroud, 1990), pp. 37f.
89. N. Rich and M. H. Fisher, eds., *The Holstein Papers*, 4 vols. (Cambridge, 1955–63), vol. 2, p. 139.
90. Longford, op. cit., p. 497.
91. Ibid., p. 510.
92. Ramm, op. cit., pp. 48, 53.
93. Vicky to Queen Victoria, 23, 26 and 29 July 1889, RA, Z45/30–2.
94. Ramm, op. cit., pp. 105f.
95. Ibid., pp. 114f., 147f., 166f., 174.
96. Longford, op. cit., p. 525.
97. See Bolitho, op. cit., pp. 275f.; Longford, op. cit., pp. 557f.

CHAPTER 6: *Vicky*

1. Woodham Smith, *Queen Victoria*, vol. 1, p. 228; Pakula, *An Uncommon Woman*, pp. 39f.
2. Fulford, *Darling Child*, p. 160.
3. Bolitho, *Further Letters*, p. 89.
4. Diary of the Crown Prince (DCP), 23 June 1858, Archiv der Hessischen Hausstiftung, Schloss Fasanerie (AHH).
5. DCP, 28 October–20 December 1858, AHH.
6. DCP, 14 December 1859–16 January 1860, AHH.
7. DCP, 10 June and 28 November 1860, AHH.
8. Fulford, *Dearest Child*, p. 335; DCP, 15 and 16 May 1861, AHH.

9. Fulford, op. cit., p. 339.
10. DCP, 21 October–10 November 1861, AHH; Pakula, op. cit., pp. 155f.
11. Fulford, op. cit., pp. 362f.
12. DCP, 11 June 1862, AHH.
13. Fulford, *Dearest Mama*, p. 75.
14. Ibid., p. 93.
15. Ibid., p. 123.
16. Ibid., p. 231.
17. Ibid., pp. 290, 293, 302.
18. Fulford, *Your Dear Letter*, p. 215n.
19. Ibid., p. 232.
20. Fulford, *Dearest Mama*, pp. 310, 317.
21. Ibid., p. 123.
22. Pakula, op. cit., p. 211; Fulford, *Your Dear Letter*, pp. 38f.
23. DCP, 7 and 18 October and 25 December 1864, AHH.
24. DCP, 6 and 11 January, 26 March, 17 September and 4 and 5 November 1865, AHH.
25. DCP, 7–9 January, 21 July, 5 and 14 November 1866, AHH; Vicky to Fritz, 14 November 1866, AHH.
26. Vicky to Fritz, 4 August 1866, AHH.
27. Fulford, op. cit., pp. 72f.; Vicky to Fritz, 11 November 1866, AHH; DCP, 9 November 1866, AHH.
28. Vicky to Fritz, 11 November 1866, AHH.
29. DCP, 6 October–25 November 1867, AHH.
30. Pakula, op. cit., p. 246.
31. Vicky to Fritz, 24 April 1868; Alice Grand Duchess of Hesse-Darmstadt to Crown Prince of Prussia, 23 April 1868; DCP, 21–24 April 1868, AHH.
32. Vicky to Fritz, 26 April 1868; DCP, 26 April 1868, AHH.
33. Vicky to Fritz, 27 April 1868, AHH.
34. Vicky to Fritz, 29 April 1868, AHH.
35. Vicky to Fritz, 1 May 1868, AHH.
36. Vicky to Fritz, 7–8 May 1868, AHH.
37. Fulford, op. cit., p. 189.
38. Vicky to Fritz, 9 May 1868, AHH.
39. Vicky to Fritz, 1 May 1868, AHH.
40. Wilbur L. Scoville, 'The Pharmaceutical Preparations of Chincona', *Proceedings of the 300th Anniversary of the First Recognized Use of Chincona* (St Louis, 1930), pp. 211–17; Frederic Rosengarten, 'The Minor Alkaloids of Chincona Bark', ibid., pp. 219–21; David Greenwood, 'Conflicts of Interest: The Genesis of Synthetic Antimalarial Agents in Peace and War', *Journal of Antimicrobial Chemotherapy*, vol. 36 (1995), pp. 857–72.
41. See Jan Waldenström, 'The Porphyrias as Inborn Errors of Metabolism', *American Journal of Medicine*, May 1957, pp. 758–73.

42. Vicky to Queen Victoria, 19 August 1868, RA, Z22/11; DCP, 16–18 August 1868, AHH.
43. DCP, 3–4 April 1869, AHH.
44. Vicky to Fritz, 9 May 1870, AHH,
45. Fulford, op. cit., p. 261.
46. Vicky to Fritz, 2 November 1870, AHH.
47. Vicky to Fritz, 1 and 27 January 1871; DCP, 15–26 April 1871, AHH.
48. Fulford, *Darling Child*, p. 23.
49. Vicky to Queen Victoria, 27 January 1872, RA, Z26/45. See also DCP, 9 and 23 May 1872, AHH.
50. Fulford, op. cit., pp. 80f.; DCP, 24–27 March, 4–15 April 1873, AHH.
51. Fulford, op. cit., p. 82.
52. Ibid., p. 84.
53. Bolitho, op. cit., pp. 195f. See also DCP, 28 August, 27 October, 25–27 November 1873, AHH.
54. Fulford, op. cit., p. 126.
55. DCP, 8–9 October 1874, AHH.
56. DCP, 16 November 1874, AHH.
57. DCP, 9–12 October 1875, AHH.
58. Fulford, op. cit., p. 196.
59. Ibid., p. 196.
60. DCP, 28 November, 20 December 1875 and 4 January 1876, AHH; Vicky to Prince Wilhelm, 29 November 1875, Geheimes Staatsarchiv Berlin, BPHA Rep. 52T Nr. 13.
61. Vicky to Queen Victoria, 29 December 1875, RA, Z29/61.
62. Vicky to Prince Wilhelm, 9 February 1876, GStA Berlin, BPHA Rep. 52T Nr. 13; DCP, 9 February 1876, AHH.
63. Vicky to Prince Wilhelm, 27 March 1876, GStA Berlin, BPHA Rep. 52T Nr. 13.
64. Vicky to Prince Wilhelm, 13 June 1876, GStA Berlin, BPHA Rep. 52T Nr. 13.
65. Vicky to Prince Wilhelm, 8 and 15 May 1876, GStA Berlin, BPHA Rep. 52T Nr. 13; DCP, 4–5 May 1876, AHH.
66. DCP, 19–20 May 1876, AHH.
67. Vicky to Prince Wilhelm, 12 December 1876; DCP, 14 December 1876, AHH.
68. DCP, 25 and 29 December 1876 and 10 April 1877, AHH.
69. DCP, 26 July–3 August 1877, 11 February and 11 August 1878, 12–14 January 1879, AHH.
70. Pakula, op. cit., pp. 374f.
71. Vicky to Fritz, 15 September 1885, AHH.
72. DCP, 2 and 7 May 1879, AHH.
73. Fritz to Vicky, 21 December 1879, AHH.
74. Fulford, *Beloved Mama*, p. 62.

75. Crown Prince to Ernst von Stockmar, 30 March 1880, AHH.
76. Vicky to Prince Wilhelm, 25 October and 25 November 1880, GStA Berlin, BPHA Rep. 52T Nr. 13; Vicky to Queen Victoria, 3 November 1880, RA, Z34/58; Crown Prince to Stockmar, 18 November 1880; DCP, 28 September and 21 November 1880, AHH.
77. Fulford, op. cit., p. 91.
78. DCP, 26 May, 3–6 June, 14 December 1881, 2–12 March 1882, AHH.
79. DCP, 13–28 March 1882, AHH.
80. Fulford, op. cit., p. 136; Fritz to Prince Wilhelm, 6 May 1883, GStA Berlin, BPHA Rep. 52J Nr. 336a.
81. Ramm, *Beloved and Darling Child*, pp. 47f.
82. Vicky to Queen Victoria, 26 March, 22 and 29 April, 11 May 1887, RA, Z39/13, 19–20, 22.
83. Vicky to Queen Victoria, 18 December 1887, RA, Z38/106.
84. Vicky to Queen Victoria, 2, 4, 5, 7 and 9 May 1888, RA, Z41/42–46. Cf. Ramm, op. cit., pp. 68ff.
85. Vicky to Queen Victoria, 27 and 30 July 1888, RA, Z42/23–4.
86. Vicky to Queen Victoria, 30 August 1888, RA, Z42/41.
87. Vicky to Queen Victoria, 13 and 18 May, 9 and 29 July 1889, RA, Z45/1–2, 25, 32.
88. Vicky to Queen Victoria, 20 October 1889, RA, Z46/26.
89. Vicky to Queen Victoria, 4 April 1890, RA, Z48/10.
90. Vicky to Queen Victoria, 15 and 17 October 1890, RA, Z49/19–20.
91. Vicky to Queen Victoria, 9 December 1890, RA, Z49/41.
92. Vicky to Queen Victoria, 24 and 26 March 1891, RA, Z50/24, 26. See her earlier worries about Edward's health in Ramm, op. cit., pp. 91, 93.
93. Vicky to Queen Victoria, 6 August 1891, RA, Z51/7.
94. Vicky to Queen Victoria, 22 August 1891, RA, Z51/14.
95. Vicky to Victoria Princess of Schaumburg-Lippe, 2–3 June 1891, AHH.
96. Vicky to Princess Victoria 8–12, 25 February 1892, AHH.
97. See her descriptions of her suffering in Ramm, op. cit., pp. 223ff.
98. Pakula, op. cit., p. 556.
99. Vicky to Queen Victoria, 4 January 1896, AHH.

CHAPTER 7: *'Charlotte the Brat'*

1. Pakula, *An Uncommon Woman* p. 335.
2. Vicky to Fritz, 9 May 1864, AHH.
3. Pakula, op. cit., p. 335.
4. Ibid.
5. Vicky to Queen Victoria, 23 May 1863, RA, Z15/25.
6. Vicky to Fritz, 8 April 1864, AHH.

7. Vicky to Queen Victoria, 23 May 1863, RA, Z15/25.
8. Vicky to Fritz, 2 May 1862, AHH.
9. Vicky to Fritz, 5 June 1866, AHH.
10. Fulford, *Darling Child*, pp. 138f. Charlotte had been suffering from severe catarrh and a small growth in the nose since 1870. Queen Victoria arranged for her to be examined by Sir William Jenner and Sir James Paget at Osborne in August 1874; ibid., p. 145; Vicky to Prince Wilhelm, 1 August 1887, GStA Berlin, BPHA Rep. 52T Nr. 13.
11. Pakula, op. cit., p. 372.
12. Vicky to Fritz, 6, 10 and 20 February, 18 and 29 March, 20 April 1864, AHH.
13. Vicky to Fritz, 28 October 1877, AHH.
14. Fritz to Vicky, 29 October 1877, AHH.
15. Vicky to Queen Victoria, 9 September 1879, RA, Z33/34.
16. Vicky, diary entry for 24 July 1888, GStA Berlin, BPH Rep. 52 Nr. 3.
17. Vicky to Fritz, 17 September 1883, AHH.
18. Vicky to Louise, Duchess of Connaught, 2 January 1885, RA, A15/4374.
19. Charlotte to EH, 16 March 1893, ThStaMgn, HA 342; Princess Victoria to her mother, 15 and 17 March 1893, AHH.
20. Vicky to Princess Victoria, 29 October 1892 and 8 January 1893, AHH.
21. Vicky to Queen Victoria, 2 November 1888, 20 August 1890 and 31 March 1891, RA, Z43/32, Z49/8 and Z50/30. See also Princess Victoria to Vicky, 30 May 1891, and Vicky to Princess Victoria, 22 July 1892, AHH.
22. Pakula, op. cit., p. 374. For the political intrigues of 'la jeune et charmante Meiningen' at this time see Rich and Fisher, *The Holstein Papers*, vol. 3, no. 238. For the bitter rivalry between Charlotte and her sister-in-law Dona see John C. G. Röhl, *The Kaiser and his Court: Wilhelm II and the Government of Germany* (Cambridge, 1984), p. 90f.
23. Hannah Pakula, *The Last Romantic: A Biography of Queen Marie of Roumania* (New York, 1984), p. 56f.
24. Feodora Princess of Reuss to EH, 28 December 1908, ThStaMgn, HA 382/IV.
25. See e.g. Charlotte to Hermann Fürst zu Hohenlohe-Langenburg, 25 March 1884, Hohenlohe Zentralarchiv Neuenstein, Hermann Hohenlohe Papers, Bü. 113; Vicky to Princess Victoria, 28 November 1890 and 24 February 1891, AHH.
26. See Pakula, op. cit., pp. 59, 109, 123; Pakula, *An Uncommon Woman*, p. 561. On the poison-letters scandal see Fritz Friedmann, *Der deutsche Kaiser und die Hofkamarilla: Der Fall Kotze* (Zürich, 1896). Friedmann voiced the suspicion that the letters were written by a woman; Philipp Eulenburg, the Kaiser's best friend, actually named Charlotte as their most likely originator. For the most recent treatment

of the scandal, see Tobias C. Bringmann, *Reichstag und Zweikampf.*
Die Duellfrage als innenpolitischer Konflikt des deutschen Kaiserreichs
1871–1918 (Freiburg, 1997), pp.152–224.

27. Vicky to Queen Victoria, 6 August 1891, RA, Z51/7.
28. Vicky to Princess Victoria, 5 December 1892, AHH.
29. Vicky to Princess Victoria, 28 April 1893, AHH; Charlotte to EH, 16 March 1893, ThStaMgn, HA 342.
30. Vicky to Princess Victoria, 30 April 1893, AHH.
31. Bernhard Hereditary Prince of Saxe-Meiningen to EH, 20 August 1894, ThStaMgn, HA 341.
32. Charlotte to EH, 13 August 1894, ThStaMgn, HA 342.
33. Charlotte to EH, 21 September 1901, ThStaMgn, HA 343.
34. Charlotte to EH, 26 February, 12 March 1896, 2 March and 27 November 1899, 29 January 1902, ThStaMgn, HA 342, 343.
35. Charlotte to EH, 29 October and 18 November 1902, ThStaMgn, HA 343.
36. Charlotte to EH, n.d., ThStaMgn, HA 207. See also Charlotte to EH, 16 May 1913, ThStaMgn, HA 345/I.
37. Charlotte to Ernst Schweninger, 14 July 1917, Bundesarchiv Berlin, Schweninger Papers (BABSP).
38. Charlotte to EH, 4 May 1896, ThStaMgn, HA 342.
39. Charlotte to Schweninger, 7 September 1896, BABSP.
40. Charlotte to EH, 11 November 1896, ThStaMgn, HA 342.
41. Charlotte to EH, 7 December 1896, ThStaMgn, HA 342.
42. Charlotte to EH, 15 March 1897, ThStaMgn, HA 342.
43. Charlotte to Vicky, 5 June 1898, AHH; Charlotte to EH, 9 October 1898, ThStaMgn, HA 343.
44. Charlotte to EH, 1 December 1898 and 18 November 1902, ThStaMgn, HA 343.
45. Charlotte to EH, 1 May, 20 June and 11 July 1899, ThStaMgn, HA 343.
46. Charlotte to EH, 4 June 1900, ThStaMgn, HA 343.
47. Charlotte to Schweninger, 8 July 1900, BABSP.
48. Charlotte to Schweninger, 12 September 1900, BABSP. Cf. Charlotte to EH, 20 March 1901, ThStaMgn, HA 343.
49. Charlotte to EH, 5 December 1900, ThStaMgn, HA 343.
50. Charlotte to EH, 8, 16 and 27 October 1901, ThStaMgn, HA 343.
51. Charlotte to EH, 13 November 1901, ThStaMgn, HA 343.
52. Charlotte to EH, 10 and 28 April, 24 November 1902, ThStaMgn, HA 343.
53. Charlotte to EH, 30 September 1900, ThStaMgn, HA 343.
54. Charlotte to EH, 28 April 1902, ThStaMgn, HA 343.
55. Feo to EH, 14 June 1904, ThStaMgn, HA 382/II.
56. Charlotte to EH, 17 June and 30 September 1902, ThStaMgn, HA 343.
57. Charlotte to EH, 18 and 24 November 1902, ThStaMgn, HA 343.

58. Charlotte to Schweninger, 26 June 1903, BABSP.
59. Charlotte to Lena Schweninger, 17 September 1903, BABSP.
60. Charlotte to EH, 22 October 1904, 14 April and 2 May 1905, ThStaMgn, HA 207. See also Bernhard to Schweninger, 11 April 1905, BABSP.
61. Siegmund Freud/Georg Groddeck, *Briefe über das Es* (Frankfurt am Main, 1988); Georg Groddeck, *Der Seelensucher* (Leipzig, Vienna and Zürich, 1921); Georg Groddeck, *Das Buch vom Es* (1923). The latter work has been translated into English as *The Book of the It: Psychoanalytical Letters to a Friend* (New York and Washington, 1928).
62. Charlotte to EH, 26 October 1904, ThStaMgn, HA 207.
63. Charlotte to EH, 28 October and 6 November 1904, ThStaMgn, HA 207.
64. Charlotte to EH, 28 October and 6 November 1904, ThStaMgn, HA 207.
65. Charlotte to EH, 2 May 1905, ThStaMgn, HA 207.
66. Charlotte to EH, 25 September 1906, ThStaMgn, HA 207.
67. ThStaMgn, Hofmarschallamt, HA 368; Charlotte to EH, 30 December 1908 and 17 February 1909, ThStaMgn, HA 345/I.
68. Charlotte to EH, 16 November 1905, ThStaMgn, HA 207.
69. Charlotte to Schweninger, 1 April 1906, BABSP.
70. Charlotte to Schweninger, 7 April 1906, BABSP.
71. Charlotte to Schweninger, 23 November 1906, BABSP. Charlotte uses the word '*Pesten*' to describe her period pains, which was evidently a Germanization of the term 'plagues' used by Queen Victoria to denote the same discomfort.
72. Charlotte to Schweninger, 3 December 1906, BABSP.
73. Charlotte to Schweninger, 24 December 1906, BABSP.
74. Charlotte to Schweninger, 25 April 1907, BABSP.
75. Charlotte to Schweninger, n.d., Groddeck Papers, Zürich. We thank Frau Margaretha Honegger for placing this document at our disposal.
76. Charlotte to Schweninger, 18 October 1907, BABSP.
77. Charlotte to Schweninger, 10 and 15 November 1907, BABSP.
78. Charlotte to Schweninger, 18 November 1907, BAPSP.
79. Charlotte to EH, 28 November and 2 December 1907, ThStaMgn, HA 207.
80. Charlotte to Schweninger, 16 December 1907, BABSP.
81. Charlotte to Schweninger, 23 December 1907, BABSP.
82. Charlotte to Schweninger, 7 January 1908, BABSP.
83. Charlotte to Schweninger, 21 January 1908, BABSP.
84. Charlotte to EH, 19 January 1908, ThStaMgn, HA 207.
85. Charlotte to Schweninger, 5 February 1908, BABSP.
86. Charlotte to Schweninger, 13 February 1908, BABSP.
87. Charlotte to EH, 4 February 1908, ThStaMgn, HA 207.
88. Charlotte to Schweninger, 20 February 1908, BABSP.

89. Charlotte to Schweninger, 7 March 1908, BABSP.
90. Charlotte to Schweninger, 13 March 1908, BABSP.
91. Charlotte to EH, 28 April and 8 May 1908, ThStaMgn, HA 345/I.
92. Charlotte to EH, 8 and 25 May 1908, ThStaMgn, HA 345/I.
93. Charlotte to EH, 15 June 1908, ThStaMgn, HA 207.
94. Charlotte to Schweninger, 18 July 1908, BABSP.
95. Feo to EH, 19 July 1908, ThStaMgn, HA 382/IV.
96. Charlotte to EH, 20 and 31 August 1908, ThStaMgn, HA 345/I.
97. Charlotte to Schweninger, 8 and 30 September 1908, BABSP.
98. Charlotte to Schweninger, 11 October 1908, BABSP.
99. Charlotte to EH, 6 November 1908, ThStaMgn, HA 207; Charlotte to
    Schweninger, 8 December 1908, BABSP.
100. Charlotte to Schweninger, 25 December 1908, BABSP.
101. Charlotte to Schweninger, 7 and 14 January 1909, BABSP.
102. Charlotte to Schweninger, 16 January 1909, BABSP.
103. Charlotte to Schweninger, 11 February 1909, BABSP. Charlotte to
    EH, 17 February 1909, ThStaMgn, HA 345/I.
104. Charlotte to Schweninger, 25 February 1909, BABSP.
105. Charlotte to Schweninger, 31 March 1909, BABSP.
106. Charlotte to Schweninger, 3 May 1909, BABSP.
107. Charlotte to EH, 10 April 1909, ThStaMgn, HA 207.
108. Bernhard to Schweninger, 15 June 1909; Charlotte to Schweninger, 4
    July 1909, BABSP.
109. Charlotte to EH, 8 October 1909, ThStaMgn, HA 207.
110. Charlotte to Schweninger, 30 October 1909, BABSP.
111. Charlotte to Schweninger, 24 October 1909, BABSP.
112. Charlotte to Schweninger, 5 November 1909, BABSP.
113. Charlotte to Schweninger, 23 November 1909, BABSP.
114. Charlotte to EH, 6 January 1910, ThStaMgn, HA 345.
115. Charlotte to Schweninger, 4 and 12 December 1909, BABSP;
    Charlotte to EH, 6 January 1910, ThStaMgn, HA 345.
116. Charlotte to Schweninger, 23 November 1909 and 28 January 1910,
    BABSP.
117. Charlotte to EH, 14 January 1910, ThStaMgn, HA 345.
118. Charlotte to Schweninger, 17 February 1910, BABSP.
119. Charlotte to EH, 26 April 1910, ThStaMgn, HA 345.
120. Charlotte to EH, 6 May 1910, ThStaMgn, HA 345.
121. Charlotte to Schweninger, 7 May 1910, BABSP.
122. Charlotte to Schweninger, 12 May 1910, BABSP.
123. Charlotte to Schweninger, 10 June and 2 July 1910, BABSP.
124. Charlotte to Schweninger, 30 July 1910, BABSP.
125. Charlotte to EH, 3 December 1910, ThStaMgn, HA 345.
126. Charlotte to Schweninger, 18 December 1910 and 20 January 1911,
    BABSP.
127. Charlotte to Schweninger, 16 February 1911, BABSP.
128. Charlotte to EH, n.d. (May 1911), ThStaMgn, HA 345.

129. Charlotte to Schweninger, 13 June 1911, BABSP.
130. Charlotte to EH, 25 July 1911, ThStaMgn, HA 345.
131. Charlotte to Schweninger, 13 and 18 July 1911, BABSP.
132. Charlotte to Schweninger, 14 September and 4 October 1911, BABSP.
133. Charlotte to Schweninger, 25 October, 9 November and 12 December 1911, BABSP.
134. Charlotte to EH, 20 May 1912, ThStaMgn, HA 207.
135. Charlotte to Schweninger, 12 and 24 June 1912, BABSP.
136. Charlotte to Schweninger, 18 July and 10 November 1912, BABSP.
137. Adelheid Princess of Prussia to EH, n.d. (November 1916), ThStaMgn, HA 410/III.
138. Charlotte to Schweninger, 14 July 1917, BABSP.
139. Charlotte to Schweninger, 12 and 21 December 1917, 12 January 1918, BABSP.
140. Charlotte to Schweninger, 2 January 1919, BABSP.
141. Charlotte to Schweninger, 6 July 1919, BABSP. See also Charlotte to Lena Schweninger, 31 August 1919, ibid.

CHAPTER 8: *Feodora, Our Last Princess*

1. The death certificates of Feodora, her husband and her companion are held in the Burgomaster's office at Kowary. We are deeply grateful to the Mayor, Mr Marek Jiruska, and his deputy, Mr Czeslaw Mikicki, for making these documents available to us.
2. Vicky to Princess Victoria, 2, 24–25 April and 18 November 1892 and 7 January 1893, AHH; Vicky to Queen Victoria, 24 May 1892, RA, Z52/53.
3. Vicky to Queen Victoria, 15 October 1890, RA, Z49/19–20.
4. Feo to EH, 8 December 1895, ThStaMgn, HA 382/I.
5. Vicky to Princess Victoria, 12 January 1893, AHH.
6. Charlotte to EH, 4 May 1896, ThStaMgn, HA 342.
7. Charlotte to EH, 25 February 1896, ThStaMgn, HA 342.
8. Since all male children of both the older and the younger line of Reuss were by tradition given the name Heinrich, the inflated dynastic numeral came to be the only way of distinguishing between them.
9. Charlotte to Schweninger, 1 October 1897, BABSP, no. 130; Charlotte to Vicky, 13 May 1898, AHH; Charlotte to EH, 16 September 1898, ThStaMgn, HA 343.
10. Feo to EH, 14 November 1898 and 27 May 1899; Charlotte to EH, 1 December 1898, ThStaMgn, HA 382/I and 343.
11. Charlotte to Vicky, 23 January 1899, AHH.
12. Charlotte to EH, 2 April 1899, ThStaMgn, HA 343.
13. Charlotte to EH, 19 May, 20 June and 11 July 1899, ThStaMgn, HA 343.

14. Feo to EH, 26 November 1899, ThStaMgn, HA 382/I.
15. Charlotte to EH, 27 November 1899, ThStaMgn, HA 343.
16. Heinrich Reuss to EH, 27 November 1899; Charlotte to Feo, 9 January 1900; Bernhard to EH, 8 April 1900, ThStaMgn, HA 381/I, HA 381/IV, HA 341.
17. Feo to EH, 5 April 1900, enclosing a copy of her father's letter and her reply, ThStaMgn, HA 382/I.
18. Charlotte to EH, 22 April, 10 and 29 May, 4 June, 23 July and 12 September 1900, ThStaMgn, HA 343; Heinrich Reuss to EH, 15 May 1900, Feo to EH, 9 August 1900, ThStaMgn, HA 383/I.
19. Feo to her grandfather, 21 September 1899, ThStaMgn, HA 382/I.
20. Feo to EH, 15 November 1899, ThStaMgn, HA 382/I.
21. Feo to EH, 9 and 25 March 1900, ThStaMgn, HA 382/I.
22. Charlotte to EH, 1 March and 13 May 1902, ThStaMgn, HA 343; Bernhard to Feo, 25 December 1902, ThStaMgn, HA 341; Charlotte to EH, 6 August 1911, ThStaMgn, HA 345/I.
23. Charlotte to EH, 3 October 1900, ThStaMgn, HA 343; Feo and Heinrich Reuss to EH, 28 May 1901, ThStaMgn, HA 382/I.
24. Feo to EH, 20 November 1900, ThStaMgn, HA 382/I.
25. Feo to EH, 10 January 1901, ThStaMgn, HA 382/I.
26. Charlotte to EH, 5 December 1900 and 28 March 1901, ThStaMgn, HA 343.
27. Charlotte to EH, 25 July, 4 and 21 September and 8 October 1901, ThStaMgn, HA 343.
28. Charlotte to EH, 4 February 1902, ThStaMgn, HA 343; Feo to EH, 12 February 1902, ThStaMgn, HA 382/I.
29. Feo to EH, 4 March 1902, ThStaMgn, HA 382/I.
30. Feo to EH, 1 April 1902, ThStaMgn, HA 382/I.
31. Feo to EH, 16 April 1902, ThStaMgn, HA 382/I.
32. Charlotte to EH, 30 November 1901, ThStaMgn, HA 343.
33. Charlotte to EH, 27 March 1902, ThStaMgn, HA 343.
34. Feo to EH, 13 and 28 May 1905, 15 June and 2 July 1907, ThStaMgn, HA 382/II, HA 382/IV.
35. Feo to EH, 31 July 1910, ThStaMgn, HA 383/I. In 1907, Prince Heinrich of Prussia told Feo that he had known of this matter 'for four years' and had broken with his sister Charlotte over this very scandal: Feo to EH, 12 July 1907, ThStaMgn, HA 382/IV. See also Feo to EH, 26 and 27 October and 28 December 1908, ibid.
36. Feo to EH, 29 October 1902, ThStaMgn, HA 382/II.
37. Feo to EH, 27 November 1902, ThStaMgn, HA 382/I.
38. Feo to EH, 31 December 1902, ThStaMgn, HA 382/II.
39. Feo to EH, 14 May and 23 June 1903, ThStaMgn, HA 382/II; Heinrich Reuss to EH, 25 November 1903, ThStaMgn, HA 381/I.
40. When Charlotte and Bernhard of Saxe-Meiningen visited Prince Heinrich of Prussia at the latter's nearby estate of Hemmelmark in November 1906, they openly refused to meet their daughter, nor

would they go to visit her at Flensburg. Charlotte also returned Feo's registered letters to her father unopened. Feo to EH, 1 and 8 November 1906, 14 June 1907, ThStaMgn, HA 382/III; Heinrich Reuss to EH, 26 November 1906, ThStaMgn, HA 381/I.

41. Feo to EH, 5 February, 28 and 30 May, 14 June, 13 July, 26 October, 28 November 1904, 3 and 14 March, 6 April and 28 November 1905, ThStaMgn, HA 382/II.

42. Feo to EH, 12 June and 2 August 1905, ThStaMgn, HA 382/II. When Charlotte heard of her daughter's attempts to have children, she exclaimed: 'No *thanks*, I can live without the *damned* brood!', Feo to EH, 15 May 1905, ThStaMgn, HA 382/II.

43. Feo to EH, 14 June 1904, ThStaMgn, HA 382/II.

44. Heinrich Reuss to EH, 28 May 1904, ThStaMgn, HA 382/I.

45. Feo to EH, 14 June 1904, ThStaMgn, HA 382/II.

46. Feo to EH, 7 November 1905, ThStaMgn, HA 382/II.

47. Feo to EH, 10 March 1906, ThStaMgn, HA 382/II.

48. Feo to EH, 4 and 7 July 1906, ThStaMgn, HA 382/III.

49. Feo to EH, 14 June and 2 July 1907, ThStaMgn, HA 382/III, HA 382/IV.

50. Feo to EH, 5 August 1907, ThStaMgn, HA 382/IV.

51. Feo to EH, 26 August and 23 September 1907, ThStaMgn, HA 382/IV.

52. Feo to EH, 15 October 1907, ThStaMgn, HA 382/IV.

53. Feo to EH, 6 July 1909, ThStaMgn, HA 383/I.

54. Feo to EH, 4 and 19 August 1909, ThStaMgn, HA 383/I.

55. Feo to EH, 6 July 1909, ThStaMgn, HA 383/I.

56. Feo to EH, 10 January 1910, ThStaMgn, HA 383/I.

57. Prof. Döderlein to EH, 4 February 1910, ThStaMgn, HA 383/IV.

58. Heinrich Reuss to EH, 12 and 13 February 1910, ThStaMgn, HA 383/IV.

59. Katharina Freifrau von Saalfeld to EH, 20 February 1910, ThStaMgn, HA 383/IV. See also Heinrich Reuss to EH, 27 February 1910, ThStaMgn, HA 381/I.

60. Feo to EH, 23 March 1910, ThStaMgn, HA 383/I.

61. Feo to EH, 2 May 1910, ThStaMgn, HA 383/I.

62. Feo to EH, 15 May and 2 July 1910, ThStaMgn, HA 383/I.

63. Feo to EH, 20 April 1910, ThStaMgn, HA 383/I.

64. Feo to EH, 2 May 1910, ThStaMgn, HA 383/I.

65. Ibid.; Feo to Duke Georg II of Saxe-Meiningen, 1 May 1910, ThStaMgn, HA 383/I.

66. Feo to Duke Georg II, 18 June 1910, ThStaMgn, HA 383/I.

67. Feo to EH, 18 June 1910, ThStaMgn, HA 383/I.

68. Feo to EH, 13 September 1910, ThStaMgn, HA 383/I.

69. Feo to EH, 8 February and 25 March 1911, ThStaMgn, HA 383/II.

70. Feo to EH, 29 May and 27 June 1911, ThStaMgn, HA 383/II.

71. Prof. Albert Döderlein, 'Kranken- und Operationsbericht von Ihrer

Durchlaucht der Prinzessin Heinrich XXX von Reuss', 9 September 1911, ThStaMgn, HA 383/II; Heinrich Reuss to EH, 9 and 10 September 1911, ThStaMgn, HA 381/II.

72. Heinrich Reuss to EH, 14 and 22 September 1911; Bernhard to Heinrich Reuss, 16 September 1911; Döderlein to EH, 21 September 1911, ThStaMgn, HA 381/II.

73. Charlotte to Feo, 11 and 14 September 1911; Bernhard to Heinrich Reuss, 16 September 1911, ThStaMgn, HA 381/II; Charlotte to EH, 13 September 1911, ThStaMgn HA 207.

74. Charlotte to Feo, 17 September 1911, ThStaMgn, HA 381/II.

75. Heinrich Reuss to EH, 2 December 1911, ThStaMgn, HA 381/II.

76. Feo to EH, 22 December 1911, ThStaMgn, HA 383/II.

77. Heinrich Reuss to EH, 21 January 1912, ThStaMgn, HA 381/II.

78. Feo to EH, 16 February 1912, ThStaMgn, HA 383/II.

79. Heinrich Reuss to EH, 29 May 1912, ThStaMgn, HA 381/II.

80. Feo to EH, 18/19 May 1912, ThStaMgn, HA 383/II.

81. Heinrich Reuss to EH, 29 May 1912, ThStaMgn, HA 381/II.

82. Feo to EH, 28 May 1912, ThStaMgn, HA 383/II.

83. Feo to EH, 28 May 1912, ThStaMgn, HA 383/II.

84. Charlotte to EH, 25 and 29 May 1912, ThStaMgn, HA 207.

85. Heinrich Reuss to EH, 6 July, 9 and 26 August 1912, ThStaMgn, HA 381/II.

86. Feo to EH, 11 October 1912, ThStaMgn, HA 383/II.

87. Feo to EH, 27 January 1913, ThStaMgn, HA 383/II.

88. Heinrich Reuss to EH, 28 October and 6 November 1912, ThStaMgn, HA 381/II.

89. Heinrich Reuss to EH, 22 December 1912; Heinrich Reuss to Duke Georg II, 25 December 1912, ThStaMgn, HA 381/II.

90. Feo to Duke Georg II, 27 December 1912, ThStaMgn, HA 383/II.

91. Feo to EH, 5 May 1913, ThStaMgn, HA 383/II.

92. Feo to Duke Georg II, 15 May 1913; Feo to EH, 19 May 1913, ThStaMgn, HA 383/II.

93. See Cavalier Hargrove Joüet, *Index to the Literature on Thorium, 1817–1902* (Washington, 1903).

94. Heinrich Reuss to EH, 24 May 1913, ThStaMgn, HA 381/II.

95. Charlotte to EH, 17 May and 2 June 1913, ThStaMgn, HA 345/I.

96. Feo to Duke Georg II, 23 December 1913, ThStaMgn, HA 383/III. See also Heinrich Reuss to EH, 28 November 1913, ThStaMgn, HA 381/III.

97. Heinrich Reuss to EH, 1 February 1914, ThStaMgn, HA 381/III; Feo to EH, 18 February 1914, ThStaMgn, HA 383/III.

98. Feo to EH, 30 March 1914, ThStaMgn, HA 383/III.

99. Charlotte to EH, 14 May 1914, ThStaMgn, HA 345/I; Heinrich Reuss to EH, 2 October and 2 December 1914, ThStaMgn, HA 381/III.

100. Heinrich Reuss to EH, 25 September 1915, ThStaMgn, HA 381/III.

101. Feo to EH, 6 December 1914, ThStaMgn, HA 383/III.

102. Feo to EH, 1 April 1915, ThStaMgn, HA 383/III.

103. Heinrich Reuss to EH, 19 March 1915, ThStaMgn, HA 381/III.
104. Feo to EH, 28 May 1915, ThStaMgn, HA 383/III.
105. Heinrich Reuss to EH, 2 June 1915, ThStaMgn, HA 381/III.
106. Feo to EH, 16 August 1915, ThStaMgn, HA 383/III.
107. Feo to EH, 19 October 1915, ThStaMgn, HA 383/III.
108. Heinrich Reuss to EH, 27 October, 20 November and 29 December 1915, ThStaMgn, HA 381/III.
109. Dr Haedke to EH, 16 January 1916, ThStaMgn, HA 383/IV.
110. Feo to EH, 7 January 1916, ThStaMgn, HA 383/IV.
111. Feo to EH, 8 January 1916, ThStaMgn, HA 383/IV.
112. Feo to EH, 4 and 10 February, 6 March 1916, ThStaMgn, HA 383/V.
113. Heinrich Reuss to EH, 16 February and 2 March 1916, ThStaMgn, HA 381/III.
114. Dr Haedke to EH, 14 February 1916, ThStaMgn, HA 383/IV.
115. Adelheid Princess of Prussia to EH, ThStaMgn, HA 410/III. On Adelheid's own medical history see pp. 30–4.
116. Heinrich Reuss to EH, 2 March 1916, ThStaMgn, HA 381/III.
117. Heinrich Reuss to EH, 3 February 1916, ThStaMgn, HA 381/III.
118. Heinrich Reuss to EH, 16 February 1916, ThStaMgn, HA 381/III.
119. Feo to EH, 15, 16 and 21 February 1916, ThStaMgn, HA 383/IV.
120. Heinrich Reuss to EH, 2 March 1916, ThStaMgn, HA 381/III.
121. Heinrich Reuss to EH, 16 February 1916, ThStaMgn, HA 381/III.
122. Feo to EH, 13 March 1916, ThStaMgn, HA 383/II.
123. Feo to EH, 29 May 1916, ThStaMgn, HA 383/V.
124. Heinrich Reuss to EH, 24 May 1916, ThStaMgn, HA 381/III.
125. Heinrich Reuss to EH, 25 June 1916, ThStaMgn, HA 381/III.
126. Heinrich Reuss to EH, 15 July 1916, ThStaMgn, HA 381/III.
127. Feo to EH, 9 October 1916, ThStaMgn, HA 383/V.
128. Heinrich Reuss to EH, 29 November 1916, ThStaMgn, HA 381/III.
129. Heinrich Reuss to EH, 25 December 1916, ThStaMgn, HA 381/III.

CHAPTER 9: *Ancient DNA*

1. S. Pääbo. 'Molecular Cloning of Ancient Egyptian Mummy DNA', *Nature*, vol. 314 (1985), pp 644–5.
2. K. B. Mullis, 'The Unusual Origin of the Polymerase Chain Reaction', *Scientific American*, April 1990, pp. 56–61.
3. S. Pääbo, 'Ancient DNA', *Scientific American*, November 1990, pp. 60–6.
4. M. Höss, S. Pääbo, and N. K. Vereshchagin, 'Mammoth DNA Sequences', *Nature*, vol. 370 (1994), p. 333; E. Hagelberg, M. G. Thomas, C. E. Cook Jr, A. V. Sher, G. F. Baryshnikov and A. M. Lister, 'DNA From Ancient Mammoth Bones', ibid., pp. 333–4.
5. R. DeSalle, J. Gatesy, W. Wheeler and D. Grimaldi, 'DNA Sequences From a Fossil Termite in Oligo-Miocene Amber and Their Phylogenetic

Implications', *Science*, vol. 257 (1992), pp. 1933–6.

6. S. R. Woodward, N. J. Weyand and M. Bunnell, 'DNA Sequence From Cretaceous Period Bone Fragments', *Science*, vol. 266 (1994), pp. 1229–32.

7. 'Detecting Dinosaur DNA', *Science*, vol. 268 (1994), pp. 1191–4.

8. E. Beraud-Colomb, R. Roubin, J. Martin, N. Maroc, A. Gardeisen, G. Trabuchet and M. Goossens, 'Human Beta-Globin Gene Polymorphisms Characterized in DNA Extracted From Ancient Bones 12,000 Years Old', *American Journal of Human Genetics*, vol. 57 (1995), pp. 1267–74.

9. D. A. Lawlor, C. D. Dickel, W. W. Hauswirth and P. Parham. 'Ancient HLA Genes From 7,500-Year-Old Archaeological Remains', *Nature*, vol. 349 (1991), pp. 785–8.

10. R. L. Parr, S. W. Carlyle and D. H. O'Rourke, 'Ancient DNA Analysis of Freemont Amerindians of the Great Salt Lake Wetlands', *American Journal of Physiological Anthropology*, vol. 99 (1996), pp. 507–18.

11. J. Klier and H. Mingay, *The Quest for Anastasia* (London, 1996).

12. P. Gill, P. L. Ivanov, C. Kimpton, R. Piercy, N. Benson, G. Tully, I. Evett, E. Hagelberg and K. Sullivan, 'Identification of the Remains of the Romanov Family by DNA Analysis', *Nature Genetics*, vol. 6 (1994), pp. 130–5; P. L. Ivanov, M. J. Wadhams, R. K. Roby, M. M. Holland, V. W. Weedn and T. J. Parsons, 'Mitochondrial DNA Sequence Heteroplasmy in the Grand Duke of Russia Georgij Romanov Establishes the Authenticity of the Remains of Tsar Nicholas II', *Nature Genetics*, vol. 12 (1996), pp. 417–20.

13. M. Stoneking, T. Melton, J. Nott, S. Barritt, R. Roby, M. Holland, V. W. Weedn, P. Gill, C. Kimpton, R. Aliston-Greiner and K. Sullivan, 'Establishing the Identity of Anna Anderson Manahan', *Nature Genetics*, vol. 9 (1995), pp. 9–10.

14. J. Dalton, 'Extraordinary Facts Relating to the Vision of Colours', *Memoirs of Manchester Literary and Philosophical Society*, vol. 5 (1798), pp. 28–45.

15. D. M. Hunt, K. S. Dulai, J. K. Bowmaker and J. D. Mollon, 'The Chemistry of John Dalton's Color Blindness', *Science*, vol. 267 (1995), pp. 984–8.

16. W. C. Henry, *Memoirs of the Life and Scientific Researches of John Dalton* (London, 1854); D. Brewster, *Letters on Natural Magic, Addressed to Sir Walter Scott* (London, 1842).

CHAPTER 10: *Blood and Bones: The Search for the Royal Mutation*

1. J. A. Petit, *History of Mary Stuart*, vol. 1 (Edinburgh, 1883), pp 120–2; C. Nau, *The History of Mary Stuart*, ed. J. Stevenson (Edinburgh, 1883), pp.31–2; R. Keith, *History of the Affairs of Church and State in Scotland*, vol. 3 (Edinburgh, 1844–50), p. 286.

2. Fraser, *Mary Queen of Scots*, p. 445.

3. T. B. Macaulay, *The History of England From the Accession of James II*, (1858) vol. 7, p. 76.

4. A. W. Beasley, 'The Disability of James VI & I', *Seventeenth Century*, vol. X, no. 2 (1995) pp. 151–62.

5. M. A. E. Green, *Lives of the Princesses of England* (London, 1855), vol. 6, pp. 543–90.

6. R. F. Whistler, 'The Relics of King Charles I at Ashburnham Place', *Sussex Archaeological Collections*, XXXVI (1888).

7. Stiftung Thüringer Schlösser und Gärten to the authors, 12 May 1996.

8. P. Gill, P. L. Ivanov, C. Kimpton, R. Piercy, N. Benson, G. Tully, I. Evett, E. Hagelberg and K. Sullivan, 'Identification of the Remains of the Romanov Family by DNA Analysis', *Nature Genetics*, vol. 6 (1994), pp. 130–5.

9. A. G. Roberts, S. D. Whatley, J. Daniels, P. Holmans, I. Fenton, M. J. Owen, P. Thompson, C. Long and G. H. Elder, 'Partial Characterization and Assignment of the Gene for Protoporphyrinogen Oxidase and Variegate Porphyria to Human Chromosome 1q23', *Human Molecular Genetics*, vol. 4 (1995), pp. 2387–90.

10. S. Taketani, J. Inazawa, T. Abe, T. Furukawa, H. Kohno, R. Tokunaga, K. Nishimura and H. Inokuchi, 'The Human Protoporphyrinogen Oxidase Gene (PPOX): Organization and Location on Chromosome 1', *Genomics*, vol. 29 (1995), pp. 698–703.

11. L. Warnich *et al.*, 'Identification of Three Mutations and Associated Haplotypes in the Protoporphyrinogen Oxidase Gene in South African Families with Variegate Porphyria', *Human Molecular Genetics*, vol. 5 (1996), pp. 981–4; H. Lam *et al.*, 'Molecular Basis of Variegate Porphyria: A De Novo Insertion Mutation in the Protoporphyrinogen Oxidase Gene', *Human Genetics*, vol. 99 (1997), pp. 126–9.

12. J.-C. Deybach and H. Puy, 'Porphobilinogen Deaminase Gene Structure and Molecular Defects', *Journal of Bioenergetics and Biomembranes*, vol. 27 (1995), pp. 197–205.

13. Professor George Elder to the authors, March 1988.

CHAPTER 11: *The Ghosts of Windsor*

1. Brooke, *King George III*, p. 392.

2. Ibid., p. vii–ix.

3. M. Gillen, *The Prince and His Lady* (New York, 1971), p. 130.

4. D. M. Potts and W. T. W. Potts, *Queen Victoria's Gene: Haemophilia and the Royal Family* (Stroud, 1995), p. 59.

5. Ibid.

6. Col. Richard Symes to Gen. R. Grenville, RA, 45412–7.

7. Ian R. Christie, 'George III and the Historians – Thirty Years On', *Journal of Historical Associations*, vol. 71 (1985), pp. 205–8.

8. James Brough, *Margaret: The Tragic Princess* (London, 1978), pp. 236–49.

9. H. E. Bellringer to the authors, 5 February 1996.

10. This account is based on Giles St Aubyn, ed., *William of Gloucester*,

Pioneer Prince (London, 1977).
11. Ibid., p. 90.
12. Ibid.
13. H. E. Bellringer to the authors, 5 February 1996.
14. Green, *The Madness of Kings*, p. 203.

CONCLUSION

1. John C. G. Röhl, *The Kaiser and his Court*, p. 23.
2. Ibid., p. 21.
3. The Diary of Lord Esher, 21 November 1908, Esher Papers, Churchill Archives Centre, Cambridge.

APPENDIX

1. A more detailed account can be obtained from any biochemistry or genetics textbook, for example B. Lewin, *Genes V* (Oxford, 1995).
2. J. D. Watson and F. H. C. Crick, 'Genetical Implications of the Structure Deoxyribonucleic Acid', *Nature*, vol. 171 (1953), pp. 737–8; M. H. F. Wilkins, A. R. Stokes and H. R. Wilson, 'Molecular Structure of Deoxypentose Nucleic Acids', ibid., pp. 738–40.
3. O. T. Avery, C. M. Macleod and M. McCarty, 'Studies on the Chemical Nature of the Substance Inducing Transformation of Pneumococcal Types: Induction of Transformation by a Deoxyribonucleic Acid Fraction Isolated From Pneumococcus Type III', *Journal of Experimental Medicine*, vol. 79 (1944), pp. 137–58.
4. This phrase was coined by Prof. Sir Alan Battersby, see A. R. Battersby, *Science*, vol. 264 (1994), pp. 1551–7; for an account of the biology and chemistry of these pigments see L. M. Milgrom, *The Colours of Life* (Oxford, 1997).
5. Detailed reviews of haem biosynthesis can be found in H. A. Dailey, ed., *Biosynthesis of Heme and Chlorophyll* (New York, 1990), and P. M. Jordan, *Biosynthesis of Tetrapyrroles* (London, 1991).
6. P. T. Erskine N. Senior, S. Awan, R. Lambert, G. Lewis, I. J. Tickle, M. Sarwar, P. Spencer, P. Thomas, M. J. Warren, P. M. Shoolingin-Jordan, S. P. Wood and J. B. Cooper, 'Structure of yeast 5-aminolaevulinic acid to 2.4Å', *Nature Structural Biology*, vol. 4, pp. 1025–31 (1997).
7. P. D. Brownlie, R. Lambert, G. V. Lonie, P. M. Jordan, T. L. Blundell, M. J. Warren, J. B. Cooper and S. P. Wood, 'The three-dimensional structures of mutants of porphobilinogen deaminase: Towards an understanding of the structural basis of acute intermittent porphyria', *Protein Science*, vol. 3 (1994), pp. 1644–50.
8. S. Taketani, J. Inazawa, T. Abe, T. Furukawa, H. Kohno, R. Tokunaga, K. Nishimura and H. Inokuchi, 'The Human Protoporphyrinogen Oxidase

Gene (PPOX): Organization and Location on Chromosome 1', *Genomics*, vol. 29 (1995), pp 698–703; A. G. Roberts, S. D. Whately, J. Daniels, P. Holmans, I. Fenton, M. J. Owen, P. Thompson, C. Long and G. H. Elder, 'Partial Characterization and Assignment of the Gene for Protoporphyrinogen Oxidase and Variegate Porphyria to Human Chromosome 1q23', *Human Molecular Genetics*, vol. 4 (1995), pp. 2387–90; H. Puy, A. Robreau, R. Rosipal, Y. Nordmann and J.-C. Deybach, *Biochemical and Biophysical Research Communications*, vol. 226 (1996), pp. 226–30.

9. For a comprehensive review of the porphyrias see, A. Kappas, S. Sassa, R. A. Galbraith and Y. Nordmann, in C. R. Scriver, A. L. Beaudet and W. S. Sly, eds., *The Metabolic Basis of Inherited Disease* (New York, 1995), pp. 2103–59.

10. Sir G. Baker, *Medical Transactions of the College of Physicians, London*, vol. 1, (1767), p. 175.

11. J. H. Dagg, A. Goldberg, A. Lochhead and J. A. Smith, *Quarterly Journal of Medicine*, vol. 134 (1965), pp. 163–75.

12. D. B. Stewart, 'The Fate of the Franklin Expedition, Part One: In the Wake of the Erebus and Terror', *Beaver*, vol. 68 (1988), pp. 13–18; 'Was the Ill-Fated Franklin Expedition a Victim of Lead Poisoning?' *Nutrition Reviews*, vol. 47 (1989), pp. 322–3; see also A. Keenleyside, M. Bertulli and H. C. Fricke, 'The Final Days of the Franklin Expedition: New Skeletal Evidence', *Arctic*, vol. 50 (1997), pp. 36–46.

13. S. C. Gilfillan, *Journal of Occupational Medicine*, vol. 7 (1965), p. 53.

14. C. Cam and G. Nigogosyan, 'Acquired Toxic Porphyria Cutanea Tarda Due to Hexachlorobenzene', *Journal of the American Medical Association*, vol. 183 (1963), pp. 88–91.

15. Based on Ann M. Cox, 'Porphyria and Vampirism: Another Myth in the Making', *Postgraduate Medical Journal*, vol. 71 (1995), pp. 643–4.

16. Macalpine and Hunter, 'The Insanity of King George III'.

17. Macalpine, Hunter and Rimington, 'Porphyria in the Royal Houses'.

18. Dean, *The Porphyrias*, pp. 103–13.

19. P. N. Meissner, T. A. Dailey, R. J. Hift, M. Ziman, A. V. Corrigal, A. G. Roberts, D. M. Meissner, R. E. Kirsch and H. A. Dailey, *Nature Genetics*, vol. 13 (1996), pp. 95–7.

20. See also Michael R. Moore, 'Historical Introduction to Porphyrins and Porphyrias', in Dailey, op. cit., pp. 1–54; T. K. With, 'A Short History of Porphyrins and the Porphyrias', *International Journal of Biochemistry*, vol. 11 (1980), pp. 189–200.

21. P. Voswinckel, *History of Psychiatry*, vol. 1 (1990), pp. 159–68; C. R. Rimington, *International Journal of Biochemistry*, vol. 25 (1993), pp. 1351–2.

22. See R. L. P. Lindberg, C. Porcher, B. Grandchamp, B. Ledermann, K. Bürki, S. Brander, A. Aguzzi and U. A. Meyer, 'Porphobilinogen Deaminase Deficiency in Mice Causes a Neuropathy Resembling that of Human Hepatic Porphyria', *Nature Genetics*, vol. 12 (1996), pp. 195–9.

List of Archives

Royal Archives, Windsor Castle (RA)
Archive of the Hessische Hausstiftung, Schloss Fasanerie (AHH)
Thuringian State Archive, Meiningen (ThStaMgn)
Bundesarchiv Berlin (BA)
Cambridge University Library Manuscripts Department (CUL)
Churchill Archives Centre, Cambridge
State Archive of Lower Saxony, Hanover
State Library of Lower Saxony Manuscripts Department, Hanover
Municipal Museum, Bad Homburg
Württemberg State Archive, Stuttgart

Bibliography

Abbot, C., ed., *The Diary and Correspondence of Charles Abbot, Lord Colchester*, vol. 1 (1861).

Andreas, W., and von Scholz, W., *Die Grossen Deutschen, Neue Deutsche Biographie* (Berlin, 1935), vol. 2.

Aspinall, A., ed., *The Letters of King George IV* (Cambridge, 1938), vol. 2.

—, ed., *Letters of the Princess Charlotte* (London, 1949).

—, ed., *Mrs Jordan and Her Family, Being the Unpublished Correspondence of Mrs Jordan and the Duke of Clarence, Later William IV* (London, 1951).

—, ed., *The Correspondence of George, Prince of Wales, 1770–1812* (London, 1963–71).

—, ed., *The Later Correspondence of George III* (Cambridge, 1962).

Ayling, S., *George the Third* (London, 1972).

Beasley, A. W., 'The Disability of James VI & I', *Seventeenth Century*, vol. X, no. 2 (1995).

Bernard, J., *Le Sang et l'Histoire* (Paris, 1983).

Bladon, F. M., ed., *The Diaries of Colonel the Hon. Robert Fulke Greville* (London, 1930).

Bolitho, H., *The Prince Consort and His Brother* (London, 1933).

—, ed., *Further Letters of Queen Victoria* (London, 1938).

Brewster, D., *Letters on Natural Magic, Addressed to Sir Walter Scott* (London, 1842).

Bringmann, T. C., *Reichstag und Zweikampf: Die Duellfrage als Innenpolitischer Konflikt des Deutschen Kaiserreichs 1871–1918* (Freiburg, 1997).

Brooke, J., *King George III* (London, 1972).

Brough, J., *Margaret: The Tragic Princess* (London, 1978).

Dailey, H. A., ed., *Biosynthesis of Heme and Chlorophyll* (New York, 1990).

Dean, G., *The Porphyrias: A Story of Inheritance and Environment* (London, 1971).

Broughton, V. Delves, *Court and Private Life in the Time of Queen Charlotte: Being the Journals of Mrs Papendiek* (London, 1887), vol. 1.

Duncan, G. G., ed., *Duncan's Diseases of Metabolism* (Philadelphia, 1974).

Feduccia, A., *The Origin and Evolution of Birds* (New Haven and London, 1996).

Fitzgerald, P., *Royal Dukes and Princesses of the Family of George III: A View of Court Life and Manners for Seventy Years, 1760–1830* (London, 1882), vol. 1.

Fraser, A., *Mary Queen of Scots* (London, 1969).

Friedmann, F., *Der Deutsche Kaiser und die Hofkamarilla: Der Fall Kotze* (Zürich, 1896).

Fulford, R., *Royal Dukes: The Father and Uncles of Queen Victoria* (London, 1933).

—, *George the Fourth* (London, 1935)

—, ed., *Dearest Child: Private Correspondence of Queen Victoria and the Princess Royal, 1858–1861* (London, 1964).

—, ed., *Dearest Mama: Private Correspondence of Queen Victoria and the Crown Princess of Prussia, 1861–1864* (London, 1968).

—, ed., *Your Dear Letter: Private Correspondence of Queen Victoria and the German Crown Princess, 1865–1871* (London, 1971).

—, ed., *Darling Child: Private Correspondence of Queen Victoria and the German Crown Princess* (London, 1976).

—, ed., *Beloved Mama: Private Correspondence of Queen Victoria and the German Crown Princess, 1878–1885* (London, 1981).

Gillen, M., *The Prince and His Lady* (London, 1970).

Gore, J. ed., *Creevey* (London, 1948).

Gore Allen, W., *King William IV* (London, 1960).

Granville, C., ed., *Lord Granville Leveson Gower (First Earl Granville): Private Correspondence, 1781–1821* (London, 1916), vol. 2.

Green, M. A. E., *Lives of the Princesses of England* (London, 1855), vol. 6.

Green, V. H. H., *The Madness of Kings: Personal Trauma and the Fate of Nations* (Stroud, 1993).

Grieg, J., ed., *The Farington Diary* (London, 1922–8).

Guttmacher, M., *America's Last King: An Interpretation of the Madness of George III* (New York, 1941).

Harris, J. H., ed., *Diaries and Correspondence of James Harris, First Earl of Malmesbury* (London, 1844).

Harrison, M., *Clarence: The Life of HRH the Duke of Clarence and Avondale (1864–1892)* (London, 1972).

Hauck, K., ed., *Briefe der Kinder des Winterkönigs* (Heidelberg, 1908).

Helmholtz, H. von, *Handbuch der Physiologischen Optik* (Hamburg, 1896).

Henry, W. C., *Memoirs of the Life and Scientific Researches of John Dalton* (London, 1854).

Hessen, R. von, ed., *Wir Wilhelm von Gottes Gnaden: Die Lebenserinnerungen Kurfürst Wilhelms I. von Hessen 1743–1821* (Frankfurt/Main and New York, 1996).

Hibbert, C., *George IV Prince of Wales 1762–1811* (London, 1972).

Ilchester, Earl of, ed., *The Journal of Elizabeth, Lady Holland, 1791–1811* (London, 1908), vol. 2.

Jordan, P. M., *Biosynthesis of Tetrapyrroles* (London, 1991).

Joüet, C. H., *Index to the Literature on Thorium, 1817–1902* (Washington, 1903).

Keith, R., *History of the Affairs of Church and State in Scotland* (Edinburgh, 1844–50), vol. 3.

Klier, J., and Mingay, H., *The Quest for Anastasia* (London, 1996).

Law, E., ed., *Lord Ellenborough, A Political Diary, 1828–1850* (London, 1881), vols. 1 and 2.

Lewin, B., *Genes V* (Oxford, 1995).

Lindsey, J., *The Lovely Quaker* (London, 1998).

Longford, E., *Victoria R.I.* (London, 1964).

Macalpine, I., and Hunter, R., 'The Insanity of King George III: A Classic Case of Porphyria', *BMJ* (1966).

—, 'A Clinical Reassessment of the Insanity of George III and some of its Historical Implications', *Bulletin of the Institute of Historical Research*, vol. 40 (1967).

—, 'Porphyria and King George III', *Scientific American*, July 1969.

—, *George III and the Mad Business* (London, 1969).

Macalpine, I., Hunter, R., and Rimington, C., 'Porphyria in the Royal Houses of Stuart, Hanover and Prussia: A Follow-up Study of George III's Illness', *BMJ* (1968).

Macaulay, T. B., *The History of England From the Accession of James II* (1858), vol. 1.

Magnus, P. M., *King Edward the Seventh* (London, 1964).

Maltzahn, A. A. F. von, *Elisabeth Landgräfin von Hessen-Homburg, Königl. Prinzessin von Grossbritannien und Irland* (Homburg, 1908).

Marchesseau, R., *Une Urgence Abdominale: La Mort de Madame Henriette d'Angleterre* (Bordeaux, 1947).

McKenna, P. J., *Schizophrenia and Related Syndromes* (London, 1997).

Midelfort, H. C. E., *Mad Princes of Renaissance Germany* (Charlottesville and London, 1994).

Milgrom, L. M., *The Colours of Life* (Oxford, 1997).

Moore, M. R., McColl, K. E. L., Rimington C. and Goldberg, A., *Disorders of Porphyrin Metabolism* (New York, 1987).

Munk, W., *The Life of Sir Henry Halford* (London and New York, 1895).

Nesse, R. M. and Williams, G. C., *Evolution and Healing* (London, 1995).

Neumann, H.-J., *Erbkrankheiten in Europäischen Fürstenhäusern* (Berlin, 1993).

Oestreich, G., *Friedrich Wilhelm I: Preussischer Absolutismus, Merkantilismus, Militarismus* (Göttingen, 1977).

Oman, C., *Elizabeth of Bohemia* (London, 1938).

Pain, N., *George III at Home* (London, 1975).

Pakula, H., *The Last Romantic: A Biography of Queen Maria of Roumania* (New York, 1984).

—, *An Uncommon Woman: The Empress Frederick, Daughter of Queen Victoria, Wife of the Crown Prince of Prussia, Mother of Kaiser Wilhelm* (New York, London, Toronto, Sydney, Tokyo, Singapore, 1995).

Perutz, M., *Protein Structure: New Approaches to Disease and Therapy* (New York, 1992).

Pierach, C. A. and Jennewein, E., 'War der Preussische König Friedrich Wilhelm I (1688–1740) an Porphyrie Erkrankt?', in *Internationale Zeitschrift für Geschichte und Ethik der Naturwissenschaften, Technik un Medizin*, forthcoming.

Plumb, J. H., *The First Four Georges* (London, 1956).

Ponsonby, A., *Henry Ponsonby, Queen Victoria's Private Secretary: His Life From His Letters* (London, 1942).

Post, J. M., and Robins, R. S., *When Illness Strikes the Leader: The Dilemma of the Captive King From George III to Ronald Reagan* (New Haven, 1993).

Potts, D. M. and Potts, W. T. W., *Queen Victoria's Gene: Haemophilia and the Royal Family* (Stroud, 1995).

Quennell, P., ed., *The Private Letters of Princess Lieven to Prince Metternich 1820–26* (London, 1948).

Ramm, A., ed., *Beloved and Darling Child: Last Letters Between Queen Victoria and Her Eldest Daughter 1886–1901* (Stroud, 1990).

Ray, I., 'Insanity of King George III', *American Journal of Insanity* (1855).

Rich, N. and Fisher, M. H., eds., *The Holstein Papers: The Memoirs, Diaries and Correspondence of Friedrich von Holstein, 1837–1919* (Cambridge, 1955–63), vols. 2 and 3.

Richardson, J., *George IV: A Portrait* (London, 1966).

Röhl, J. C. G., *The Kaiser and His Court: Wilhelm II and the Government of Germany* (Cambridge, 1984).

—, *Young Wilhelm: The Kaiser's Early Life 1859–1888* (Cambridge, 1998).

St Aubyn, G., ed., *William of Gloucester, Pioneer Prince* (London, 1977).

Scriver, C. R., Beaudet, A. L. and Sly, W. S., eds., *The Metabolic Basis of Inherited Disease* (New York, 1995).

Spillmann, K. R. and Spillmann, K., 'Friedrich Wilhelm I und die Preussische Armee: Versuch einer Deutung auf Psychoanalytischer Basis', 16th International Historical Congress (Stuttgart, 1985).

Stanhope, P. H., *Life of the Right Honourable William Pitt*, 3rd edn

(1867), vol. 2.

Stevenson, J., ed., *History of Mary Stuart* (Edinburgh, 1883).

Strachey, L. and Fulford, R., eds., *The Greville Memoirs* (London, 1938).

Stuart, D. M., *The Daughters of George III* (London, 1939).

Van der Cruysse, D., ed., *Madame Palatine, Lettres Françaises* (Paris, 1989).

Van der Kiste, J., and Jordaan, B., *Dearest Affie ... Alfred, Duke of Edinburgh, Queen Victoria's Second Son 1844–1900* (London, 1984).

Vannotti, A., *Porphyrins: Their Biological and Chemical Importance* (London, 1954).

Villiers, G., *A Vanished Victorian: The Life of Lord Clarendon by His Grandson* (London, 1938).

Wheatley, H. B., ed., *The Historical and Posthumous Memoirs of Sir Nathanial William Wraxall* (London, 1884), vol. 5.

Wilson, P. W., ed., *The Greville Diary* (London, 1927), vol. 1.

Woodham Smith, C., *Queen Victoria: Her Life and Times* (London, 1972), vol. 1.

Wormald, J., *Court, Kirk and Community in Scotland* (Edinburgh, 1991).

Wright, W. D., *The Rays Are Not Coloured* (London, 1967).

Yorke, P. C., ed., *Letters of Princess Elizabeth of England, Daughter of King George III, and Landgravine of Hesse-Homburg* (London, 1898).

Young, T. A., *Course of Lectures on Natural Philosophy and the Mechanical Arts* (London, 1807).

Ziegler, P., *King William IV* (London, 1971).

Index